Surgical Oncology: A Practical and Comprehensive Approach

Surgical Oncology: A Practical and Comprehensive Approach

Edited by Jerome Baker

hayle
medical

New York

Hayle Medical,
750 Third Avenue, 9th Floor,
New York, NY 10017, USA

Visit us on the World Wide Web at:
www.haylemedical.com

ISBN: 978-1-63241-701-5

Cataloging-in-Publication Data

Surgical oncology : a practical and comprehensive approach / edited by Jerome Baker.
    p. cm.
Includes bibliographical references and index.
ISBN 978-1-63241-701-5
1. Cancer--Surgery. 2. Oncology. 3. Cancer. 4. Cancer--Treatment. I. Baker, Jerome.
RD651 .S877 2019
616.994--dc23

Table of Contents

Preface

This book has been a concerted effort by a group of academicians, researchers and scientists, who have contributed their research works for the realization of the book. This book has materialized in the wake of emerging advancements and innovations in this field. Therefore, the need of the hour was to compile all the required researches and disseminate the knowledge to a broad spectrum of people comprising of students, researchers and specialists of the field.

Surgical interventions used for the treatment of cancer are under the scope of surgical oncology. Palliative surgery, minimally invasive procedures and neo-adjuvant treatments characterize modern surgical oncology. Surgical procedures can be palliative or curative. Palliative surgery is the surgical intervention that is targeted at relieving a patient's symptoms and making a positive impact on the patient's quality of life. It can involve simpler procedures to extensive debulking. Tumor debulking can also be performed for curative intent, as in cytoreduction or cytoreductive surgery. It is also performed to enhance the efficacy of radiotherapy or chemotherapy. Adrenalectomy, clitoridectomy, coccygectomy, cystoprostatectomy, colectomy, esophagectomy, etc. are some surgical procedures concerned with the removal of certain body parts where a tumor has developed. This book discusses the fundamentals as well as modern approaches of surgical oncology. It includes some of the vital pieces of work being conducted across the world, on various topics related to surgical oncology. The extensive content herein provides the readers with a thorough understanding of the subject.

At the end of the preface, I would like to thank the authors for their brilliant chapters and the publisher for guiding us all-through the making of the book till its final stage. Also, I would like to thank my family for providing the support and encouragement throughout my academic career and research projects.

Editor

The diagnostic ureteroscopy before radical nephroureterectomy in upper urinary tract urothelial carcinoma is not associated with higher intravesical recurrence

Hsiang-Ying Lee[1,2,3], Hsin-Chih Yeh[1,3,4,5], Wen-Jeng Wu[1,3,4,5], Jiun-Shiuan He[6], Chun-Nung Huang[3,4,5], Hung-Lung Ke[3,4,5], Wei-Ming Li[3,4,5,7], Chien-Feng Li[8,9,10,11,12] and Ching-Chia Li[1,3,4,5*]

Abstract

Background: To clarify if diagnostic ureteroscopy (URS) before radical nephroureterectomy for patients with upper tract urothelial carcinoma (UTUC) will increase the risk of intravesical recurrence.

Methods: From retrospective review of cohort at our institution, 502 patients with UTUC who underwent radical nephroureterectomy with bladder cuff excision were enrolled from 1990 to 2013. Cox proportional hazards model was used to analyze the overall survival (OS), disease-free survival (DFS), metastasis-free survival (MFS), and intravesical recurrence-free survival (IVRFS). The log-rank test was used for comparing survival curves. All potential risk factors were included in the multivariate Cox proportional hazards model to recognize independent predictors. From NHI database, we included patients of UTUC without bladder cancer history using population-based database in Taiwan from 1996 to 2013. In total, 3079 URS and 2634 non-URS patients with UTUC were identified. Univariate and multivariate Cox proportional hazards regressions were performed to measure the risk of IVRFS and all-cause mortality.

Results: From our database, the comparison of clinicopathological characteristics in UTUC patients between with URS biopsy group (URS+) ($n = 206$, 41%) and without URS biopsy group (URS−) ($n = 296$, 59%) was insignificantly different excluding surgical method. URS biopsy is not associated with worse OS ($p = 0.720$), DFS ($p = 0.294$), MFS ($p = 0.808$), and IVRFS ($p = 0.560$) by multivariate analysis. Only bladder cancer history is an independent significant factor to predict IVR ($p < 0.001$). The same result from NHI database, URS before radical surgery will not increase the risk of IVRFS [adjusted HR 1.136, 95% CI 1.00–1.30; $P = 0.059$] and OS [adjusted HR 0.919, 95% CI 0.82–1.04; $P = 0.164$].

Conclusions: Preoperative URS manipulation is not associated with higher risk of IVRFS even in patients without bladder cancer history. Diagnostic URS is feasible to compensate the insufficient information of image in patients with UTUC.

Keywords: Diagnostic ureteroscopy, Upper urinary tract urothelial carcinoma, Intravesical recurrence

Background

Upper tract urothelial carcinoma (UTUC), involving renal pelvis and ureter, is rare in western countries but presents an unusual feature in Taiwan. The US National Cancer Database identifies a ratio of bladder cancer to UTUC of 93 to 7%. The male-to-female and pyelocaliceal-to-ureter tumor ratio incidence of UTUC are both about 2–3:1 [1, 2]. However, UTUC comprises up to 30% of all UCs in Taiwan, and the male-to-female ratio incidence is approximately equal, as well as in renal pelvis and ureter [3, 4]. The standard treatment of UTUC is radical nephroureterectomy with ipsilateral bladder cuff excision. However, minimally invasive uretereorenoscopic (URS) therapy in selected cases is also considered because it can preserve renal function and reduce morbidity. It also provides effective oncologic

* Correspondence: ashum1009@gmail.com
[1]Department of Urology, Kaohsiung Municipal Ta-Tung Hospital, Kaohsiung, Taiwan
[3]Department of Urology, Kaohsiung Medical University Hospital, Kaohsiung, Taiwan
Full list of author information is available at the end of the article

outcomes [5]. Because URS allows direct visualization of the entire collecting system, when combined with biopsies, it can increase the detection rate of UTUC lesions [6, 7]. However, pyelolymphatic, pyelotubular, and pyelovenous backflow of irrigation can occur during diagnostic URS [8, 9]. The raising about the possibility of backflow of malignant urothelial cells and tumor seeding during URS evaluation is to be considered to induce higher risk of intravesical recurrence (IVR). Although URS has been reported to be safe [10–12], more evidences are needed to establish that this procedure is not harmful for patients with UTUC. Besides, the impact of delay radical treatment because of previous URS biopsy is still controversial.

The primary recognized prognostic factors of survival for UTUC are tumor stage and grade. UTUC that invade the muscle layer usually have a relatively poor prognosis. The 5-year disease-specific survival of UTUC is < 50% for pT2/pT3 and < 10% for pT4 [13]. Based on the possibility of occult micrometastases before the surgery, metastases are often discovered after nephroureterectomy [14]. In addition, previous studies showed that after nephroureterectomy for UTUC, 25 to 69% of patients would develop a metachronous bladder tumor recurrence. Therefore, to figure out the potential risk factors of survival, metastasis and subsequent IVR for UTUC are important and will affect our clinical decision in further treatment and surveillance.

In this study, we evaluated the influence of URS biopsy on survival, metastasis, and especially focus on IVR and to analyze if delay of the curative treatment will cause worse survival. We aim to provide a more precise comparison and, therefore, also assess the impact by calculating our National Health Insurance (NHI) database. Besides, we attempted to identify the significant prognostic factors to predict disease-specific survival, metastasis-free survival, and intravesical recurrence-free survival for UTUC after nephroureterectomy.

Methods
Patient collection and methods of cohort in our institution
We enrolled 502 patients who underwent radical nephroureterectomy with bladder cuff excision with retrospective review of the medical records and were histologically confirmed to have UTUC from 1990 to 2013 at our institution. This study was approved by our Institutional Review Board (KMUH-IRB-20120138). None of all patients received immediate intravesical chemotherapy after radical surgery. Parameters including age, gender, smoking, bladder cancer history, estimated renal function before radical surgery, type of operation, tumor multifocality, tumor grade, pathological T stage, pathological N stage, previous diagnostic URS biopsy or none were recorded. All tumor specimens were graded by the 2004 WHO/International Society of Urologic Pathology consensus classification and

staged according to the 2002 TNM classification for UCC. The decision to perform diagnostic URS or not was based on the surgeon's judgment. The definition of metastasis progression is tumor local recurrence over tumor bed, regional lymph nodes, and distant metastasis.

Regular surveillance consisted of physical examination, cystoscopy, urine cytology, and periodic imaging studies were organized following the institutional guidelines. The schedule of cystoscopy is every 3 months for the first 2 years, every 6 months for the next 3 years, and annually thereafter. IVR was defined as pathologically identified UC in the urinary bladder after radical surgery.

Statistical analysis of cohort in our institution
Demographic and clinicopathological factors between those with URS biopsy (URS+) and those without URS biopsy (URS–) were compared using independent sample t test for continuous variables and chi-square test for categorical variables. We estimated the impact of URS biopsy on overall survival (OS), disease-free survival (DFS), metastasis-free survival (MFS), and intravesical recurrence-free survival (IVRFS) by the Kaplan-Meier method. The duration of radical surgery to the cancer-specific death, metastatic progression, and intravesical recurrence or last visit was calculated to survival rates. The log-rank test was used for comparing survival curves. All potential risk factors were included in the multivariate Cox proportional hazards model to recognize independent predictors. The impact of URS biopsy was further analyzed in IVR based on tumor grade, bladder cancer history, and tumor location. In all analysis, $P < 0.05$ was considered statistically significant. Statistical analyses were performed with SPSS software, version 19 (IBM Corp., Somers, NY, USA).

NHI database
Study design and data source
A longitudinal observational cohort study was conducted by using a population-based database in Taiwan from 1996 to 2013. Database contains catastrophic illness registry data, which includes most cancer, autoimmune disease, chronic psychosis, and dialysis patients. The database includes outpatients, inpatient, and enrollment data for catastrophic illness patients, so we could use the database to obtain information about patient comorbidities. All data was acquired from the National Health Insurance Research Database (NHIRD).

Study population
Over 99% of the 23.74 million residents of Taiwan were included in the Taiwan NHI program. Nearly one million patients are included in the Registry for catastrophic illness. UTUC patients were identified if they had a primarily UTUC diagnosis (ICD-9-CM code with 189) in inpatient hospitalization between 2000 and 2010. We

exclude patients who had bladder cancer (ICD-9-CM code with 188) history before UTUC was diagnosed. All patients included received radical nephroureterectomy (ICD-9-OP 55.5). We identified patients who receive diagnostic URS (URS+) before radical nephroureterectomy as the URS cohort. Then, we identified non-URS (URS−) patients for the comparison group. All patients defined the date of receiving radical nephroureterectomy as index date. In total, 3079 URS+ and 2634 URS− patients with UTUC were identified.

Variable definitions

The major endpoints were to compare the risk of bladder cancer and all-cause mortality between URS and non-URS patients. Bladder cancer occurrences were identified using ICD-9 CM diagnosis code in the national catastrophic illness registry data. We defined death occurrences using the enrollment data. Several baseline characteristics were included as control variables, because they may affect outcomes. Demographic covariates included age and gender. Charlson Comorbidity Index (CCI) within 1 year before index date was used to measure patients' baseline comorbidities. The comorbidities were diabetes mellitus (ICD-9-CM code with 250), hypertension (ICD-9-CM code with 401−405), hyperlipidemia (ICD-9-CM code with 272), ESRD (ICD-9-CM code with 585) diagnosed within 1 year before index date, and other cancers (ICD-9-CM code with 140−208) diagnosed before index date.

Statistical analysis

The χ^2 test was used to evaluate the differences in gender, age, CCI score, and comorbidities between URS+ and URS− patients, except for mean age and mean CCI score, which were examined through independent sample t test. Univariate and multivariate Cox proportional hazards regressions were performed to measure the risk of bladder cancer and all-cause mortality. Hazard ratios (HRs) and 95% confidence intervals (CIs) were reported. Potential confounding variables as shown in Table 4 were controlled for multivariate models. The impact of time factors on bladder cancer incidence and UTUC cumulative survival rate was estimated with Kaplan-Meier survival curves, and differences were assessed by means of the log-rank statistic. All statistical calculations were analyzed using SAS version 9.3 (SAS institute, Cary, NC) and Stata version SE 11. A two-tailed P value lower than 0.05 was considered significant.

Results

Cohort in our institution

Table 1 lists the comparison of clinicopathological characteristics in UTUC patients between URS+ ($n = 206$, 41%) and URS− ($n = 296$, 59%). In all patients, the mean age

was 65.8 years, and female ($n = 282$, 56.2%) is more than male ($n = 220$, 43.8%). One hundred five (20.9%) patients have smoking habit, and 148 (29.5%) patients have bladder cancer history. More patients ($n = 327$, 65.1%) present impaired estimated renal function, and 76 (15.1%) patients underwent dialysis before radical nephroureterectomy. The distribution of UTUC pathological T stage in this cohort was as follows: 71 (14.1%) patients had pTis-Ta, 131 (26.1%) patients had pT1, 127 (25.3%) patients had pT2, 144 (28.7%) patients had pT3, and 29 (5.8%) patients had pT4, respectively. Three hundred ninety-one (77.9%) patients have high tumor grade. Only surgical modality is the significant difference among two groups.

Overall survival

During mean the follow-up duration of 6.4 years, the 5-year OS rate (SD) was 89.5% (1.8) in the URS− group and 90.3% (2.2) in the URS+ group. Patients with diagnostic URS showed no negative impact on OS ($P = 0.76$) (Table 2). Excluding age, advanced T stage, higher tumor grade, lymph node involvement, and multifocality were also significantly associated with lower OS rates. Multivariate analysis showed that high tumor grade, advanced tumor T stage, and lymph node involvement were independent prognostic factors for OS [Cox regression hazard ratio (HR) 2.048, 95% CI 1.023−4.100, $P = 0.043$; HR 2.339, 95% CI 1.378−3.972, $P = 0.002$; and HR 6.342, 95% CI 3.950−10.183, $P < 0.001$, respectively; Table 2).

Disease-specific survival

The DSS rate (SD) at 5 years was 92.0% (1.6) in the URS− group and 91.8% (2.0) in the URS+ group. From the univariate analysis indicated that advanced T stage, higher tumor grade, lymph node involvement, and multifocality were significantly related to lower DSS rates. In a multivariate analysis, only advanced T stage and lymph node involvement were independent risk factors of worse survival [Cox regression hazard ratio (HR) 5.242, 95% CI 2.208−12.442, $P < 0.001$; and HR 8.084, 95% CI 4.804−13.602, $P < 0.001$, respectively; (Table 2). Diagnostic URS biopsy remains not associated with worse DSS ($P = 0.294$ in multivariate analysis).

Metastasis-free survival

One hundred thirty-five (26.9%) patients experienced cancer progression in this cohort. The MFS rates (SD) after 5 years were 87.4% (2.0) in the URS− group and 83.8% (2.7) in the URS+ group. In multivariate analysis, multifocality, advanced T stage, and lymph node involvement were significant predictors of MFS [Cox regression hazard ratio (HR) 1.474, 95% CI 1.014−2.143, $P = 0.042$; HR 2.983, 95% CI 1.701−5.230, $P < 0.001$; and HR 5.786, 95% CI 3.696−9.058, $P < 0.001$, respectively; (Table 3).

Table 1 Clinicopathological characteristics of 502 patients with upper tract urothelial carcinoma

	All patients (n=502)	URS or not		
		Yes (n=206)	No (n=296)	p value
	No. (%)	No. (%)	No. (%)	
Age(years)(mean [SD])	65.8 (11.0)	66.1 (10.1)	65.7 (11.6)	0.705
Gender				0.334
Male (%)	220 (43.8)	85 (41.3)	135 (45.6)	
Female (%)	282 (56.2)	121 (58.7)	161 (54.4)	
Smoking				0.984
Yes (%)	105 (20.9)	43 (20.9)	62 (20.9)	
No (%)	397 (79.1)	163 (79.1)	234 (79.1)	
Bladder cancer history				0.958
Yes (%)	148 (29.5)	61 (29.6)	87 (29.4)	
No (%)	354 (70.5)	145 (70.4)	209 (70.6)	
eGFR (mL/min/1.73 m2) (median [range])	49.4 (2.9-154.3)			0.544
$\geqq$ 60 (%)	175 (34.9)	75 (36.4)	100 (33.8)	
<60 (%)	327 (65.1)	131 (63.6)	196 (66.2)	
Dialysis				0.476
Yes (%)	76 (15.1)	34 (16.5)	42 (14.2)	
No (%)	426 (84.9)	172 (83.5)	254 (85.8)	
Surgical modality				*< 0.001
Open (%)	329 (65.5)	110 (53.4)	219 (74.0)	
Laparoscopy (%)	155 (30.9)	90 (43.7)	65 (22.0)	
Segmental resection (%)	18 (3.6)	6 (2.9)	12 (4.1)	
Tumor location				0.711
Pelvis (%)	190 (37.8)	76 (36.9)	114 (38.5)	
Ureter (%)	221 (44.0)	95 (46.1)	126 (42.6)	
Both (%)	91 (18.1)	35(17.0)	56 (18.9)	
Multifocality				0.389
Yes (%)	117 (23.3)	44 (21.4)	73 (24.7)	
No (%)	385 (76.7)	162 (78.6)	223 (75.3)	
Tumor grade				0.592
Low (%)	111 (22.1)	48 (23.2)	63 (21.3)	
High (%)	391 (77.9)	158 (76.7)	233 (78.7)	
Pathologic T stage				0.319
pTa-Tis (%)	71 (14.1)	36 (17.5)	35 (11.8)	
pT1 (%)	131 (26.1)	54 (26.2)	77 (26.0)	
pT2 (%)	127 (25.3)	47 (22.8)	80 (27.0)	
pT3 (%)	144 (28.7)	55 (26.7)	89 (30.1)	
pT4 (%)	29 (5.8)	14 (6.8)	15 (5.1)	
Pathologic N				0.999
N0 or Nx (%)	463 (92.2)	190 (92.2)	273 (92.2)	
N1-3 (%)	39 (7.8)	16 (7.8)	23 (7.8)	

*$p<0.05$

Table 2 Overall survival and disease-specific survival in univariate analysis and multivariate analysis by Cox proportional hazard model

	Overall survival				Disease-specific survival			
	Univariate analysis		Multivariate analysis		Univariate analysis		Multivariate analysis	
	HR 95% CI	p-value	HR 95% CI	p-value	HR 95% CI	p-value	HR 95% CI	p-value
Age, years	1.019 (1.002-1.036)	0.027*	1.011(0.994-1.029)	0.201	1.012 (0.993-1.032)	0.223	1.004 (0.984-1.024)	0.723
Gender (male vs female)	0.963 (0.690-1.344)	0.825	0.909 (0.633-1.393)	0.755	0.881 (0.590-1.316)	0.536	0.870(0.534-1.415)	0.574
Smoking (yes vs no)	1.073 (0.716-1.608)	0.731	0.994 (0.611-1.617)	0.981	1.182 (0.734-1.903)	0.490	0.955 (0.525-1.736)	0.880
Bladder cancer history (yes vs no)	1.041 (0.730-1.486)	0.823	0.984 (0.675-1.435)	0.932	0.928 (0.597-1.441)	0.739	0.858 (0.536-1.374)	0.523
Estimated GFR (<60 vs ≥60)	1.240 (0.865-1.777)	0.241	0.934 (0.638-1.368)	0.727	1.252 (0.809-1.937)	0.312	0.982 (0.614-1.571)	0.941
Operation method		0.098		0.184		0.078		0.101
Open	1 (reference)	-	1 (reference)	-	1 (reference)	-	1 (reference)	-
Laparoscopy	0.632 (0.415-0.963)	0.033*	0.705 (0.453-1.096)	0.121	0.558 (0.333-0.937)	0.027*	0.615 (0.356-1.063)	0.082
Segmental resection	1.028 (0.419-2.524)	0.952	1.459 (0.589-3.616)	0.414	1.141 (0.417-3.121)	0.798	1.723 (0.620-4.792)	0.297
Multifocality (yes vs no)	1.741 (1.220-2.486)	0.002*	1.319 (0.904-1.926)	0.151	1.847 (1.207-2.826)	0.005*	1.337 (0.851-2.101)	0.207
Grade (high vs low)	4.243 (2.339-7.696)	< 0.001*	2.048 (1.023-4.100)	0.043*	8.450 (3.103-23.014)	< 0.001*	2.459 (0.813-7.437)	0.111
Pathologic T stage (pT2-4 vs pTa/Tis/T1)	4.188 (2.695-6.507)	< 0.001*	2.339 (1.378-3.972)	0.002*	10.691 (4.949-23.095)	< 0.001*	5.242 (2.208-12.442)	< 0.001*
Pathologic N stage (pN1-3 vs pN0/Nx)	9.720 (6.234-15.154)	< 0.001*	6.342 (3.950-10.183)	< 0.001*	13.236 (8.144-21.510)	< 0.001*	8.084 (4.804-13.602)	< 0.001*
URS biopsy (yes vs no)	0.946 (0.664-1.348)	0.760	1.069 (0.742-1.541)	0.720	1.085 (0.717-1.644)	0.699	1.260 (0.818-1.941)	0.294

*p<0.05

Table 3 Metastasis-free survival and intravesical recurrence-free survival in univariate analysis and multivariate analysis by Cox proportional hazard model

	Metastasis-free survival				Intravesical recurrence-free survival			
	Univariate analysis		Multivariate analysis		Univariate analysis		Multivariate analysis	
	HR 95% CI	p-value	HR 95% CI	p-value	HR 95% CI	p-value	HR 95% CI	p-value
Age, years	1.006 (0.990-1.022)	0.485	0.997 (0.980-1.014)	0.722	1.007 (0.991-1.023)	0.417	1.010 (0.993-1.027)	0.260
Gender (male vs female)	0.969 (0.690-1.360)	0.854	0.901 (0.598-1.357)	0.616	0.706 (0.506-0.987)	0.041*	0.721 (0.490-1.063)	0.099
Smoking (yes vs no)	1.025 (0.676-1.554)	0.908	0.850 (0.509-1.420)	0.534	1.244 (0.837-1.848)	0.281	1.068 (0.672-1.697)	0.782
Bladder cancer history (yes vs no)	0.985 (0.683-1.422)	0.936	0.969 (0.660-1.424)	0.874	4.850 (3.440-6.837)	< 0.001*	5.085 (3.571-7.241)	< 0.001*
Estimated GFR (<60 vs ≧60)	1.153 (0.802-1.658)	0.442	1.037 (0.702-1.532)	0.853	0.998 (0.703-1.417)	0.993	0.898 (0.623-1.293)	0.562
Operation method		0.711		0.854		0.527		0.991
Open	1 (reference)	-	1 (reference)	-	1 (reference)	-	1 (reference)	-
Laparoscopy	0.855 (0.582-1.258)	0.427	1.021 (0.681-1.531)	0.921	0.809 (0.549-1.192)	0.284	1.024 (0.677-1.550)	0.909
Segmental resection	0.853 (0.313-2.321)	0.755	1.336 (0.486-3.668)	0.574	1.117 (0.454-2.747)	0.809	1.041 (0.413-2.624)	0.932
Multifocality (yes vs no)	1.952 (1.366-2.789)	< 0.001*	1.474 (1.014-2.143)	0.042*	1.132 (0.765-1.676)	0.536	0.885 (0.587-1.334)	0.559
Grade (high vs low)	4.613 (2.419-8.796)	< 0.001*	1.986 (0.961-4.105)	0.064	0.981 (0.670-1.437)	0.923	1.015 (0.643-1.601)	0.950
Pathologic T stage (pT2-4 vs pTa/Tis/T1)	5.183 (3.188-8.426)	< 0.001*	2.983 (1.701-5.230)	< 0.001*	1.042 (0.743-1.462)	0.810	1.178 (0.784-1.770)	0.430
Pathologic N stage (pN1-3 vs pN0/Nx)	8.895 (5.859-13.504)	< 0.001*	5.786 (3.696-9.058)	< 0.001*	0.977 (0.428-2.231)	0.977	0.930 (0.396-2.184)	0.867
URS biopsy (yes vs no)	0.963 (0.679-1.367)	0.834	1.046 (0.727-1.505)	0.808	1.093 (0.776-1.539)	0.611	1.113 (0.776-1.596)	0.560

*$p<0.05$

Presence of diagnostic URS biopsy was not associated with lower MFS in multivariate analysis ($P = 0.808$).

Intravesical recurrence-free survival
During the follow-up period, 138 (27.5%) patients were reported suffering from IVR. In multivariate analysis, only bladder cancer history is an independent significant factor to predict IVR ($P < 0.001$) (Table 3). Diagnostic URS biopsy performed before radical surgery did not appear to be a prognostic factor of IVR in Kaplan-Meier curves analysis ($P = 0.609$) (Fig. 1).

The effect of URS on IVRFS in with and without bladder cancer history
In the subgroup of patients without bladder cancer history, diagnostic URS had no negative impact on IVR ($P = 0.614$) (Fig. 2). Similarly, there was no significant difference in IVRFS between the URS+ groups and URS– groups in patients with bladder cancer history ($P = 0.829$) (Fig. 3).

NHI database
The comparison of demographics and comorbidities in UTUC patients between URS+ ($n = 3079$, 53.9%) and URS– ($n = 2634$, 46.1%) is presented in Table 4. Age and gender have similar distribution between the two groups. There were more females ($n = 3241$, 56.7%) in the study cohort. Compared with the URS– groups, significant higher prevalence of higher CCI (Charlson Comorbidity Index) score was found in URS+ (CCI $\geq$ 2: $n = 2590$ (84.12%) in URS+; $n = 2048$ (77.75%) in URS–, respectively).

Intravesical recurrence-free survival
The overall incidences of IVR were 62.79 and 70.92 per 1000 person-years in the URS– and URS+ cohorts, respectively, shown in Table 5, Fig. 4. According to multivariable Cox proportional hazard regression analysis, URS+ did not have a significantly higher risk of IVR [adjusted HR 1.136, 95% CI 1.00–1.30; $P = 0.059$]. Male patients and the patients with ESRD revealed significant higher risk of IVR [adjusted HR 1.293, 95% CI 1.13–1.48; $P < 0.001$ and HR 1.221, 95% CI 1.04–1.44; $P = 0.017$, respectively].

Overall survival
The incidence mortality rates were 76.50 and 69.31 per 1000 person-years in the URS– and URS+ cohorts, respectively (Table 6, Fig. 5). Compared with URS–, URS+ groups also have no negative impact on OS [adjusted HR 0.919, 95% CI 0.82–1.04; $P = 0.164$]. Higher mortality is found in male patients, more aged patients, and ESRD patients [adjusted HR 1.225, 95% CI 1.09–1.38, $P = 0.001$; > 74 years: HR 2.290, 95% CI 1.96–2.68, $P < 0.001$; HR 1.254, 95% CI 1.08–1.46, $P = 0.003$, respectively].

Intravesical recurrence-free survival among subgroups from our cohort
Among our subgroups of high grade and low grade, there is no significant difference between patients with URS and without URS biopsy ($P = 0.442$ in low grade; $P = 0.292$ in high grade, respectively) (Fig. 6a, b). Compared with our data, no matter where the tumor location is, URS biopsy before radical surgery do not enhance the

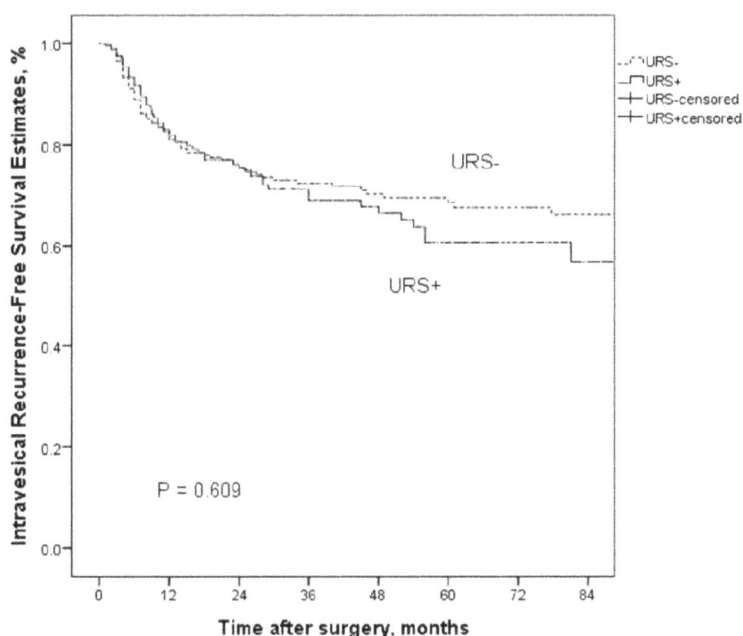

Fig. 1 Kaplan-Meier curves for IRFS according to URS status

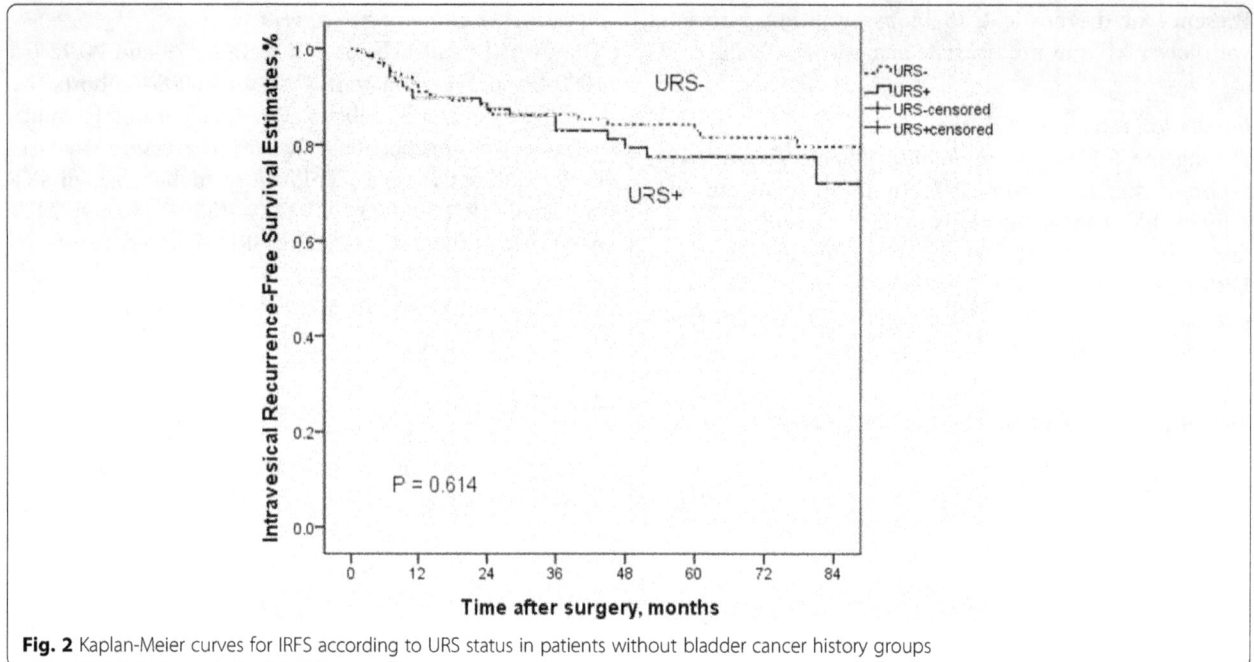

Fig. 2 Kaplan-Meier curves for IRFS according to URS status in patients without bladder cancer history groups

risk of IVR ($P = 0.186$ in renal pelvis location; $P = 0.512$ in ureter location, respectively) (Fig. 7a, b).

Discussion

Because pathological T stage and tumor grade have been established as major prognostic factors for UTUC, it is important to determine tumor architecture, grade, and stage assessment before definite treatment [15]. To compensate for the limitations of a cross-sectional image study, URS can be used as a direct visualization method for diagnosis especially combined with biopsies. Based on the analysis of previous studies, URS has been shown to have significantly higher accuracy, specificity, and positive predictive value than multiphase computed tomography urography (MCTU) [16]; however as many hospitals do not have MCTU equipment, URS evaluation is even more important. Advance in endourologic technologies improve diagnostic accuracy without severe

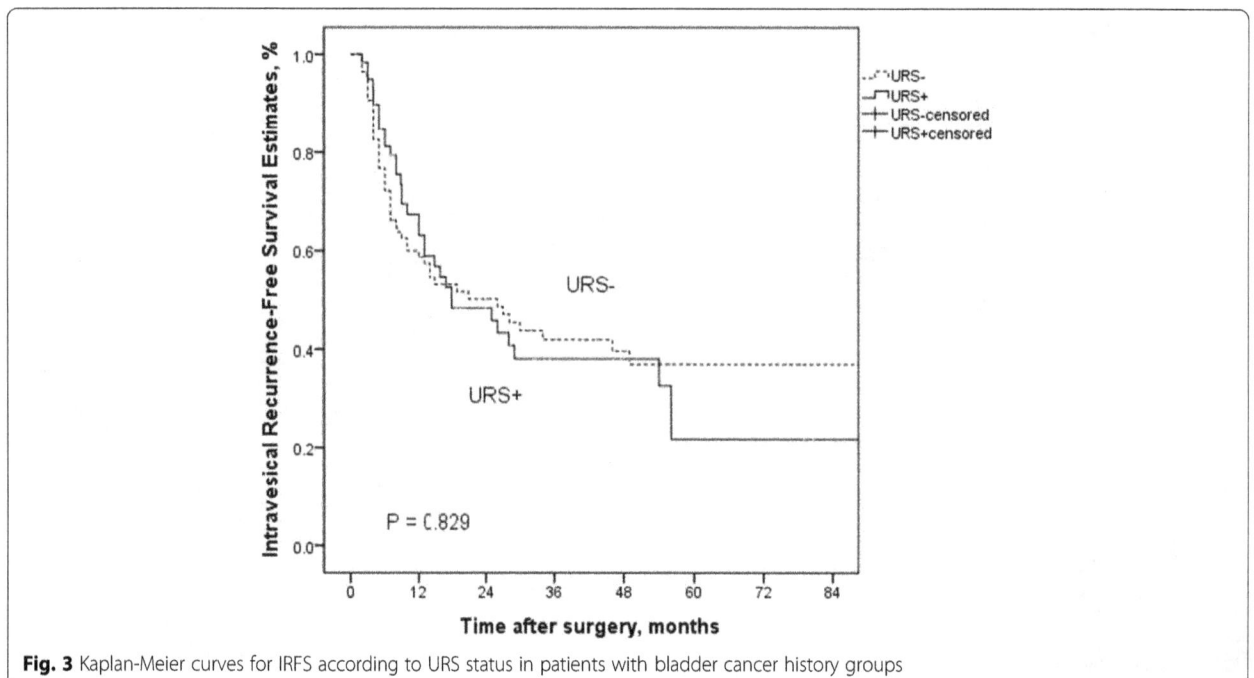

Fig. 3 Kaplan-Meier curves for IRFS according to URS status in patients with bladder cancer history groups

Table 4 Comparison of demographics and comorbidities between with and without diagnostic ureteroscopy in patients with upper tract urothelial carcinoma

	URS+ Mean±SD/ (N,%)	URS- Mean±SD/ (N,%)	P-value
	3,079 (53.9)	2,634 (46.1)	
Gender			
Male (N, %)	1,346 (43.72%)	1,126 (42.75%)	0.462
Female (N, %)	1,733 (56.28%)	1,508 (57.25%)	
Age (Mean±SD)	67.79 (±10.68)	67.63 (±11.15)	0.599
Age (N,%)			
<65 years	1,092 (35.47%)	952 (36.14%)	0.491
65-74 years	1,150 (37.35%)	944 (35.84%)	
>74 years	837 (27.18%)	738 (28.02%)	
CCI score (N,%)			
0	272 (8.83%)	341 (12.95%)	<0.001*
1	217 (7.05%)	245 (9.30%)	
$\geqq$2	2,590 (84.12%)	2,048 (77.75%)	
Comorbidity			
Hypertension			
No	1,443 (46.87%)	1,300 (49.35%)	0.061
Yes	1,636 (53.13%)	1,334 (50.65%)	
Hyperlipidemia			
No	2,371 (77.01%)	2,138 (81.17%)	<0.001*
Yes	708 (22.99%)	496 (18.83%)	
Diabetes			
No	2,345 (76.16%)	2,054 (77.98%)	0.103
Yes	734 (23.84%)	580 (22.02%)	
ESRD			
No	2,490 (80.87%)	2,072 (78.66%)	0.038*
Yes	589 (19.13%)	562 (21.34%)	

CCI Charlson Comorbidity Index, *ESRD* End-stage renal disease
*p<0.05

adverse effects and have been increasingly used for treatment purposes by direct tumor ablation with laser in selected patients. However, some previous studies have raised concerns about the possibility of intraluminal tumor seeding with manipulation during ureteroscopy and an increased incidence of IVR and metastasis [17, 18]. On the other hand, delaying radical nephroureterectomy may reduce survival rate. In order to clarify these issues and the conflicting results from several previous studies, we used both our own database and the National Health Insurance Research database to analyze the impact of pre-radical nephroureterectomy ureteroscopy on survival rate, metastasis rate, and especially the IVR rate.

Our cohort study revealed that bladder cancer history was the only risk factor for IVR after nephroureterectomy on multivariate Cox regression analysis, which is

similar to the results of previous studies [19, 20]. We found that diagnostic URS did not increase intravesical recurrence rate. In accordance with the treatment guidelines at our institution, we arranged for regular imaging studies for clinical staging before diagnostic procedure or radical surgery. For patients who had a large and obvious tumor, we considered performing radical surgery without URS biopsy. For pathology evaluation before radical surgery, we performed not only URS inspection but also simultaneous tumor biopsy. We further analyzed the subgroups of patients with and without a history of bladder cancer and noted no increase in the risk of IVR whether or not patients underwent URS before radical surgery. From the NHI database results, we included only patients with UTUC who had no previous or concurrent bladder cancer history, which is a well-known important predictive factor for IVR. This analysis also revealed that diagnostic URS was not significantly associated with increased IVR. In addition, we compared the duration of nephroureterectomy to bladder cancer recurrence between the groups with and without URSs and found that the URS group did not have significantly accelerated IVR.

Although the use of diagnostic URS followed by nephroureterectomy may raise concerns about delaying the course of curative treatment in patients with UTUC, no impact was noted on cancer-specific, bladder, or contralateral upper urinary tract recurrence and metastasis-free survival [21]. Similar to our findings, we still maintain a regular follow-up schedule based on standard guidelines instead of reducing the follow-up interval even when using diagnostic URS before radical surgery.

Early diagnosis of UTUC is still a challenging issue, especially for lower stage or flat growth pattern tumors. Although various imaging modalities are available including computed tomography urography which replaced intravenous urography owing to its higher detection rate, CT urography often cannot be used to identify carcinoma in situ or to localize superficial extensions of the tumor. Chronic inflammation can easily mimic urothelial cancer, leading to false-positive findings, which constitute a limitation of CT urography for the diagnosis of UTUC [22]. Liquid biopsy is also a popular continuing research target [23]. In addition, endoscopic management or kidney-sparing surgery can be considered for a specialized group of low-risk patients with impaired renal function; therefore, in order to avoid an unnecessary radical surgery, the imperative role of URS biopsy cannot be neglected. At a minimum, it should be included as one multimodality diagnostic option. Cutress et al. reported an analysis comparing endoscopic and laparoscopic management of noninvasive UTUC, and endoscopic treatment may provide non-inferior disease-free survival compared to radical surgery only in lower grade disease [24]. In their study, they found a significantly higher risk of IVR when patients received endoscopic

Table 5 Cox models measured incidence densities and hazard ratio of intravesical recurrence outcome

	N	Total person-year	Case	per 1000 person-year Incident rate	Crude HR (95% CI)	p-value	adjust HR (95% CI)	p-value
Main Effect								
URS- (Ref.)	2,634	6,243	392 (14.88%)	62.79	1 (Ref.)		1 (Ref.)	
URS+	3,079	7,261	515 (16.73%)	70.92	1.129 (0.99 - 1.29)	0.069	1.136 (1.00 - 1.30)	0.059
Baseline Patient Demographic Characteristics								
Gender								
Female (Ref.)	3,241	7,798	464 (14.32%)	59.50	1 (Ref.)		1 (Ref.)	
Male	2,472	5,707	443 (17.92%)	77.63	1.285 (1.13 - 1.46)	<0.001*	1.293 (1.13 - 1.48)	<0.001*
Age Categories								
<65 yr(Ref.)	2,044	5,028	332 (16.24%)	66.03	1 (Ref.)		1 (Ref.)	
65-74 yr	2,094	4,994	324 (15.47%)	64.87	0.978 (0.84 - 1.14)	0.771	0.994 (0.85 - 1.16)	0.935
>74yr	1,575	3,482	251 (15.94%)	72.09	1.067 (0.91 - 1.26)	0.440	1.087 (0.92 - 1.29)	0.334
CCI score Categories								
0 (Ref.)	613	1,467	95 (15.50%)	64.75	1 (Ref.)		1 (Ref.)	
1	462	1,105	68 (14.72%)	61.53	0.947 (0.69 - 1.29)	0.731	0.932 (0.68 - 1.28)	0.661
2+	4,638	10,932	744 (16.04%)	68.06	1.048 (0.85 - 1.30)	0.667	0.917 (0.73 - 1.15)	0.454
Hypertension								
No (Ref.)	2,743	6,560	437 (15.93%)	66.61	1 (Ref.)		1 (Ref.)	
Yes	2,970	6,944	470 (15.82%)	67.68	1.009 (0.89 - 1.15)	0.887	1.011 (0.88 - 1.16)	0.870
Hyperlipidemia								
No (Ref.)	4,509	10,591	731 (16.21%)	69.02	1 (Ref.)		1 (Ref.)	
Yes	1,204	2,913	176 (14.62%)	60.42	0.884 (0.75 - 1.04)	0.141	0.883 (0.74 - 1.05)	0.155
DM								
No (Ref.)	4,399	10,447	686 (15.59%)	65.66	1 (Ref.)		1 (Ref.)	
Yes	1,314	3,057	221 (16.82%)	72.29	1.098 (0.94 - 1.28)	0.227	1.152 (0.98 - 1.35)	0.085
ESRD								
No (Ref.)	4,562	10,876	704 (15.43%)	64.73	1 (Ref.)		1 (Ref.)	
Yes	1,151	2,628	203 (17.64%)	77.23	1.186 (1.01 - 1.39)	0.033*	1.221 (1.04 - 1.44)	0.017*

Crude HR relative hazard ratio, *Adjusted HR* adjusted hazard ratio controlling for age, gender, CCI score, Hypertension, Hyperlipidemia, diabetes and ESRD
*p<0.05

management rather than laparoscopic management in higher grade (G2 and G3) disease but not in low-grade disease. Among our high-grade and low-grade subgroups, there was no significant difference between patients with and without URS biopsy. Moreover, in a previous study, about 3% of patients with suspected UTUC who underwent radical surgery were reported to eventually have benign pathology and that they need to be prevented from unnecessary radical surgery [25]. Therefore, careful investigation in patients with previously suspected UTUC is critical.

In previous studies, about half of patients with UTUC encountered IVR after receiving radical surgery [26], which is higher than our results (around 27% (138/502)). Although IVR was not related to an increased risk of poor survival or distant metastasis, about 5–10% of recurrent bladder tumors progressed to a muscle-invasive state that

is an important risk factor for poor survival and metastasis [27]. Given the high risk of IVR, patients with UTUC after undergoing radical surgery are recommended to undergo regular endoscopic surveillance. Therefore, it is important to consider this issue to reduce the risk of IVR. Our current study indicates that bladder tumor history is the only prognostic factor for IVR. If a higher probability of IVR is suspected after radical surgery, single-dose immediate intravesical chemotherapy is reported to be a feasible and safe strategy to prevent IVR in patients with UTUC [28]. Yoo et al. hypothesized that tumor location is a key factor affecting IVR after URS with manipulation. In their assessment, the reason for bladder tumor recurrence from the ureter tumor is the previous shedding of tumor cells owing to the short distance from the ureter tumor to the bladder. They concluded that URS biopsy was an

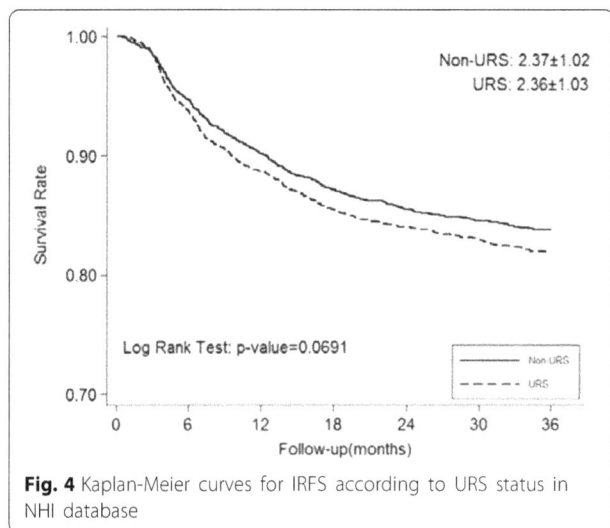

Fig. 4 Kaplan-Meier curves for IRFS according to URS status in NHI database

independent risk factor for IVR only in patients with a renal pelvis tumor which offsets the protective distance between the renal pelvis and the bladder [29]. Compared to our data, no matter where the tumor is located, URS biopsy before radical surgery does not increase the risk of IVR. Based on these results, the actual mechanism of IVR is still not clear; it may not be simply from tumor detachment induced by manipulation.

There are some limitations to the present study in addition to its retrospective design. However, in order to increase its accuracy, we also analyze the National Taiwan Insurance Database and included more patients with UTUC. The first limitation was that some possible prognostic factors for IVR including bladder cuff management method and concomitant carcinoma in situ were not included. Furthermore, we could not compare our patients with those receiving URS without biopsy or

Table 6 Cox models measured incidence densities and hazard ratio of overall survival

	N	Total person-year	Case	per 1000 person-year Incident rate	Crude HR (95% CI)	p-value	adjust HR (95% CI)	p-value
Main Effect								
URS- (Ref.)	2,634	6,941	531 (20.16%)	76.50	1 (Ref.)		1 (Ref.)	
URS+	3,079	8,195	568 (18.45%)	69.31	0.907 (0.81 – 1.02)	0.108	0.919 (0.82 – 1.04)	0.164
Baseline Patient Demographic Characteristics								
Gender								
Female (Ref.)	3,241	8,643	579 (17.86%)	66.99	1 (Ref.)		1 (Ref.)	
Male	2,472	6,493	520 (21.04%)	80.08	1.191 (1.06 – 1.34)	0.004*	1.225 (1.09 - 1.38)	0.001*
Age Categories								
<65 yr(Ref.)	2,044	5,647	266 (13.01%)	47.10	1 (Ref.)		1 (Ref.)	
65-74 yr	2,094	5,546	410 (19.58%)	73.93	1.561 (1.34 - 1.82)	<0.001*	1.597 (1.36 - 1.87)	<0.001*
>74yr	1,575	3,943	423 (26.86%)	107.28	2.245 (1.93 - 2.62)	<0.001*	2.290 (1.96 – 2.68)	<0.001*
CCI score Categories								
0 (Ref.)	613	1,637	109 (17.78%)	66.57	1 (Ref.)		1 (Ref.)	
1	462	1,209	98 (21.21%)	81.03	1.211 (0.92 – 1.59)	0.169	1.134 (0.86 – 1.49)	0.372
2+	4,638	12,289	892 (19.23%)	72.58	1.088 (0.89 – 1.33)	0.407	0.956 (0.78 – 1.18)	0.671
Hypertension								
No (Ref.)	2,743	7,322	504 (18.37%)	68.83	1 (Ref.)		1 (Ref.)	
Yes	2,970	7,814	595 (20.03%)	76.15	1.103 (0.98 – 1.24)	0.104	0.992 (0.88 – 1.12)	0.896
Hyperlipidemia								
No (Ref.)	4,509	11,883	908 (20.14%)	76.41	1 (Ref.)		1 (Ref.)	
Yes	1,204	3,253	191 (15.86%)	58.72	0.772 (0.66 – 0.90)	0.001*	0.777 (0.66 – 0.91)	0.002*
DM								
No (Ref.)	4,399	11,682	825 (18.75%)	70.62	1 (Ref.)		1 (Ref.)	
Yes	1,314	3,454	274 (20.85%)	79.32	1.122 (0.98 – 1.29)	0.099	1.141 (0.99 - 1.32)	0.072
ESRD								
No (Ref.)	4,562	12,134	862 (18.90%)	71.04	1 (Ref.)		1 (Ref.)	
Yes	1,151	3,002	237 (20.59%)	78.95	1.110 (0.96 – 1.28)	0.153	1.254 (1.08 – 1.46)	0.003*

Crude HR relative hazard ratio, *Adjusted HR* adjusted hazard ratio controlling for age, gender, CCI score, Hypertension, Hyperlipidemia, diabetes and ESRD
*p<0.05

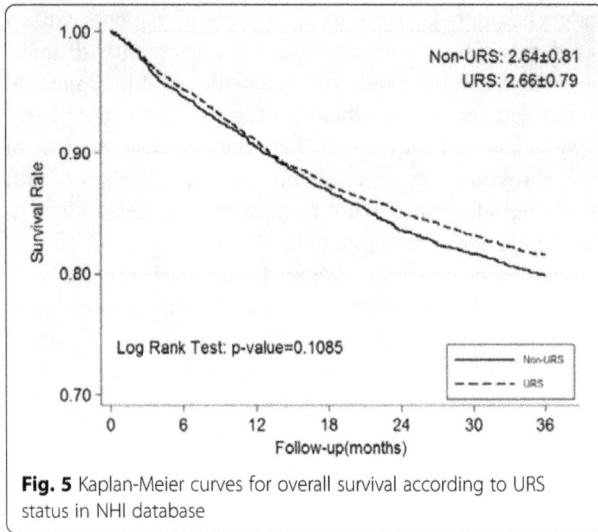

Fig. 5 Kaplan-Meier curves for overall survival according to URS status in NHI database

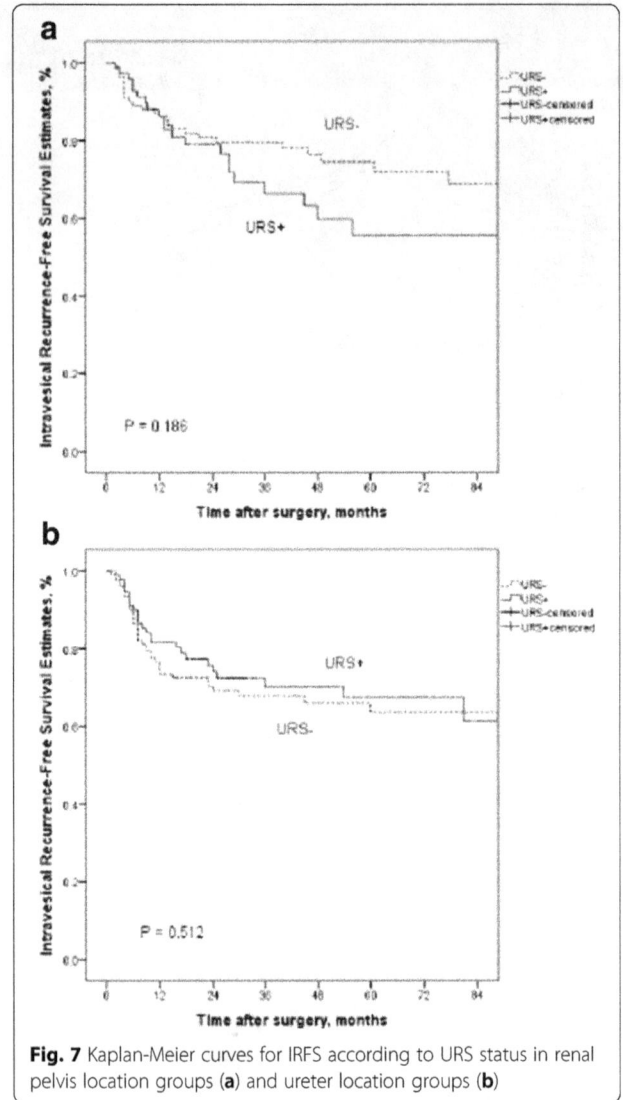

Fig. 7 Kaplan-Meier curves for IRFS according to URS status in renal pelvis location groups (**a**) and ureter location groups (**b**)

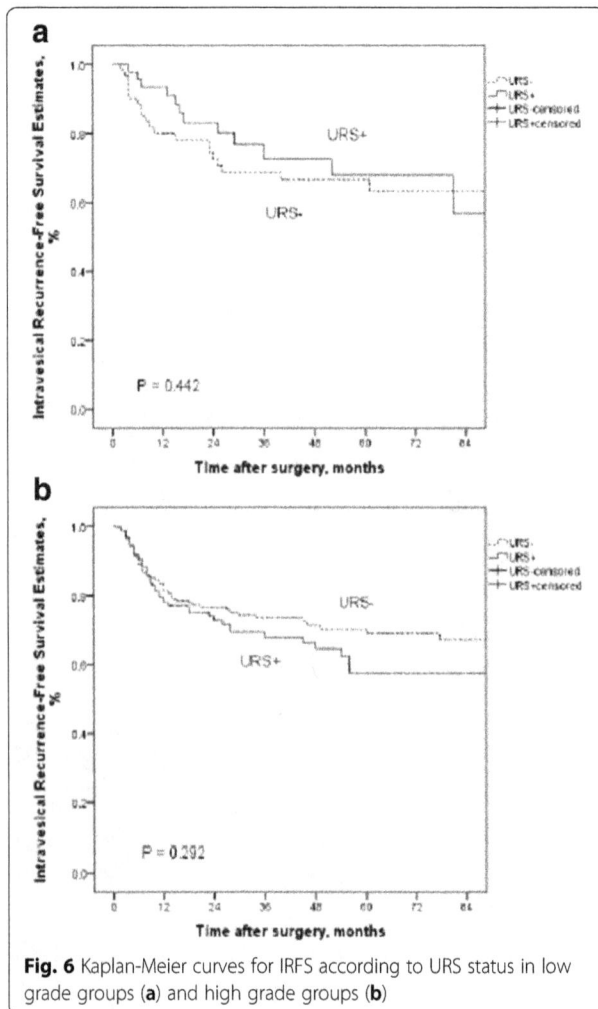

Fig. 6 Kaplan-Meier curves for IRFS according to URS status in low grade groups (**a**) and high grade groups (**b**)

with laser treatment for kidney-sparing surgery. In addition, the impact of URS on the conditional survival of IVR over time needs to be assessed because Shigeta et al. concluded that the influence of most predictive factors for IVR diminish over time [30]. A recent meta-analysis comprising six studies concluded that diagnostic URS before radical surgery seems to increase the risk of IVR after radical surgery. However, all of these six studies had the same results, and they need to be considered cautiously with various limitations. As we discussed, previous analyses have reported that diagnostic URS before radical surgery has no significant effect on IVR. On the other hand, the duration required to define bladder tumor recurrence and a primary bladder tumor event is still unclear. Nevertheless, our findings indicate that a two-session approach was not an independent risk factor for increased IVR.

Conclusion

Diagnostic URS before radical nephroureterectomy does not significantly increase the risk of worse survival, progression, and intravesical recurrence even in patients who have no history of bladder cancer. Our data from both our institution and the NHI database indicate that diagnostic URS can be part of a diagnostic strategy especially in flat, small tumors which are difficult to identify on imaging studies and when patients plan to undergo conservative treatment.

Acknowledgements

This study was supported by grants from Kaohsiung Medical University "Aim for the Top Universities" (KMU-TP105E24, KMU-TP105G00, KMU-TP105G01, KMU-TP105G02), the health and welfare surcharge of tobacco products, Ministry of Health and Welfare (MOHW106-TDU-B-212-144007), and Kaohsiung Medical University Hospital (KMUH104-4M36, KMTTH-105-006).

Funding

This research did not receive any specific grant from any funding agency in the public, commercial, or not-for-profit sector.

Authors' contributions

HY-L and CC-L analyzed and interpreted the patient data and were the major contributor in writing the manuscript. JS-H analyzed the NHI data. HC-Y, HL-K, WM-L, CF-L, CN-H, and WJ-W revised the manuscript. All authors read and approved the final manuscript.

Competing interests

The authors declare that they have no competing interests.

Author details

[1]Department of Urology, Kaohsiung Municipal Ta-Tung Hospital, Kaohsiung, Taiwan. [2]Graduate Institute of Clinical Medicine, College of Medicine, Kaohsiung Medical University, Kaohsiung, Taiwan. [3]Department of Urology, Kaohsiung Medical University Hospital, Kaohsiung, Taiwan. [4]Department of Urology, School of Medicine, College of Medicine, Kaohsiung Medical University, Kaohsiung, Taiwan. [5]Graduate Institute of Medicine, College of Medicine, Kaohsiung Medical University, No.100, Tzyou 1st Road, Kaohsiung 807, Taiwan. [6]Department of Public Health, Kaohsiung Medical University, Kaohsiung, Taiwan. [7]Department of Urology, Ministry of Health and Welfare Pingtung Hospital, Pingtung, Taiwan. [8]Department of Pathology, Chi-Mei Medical Center, Tainan, Taiwan. [9]Department of Biotechnology, Southern Taiwan University of Science and Technology, Tainan, Taiwan. [10]National Cancer Research Institute, National Health Research Institutes, Tainan, Taiwan. [11]Institute of Clinical Medicine, Kaohsiung Medical University, Kaohsiung, Taiwan. [12]Department of Internal Medicine and Cancer Center, Kaohsiung Medical University Hospital, Kaohsiung Medical University, Kaohsiung, Taiwan.

References

1. Margulis V, Shariat SF, Matin SF, et al. Outcomes of radical nephroureterectomy: a series from the Upper Tract Urothelial Carcinoma Collaboration. Cancer. 2009;115(6):1224–33.
2. Verhoest G, Shariat SF, Chromecki TF, et al. Predictive factors of recurrence and survival of upper tract urothelial carcinomas. World J Urol. 2011;29:495–501.
3. Lai MN, Wang SM, Chen PC, et al. Population-based case-control study of Chinese herbal products containing aristolochic acid and urinary tract cancer risk. J Natl Cancer Inst. 2010;102:179–86.
4. Li CC, Chang TH, Wu WJ, et al. Significant predictive factors for prognosis of primary upper urinary tract cancer after radical nephroureterectomy in Taiwanese patients. Eur Urol. 2008;54:1127–34.
5. Cutress ML, Stewart GD, Wells-Cole S, et al. Long-term endoscopic management of upper tract urothelial carcinoma: 20-year single-centre experience. BJU Int. 2012;110:1608–17.
6. Chitale S, Mbakada R, Irving S, et al. Nephroureterectomy for transitional cell carcinoma—the value of pre-operative histology. Ann R Coll Surg Engl. 2008;90:45–50.
7. Guarnizo E, Pavlovich CP, Seiba M, et al. Ureteroscopic biopsy of upper tract urothelial carcinoma: improved diagnostic accuracy and histopathological considerations using a multi-biopsy approach. J Urol. 2000;163:52–5.
8. Andersen JR, Kristensen JK. Ureteroscopic management of transitional cell tumors. Scand J Urol Nephrol. 1994;28:153–7.
9. Grasso M, McCue P, Bagley DH. Multiple urothelial recurrences of renal cell carcinoma after initial diagnostic ureteroscopy. J Urol. 1992;147:1358–60.
10. Shiraishi K, Eguchi S, Mohri J, et al. Role of ureteroscopic biopsy in the management of upper urinary tract malignancy. Int J Urol. 2003;10:627–30.
11. Ishikawa S, Abe T, Shinohara N, et al. Impact of diagnostic ureteroscopy on intravesical recurrence and survival in patients with urothelial carcinoma of the upper urinary tract. J Urol. 2010;184:883–7.
12. Hendin BN, Streem SB, Levin HS, et al. Impact of diagnostic ureteroscopy on long-term survival in patients with upper tract transitional cell carcinoma. J Urol. 1999;161:783–5.
13. Jeldres C, Sun M, Isbarn H, et al. A population-based assessment of perioperative mortality after nephroureterectomy for upper-tract urothelial carcinoma. Urology. 2010;75:315–20.
14. Shinagare AB, Fennessy FM, et al. Urothelial cancers of the upper urinary tract: metastatic pattern and its correlation with tumor histopathology and location. J Comput Assist Tomogr. 2011;35:217–22.
15. Roupret M, Babjuk M, Comperat E, et al. European guidelines on upper tract urothelial carcinomas: 2013 update. Eur Urol. 2013;63:1059–71.
16. Grahn A, Melle-Hannah M, Malm C, et al. Diagnostic accuracy of computed tomography urography and visual assessment during ureterorenoscopy in upper tract urothelial carcinoma. BJU Int. 2017;119:289–97.
17. Hafner C, Knuechel R, Zanardo L, et al. Evidence for oligoclonality and tumor spread by intraluminal seeding in multifocal urothelial carcinomas of the upper and lower urinary tract. Oncogene. 2001;20:4910–5.
18. Luo HL, Kang CH, Chen YT, et al. Diagnostic ureteroscopy independently correlates with intravesical recurrence after nephroureterectomy for upper urinary tract urothelial carcinoma. Ann Surg Onco. 2013;20:3121–6.
19. Pignot G, Colin P, Zerbib M, et al. Influence of previous or synchronous bladder cancer on oncologic outcomes after radical nephroureterectomy for upper urinary tract urothelial carcinoma. Urol Oncol. 2014;32:23.e1–8.
20. Milojevic B, Djokic M, Sipetic-Grujicic S, et al. Prognostic significance of non-muscle-invasive bladder tumor history in patients with upper urinary tract urothelial carcinoma. Urol Oncol. 2013;31:1615–20.
21. Nison L, Rouprêt M, Bozzini G, et al. The oncologic impact of a delay between diagnosis and radical nephroureterectomy due to diagnostic ureteroscopy in upper urinary tract urothelial carcinomas: results from a large collaborative database. World J Urol. 2013;31:69–76.
22. Jinzaki M, Kikuchi E, Akita H, et al. Role of computed tomography urography in the clinical evaluation of upper tract urothelial carcinoma. Int J Urol. 2016;23:284–98.
23. Zhang Z, Fan W, Deng Q, et al. The prognostic and diagnostic value of circulating tumor cells in bladder cancer and upper tract urothelial carcinoma: a meta-analysis of 30 published studies. Oncotarget. 2017; https://doi.org/10.10632/oncotarget.10521. Epub ahead of print.
24. Cutress ML, Stewart GD, Tudor EC, et al. Endoscopic versus laparoscopic management of noninvasive upper tract urothelial carcinoma: 20-year single center experience. J Urol. 2013;189:2054–60.
25. Hong S, Kwon T, You D, et al. Incidence of benign results after laparoscopic radical nephroureterectomy. JSLS. 2014;e2014.00335.

26. Azemar MD, Comperat E, Richad F, et al. Bladder recurrence after surgery for upper urinary tract urothelial cell carcinoma: frequency, risk factors, and surveillance. Urol Oncol. 2011;29:103–36.
27. Kim KH, You D, Jeong IG, et al. Muscle-invasive bladder cancer developing after nephroureterectomy for upper urinary tract urothelial carcinoma. Urol Oncol. 2013;31:1643–9.
28. Ito A, Shintaku I, Satoh M, et al. Prospective randomized phase II trial of a single early intraveiscal instillation of pirarubicin (THP) in the prevention of bladder recurrence after nephroureterectomy for upper urinary tract urothelial carcinoma: the THP Monotherapy Study Group Trial. J Clin Oncol. 2013;31:1422–7.
29. Yoo S, You D, Song C, et al. Risk of intravesical recurrence after ureteroscopic biopsy for upper tract urothelial carcinoma: does the location matter? J Endourol. 2017;31:259–65.
30. Shigeta K, Kikuchi E, Hagiwara M, et al. The over time conditional survival of intravesical recurrence in upper tract urothelial carcinoma. J Urol. 2017; 198:1278–85.

2

Comparison of clinical outcomes between mesh-reinforced pancreatojejunostomy and pancreatogastrostomy following pancreaticoduodenectomy

Junhai Pan[†], Xiaolong Ge[†], Wei Zhou[*], Xin Zhong, Lihu Gu, Hepan Zhu, Xinlong Li, Weilin Qi and Xianfa Wang[*]🅔

Abstract

Background: Postoperative complications, especially postoperative pancreatic fistulas, remain the major concern following pancreaticoduodenectomy (PD). Mesh-reinforced pancreatic anastomoses, including pancreatojejunostomy (PJ) and pancreatogastrostomy (PG), are a new effective technique in PD. This study was conducted to analyze the safety and efficacy of this new technique and to compare the results of mesh-reinforced PJ vs PG.

Methods: A total of 110 patients who underwent PD between August 2005 and January 2016 were eligible in this study. Perioperative and postoperative data of patients with a mesh-reinforced technique were analyzed. Data were also grouped according to the procedure performed: mesh-reinforced PJ and mesh-reinforced PG.

Results: Among patients undergoing PD with the mesh-reinforced technique, 42 had postoperative complications, and the comprehensive complication index (CCI) was 32.7 ± 2.5. Only 10% of patients had pancreatic fistula; three were grade A, six were grade B, and two were grade C. Biliary fistula occurred in only 8.2% of patients. Patients undergoing mesh-reinforced PG showed a significantly lower rate of CCI than did mesh-reinforced PJ patients (27.0 ± 2.1 vs 37.0 ± 3.9, $p < 0.05$). The mesh-reinforced PG was also favored over mesh-reinforced PJ because of significant differences in intra-abdominal fluid collection (5.9% vs 18.6%, $p < 0.05$) and delayed gastric emptying (3.9% vs 15.3%, $p < 0.05$).

Conclusions: PD with the mesh-reinforced technique was a safe and effective method of decreasing postoperative pancreatic fistula. Compared with mesh-reinforced PJ, mesh-reinforced PG did not show significant differences in the rates of pancreatic fistula or biliary fistula. However, CCI, intra-abdominal fluid collection, and delayed gastric emptying were significantly reduced in patients with mesh-reinforced PG.

Keywords: Pancreatogastrostomy, Pancreatojejunostomy, Pancreaticoduodenectomy, Mesh, Pancreatic fistula

Background

Pancreaticoduodenectomy (PD) is considered to be one of the most difficult and complex surgery since Whipple and colleagues published the first report of patients undergoing PD in 1935 [1]. In addition, PD has been regarded to be a standard surgical procedure in pancreatic cancer and other lesions which are located in periampullary region, while it is always with high postoperative complications

rates [2–5]. Generally, postoperative pancreatic fistula (POPF), biliary fistula, intra-abdominal fluid collection, intra-abdominal hemorrhage, and delayed gastric emptying are common post-pancreaticoduodenectomy complications even there are advances in surgical techniques in recent years, and it leads to prolonged hospital stays and increased medical costs [6, 7]. Among all the postoperative complications, POPF is regarded as Achilles heel of PD. To prevent complications, various strategies have been tried including pharmacologic prophylactic approaches and surgical techniques [8, 9]. These include octreotide, occluding the main duct with rubber or fibrin glue, pancreatic duct stenting, suture ligation of the

---
* Correspondence: zhouw@srrsh.com; 3195011@zju.edu.cn
†Junhai Pan and Xiaolong Ge contributed equally to this work.
Department of General Surgery, School of Medicine, Sir Run Run Shaw Hospital, Zhejiang University, 3 East Qingchun Road, Hangzhou 310016, Zhejiang, China

pancreatic duct, pancreaticoenterostomy with the jejunum or stomach, modification of suturing techniques, and others [10–12]. Although the rate of mortality after PD has decreased to less than 5%, the morbidity rate is still higher, ranging from 40 to 60% [13]. As the most harmful complications, the incidence of POPF has been reported, with highly variable rates depending on various definitions, ranging from 10 to 29% [14]. Postoperative complications at or around the anastomosis following PD were the most frequent and dangerous, occurring almost 25 times with five deaths [15]. Therefore, improvements in perioperative management and surgical technique remain crucial to decrease complications following PD.

For almost 10 years, we have used the new mesh-reinforced technique described by Peng and his colleagues to minimize postoperative complications after PD [16–18]. This safe and simple technique is characterized by a strip of polypropylene mesh, and it is wrapped around the pancreatic stump. Wang et al. [17] reported that no leakage occurred in 10 patients undergoing mesh-reinforced pancreaticojejunostomy (PJ) in PD. Only one patient developed grade A pancreatic leakage after mesh-reinforced pancreaticogastrostomy (PG) in a series of 13 initial cases [14, 18]. However, a large sample analysis is needed to evaluate whether the mesh-reinforced technique is safe and effective following PD. Some studies suggested that PG reduced biliary fistula and delayed gastric emptying and postoperative collections in patients following PD more so than did PJ [19, 20]. Therefore, whether mesh-reinforced PG is better than mesh-reinforced PJ in postoperative complications following PD remains unknown.

In this study, we evaluated the outcomes of the mesh-reinforced technique in 110 patients undergoing PD. Either PG or PJ was performed depending on the surgeon's preference. Postoperative complications were assessed for both types of reconstruction.

Methods

Study patients

Consecutive patients undergoing pancreatoduodenectomy because of malignant or non-malignant disease were included and analyzed in a tertiary referral hospital between August 2005 and January 2016. Written informed consent which was associated with the potential surgical risks was signed by all the patients. The present research was approved by the ethics committee of our hospital.

Surgical techniques

In our institution, we used the mesh-reinforced technique of pancreaticogastrostomy described by Professor Peng [16]. During the entire surgical procedure, non-absorbable (polypropylene mesh, large pore, Ethicon, New Jersey, USA) or absorbable (Cook, Limerick, Ireland) hernia grafts were used to reconstruct the pancreatic remnant. Pancreatojejunostomy and pancreatogastrostomy were the techniques used in reconstruction of pancreatic anastomosis. The mesh-reinforced technique in pancreaticogastrostomy was designed such that the pancreatic remnant wrapped in a mesh strip was embedded into the stomach and was bound to its posterior wall by a single layer of continuous sutures [18]. The mesh-reinforced technique in pancreaticojejunostomy was designed such that the sheath of the jejunum was bound to the pancreatic remnant which was wrapped by a strip of mesh. In our institution, this mesh-reinforced technique was the first choice for reconstruction following PD; it has been shown to be safe and effective for PG or PJ as described previously by Wang and Zhu [17, 18].

Data collection

The data collection was performed retrospectively including baseline characteristics and laboratory data from the database in our hospital. In addition, baseline characteristics mainly included gender, age, body mass index (BMI), comorbidities, pancreatic gland texture, mesh materials, American Society of Anesthesiologists (ASA), and the surgical indication. Other data about surgery included operative time, intraoperative blood transfusion, intraoperative bleeding, and the size of pancreatic duct.

Definition of outcomes

The primary outcome was pancreatic fistula after surgery according to the definition by International Study Group of Pancreatic Fistula (ISGPF). A clinical grading system of POPF was proposed as grades A, B, and C [14]. The comprehensive complication index (CCI) was created to evaluate postoperative complications, and the CCI was a score calculated based on the Clavien-Dindo system [21, 22]. Mild complications included grades I and II according to the Clavien-Dindo system, and the major complications included grades III to IV. Furthermore, the CCI system was reported to be more sensitive than the existing morbidity endpoints [21, 23]. The website of http://www.assessurgery.com was used to calculate the CCI in each patient [24]. Other outcomes included postoperative stay, biliary fistula, abdominal bleeding, intra-abdominal fluid collection, delayed gastric emptying, and reoperations [25].

Statistical analysis

SPSS version 23.0 software was used in analyzing all the data. Continuous data were presented as mean ± SD, and categorical data were presented as number (%). The continuous variables were analyzed by Mann-Whitney U test or Student's t test, and Pearson's chi-square test or the Fisher exact test was used to analyze categorical variables. The statistically significance was defined as P value < 0.05.

Results

Patients

In total, 110 patients underwent pancreatic resections by the mesh-reinforced technique and were included in this retrospective observational analysis, of which 84.5% were confirmed to be soft parenchyma. Among 110 patients following PD, 25.5% had a dilated pancreatic duct with the diameter larger than 4 mm. Fifty-one patients underwent PG, and 59 patients underwent PJ with the new mesh-reinforced technique. In the PG group, there were 27 males and 24 females, and their mean age was 60.9 years. In the PJ group, the patients' mean age was 57.1 years, and 38 patients were male. No statistically significant differences was found in the distributions of comorbidities, ASA, pancreatic gland texture, pancreatic duct size, age, and gender between the PG group and PJ group (Table 1). A total of 35 patients underwent PD due to ampullary carcinoma, 16 patients had duodenal cancer, 16 patients had distal biliary cancer, and 15 patients were diagnosed with ductal cancer. The remaining 28 patients had other conditions, primarily cystic tumors (9 patients), endocrine tumors (5 patients), and intraductal papillary mucinous tumors (5 patients). There was no significant difference between the PG group and the PJ group in terms of surgical indications (Table 2).

Postoperative outcomes

After PD with the mesh-reinforced technique, 68 patients recovered uneventfully, and 42 patients suffered postoperative complications. Some patients were found to have more than two complications after surgery. According to the Clavien-Dindo system, there were 7 patients (6.4%) with mild complications (Clavien-Dindo grade I to II) and 35 patients (31.8%) with major complications (Clavien-Dindo grade III to IV). The mean CCI based on Clavien-Dindo classification was 32.7 ± 2.5. The mean operative time was 368.0 ± 8.2 min, with estimated blood loss of 502.4 ± 48.3 mL. The mean anastomosis time of PD with this mesh-reinforced technique was 27.4 ± 0.4 min. A total of 37.3% of all the patients received intraoperative blood transfusions, and the length of the postoperative stay was 23.2 ± 0.9 days.

Postoperative pancreatic fistula

Various improvements in surgical technique were developed to avoid postoperative pancreatic fistula in studies regarding PD [13]. In our study, with the new mesh-reinforced technique, the rate of pancreatic fistula decreased to 10% in all the patients. According to the ISGPF definition [14], only three patients (2.7%) had grade A pancreatic fistula, six patients (5.5%) had grade B, and two patients (1.8%) had grade C (Table 3). In addition, only nine patients (8.2%) suffered biliary fistula, and eight patients (7.3%) had abdominal bleeding

Table 1 Baseline demographics in patients undergoing pancreatectomy

Characteristic	All ($n = 110$)	PG group ($n = 51$)	PJ group ($n = 59$)	P value
Age*	58.9 ± 1.0	60.9 ± 1.3	57.1 ± 1.5	0.07
Men, n (%)	65 (59.1)	27 (52.9)	38 (64.4)	0.22
BMI*, kg/m^2	23.0 ± 0.3	22.6 ± 0.6	23.3 ± 0.4	0.28
Comorbidities, n (%)				
Diabetes mellitus, n (%)	22 (20)	9 (17.6)	13 (22.0)	0.57
Hypertension, n (%)	27 (24.5)	13 (25.5)	14 (23.7)	0.83
Operation time*, min	368.0 ± 8.2	342.4 ± 11.7	390.0 ± 10.8	< 0.01
ASA ≥ 3, n (%)	19 (17.3)	9 (17.6)	10 (16.9)	0.92
Intraoperative blood transfusion, n (%)	41 (37.3)	14 (27.5)	27 (45.8)	0.048
Estimated blood loss*, mL	502.4 ± 48.3	392.2 ± 31.8	597.6 ± 84.2	0.03
Pancreatic gland texture, n (%)				0.55
Soft, n (%)	93 (84.5)	42 (82.4)	51 (86.4)	–
Hard, n (%)	17 (15.5)	9 (17.6)	8 (13.6)	–
Mesh materials, n (%)				< 0.01
Non-absorbable, n (%)	59 (53.6)	10 (19.6)	49 (83.1)	–
Absorbable, n (%)	51 (46.4)	41 (80.4)	10 (16.9)	–
Pancreatic duct size (> 4 mm), n (%)	28 (25.5)	14 (27.5)	14 (23.7)	0.66
The time of anastomosis*, min	27.4 ± 0.4	29.1 ± 0.7	27.9 ± 0.6	0.21

PG pancreatogastrostomy, *PJ* pancreatojejunostomy
*Value are expressed as the mean ± SE

Table 2 Surgical indications in 110 pancreaticoduodenectomies

	All (n = 110)	PG group (n = 51)	PJ group (n = 59)	P value
Ampullary carcinoma*	35 (31.8)	17 (33.3)	18 (30.5)	0.75
Distal biliary cancer*	16 (14.5)	7 (13.7)	9 (15.3)	0.82
Duodenal cancer*	16 (14.5)	7 (13.7)	9 (15.3)	0.82
Ductal cancer*	15 (13.6)	7 (13.7)	8 (13.6)	0.98
Cystic tumors*	9 (8.2)	4 (7.8)	5 (8.5)	0.90
Endocrine tumors*	5 (4.5)	3 (5.9)	2 (3.4)	0.53
Intraductal papillary mucinous tumor*	5 (4.5)	2 (3.9)	3 (5.1)	0.77
Other indications*	9 (8.2)	4 (7.8)	5 (8.5)	0.90

PG pancreatogastrostomy, PJ pancreatojejunostomy
*Values are expressed as n (%)

following PD. In addition, there were 14 patients (12.7%) with intra-abdominal fluid collections, and 11 patients (10.0%) had delayed gastric emptying. Finally, three patients (2.7%) underwent the reoperation due to serious complications associated with the pancreatic fistula (Table 3).

Comparison between PJ and PG with mesh-reinforced technique

At present, PJ and PG are both widely used following PD, and many studies have been published in order to compare the safety and efficacy of these two methods. Similarly, when the mesh-reinforced technique was performed during reconstruction in our study, the postoperative outcomes were compared between PJ and PG. The postoperative course showed that 18 (35.3%)

patients had complications in the PG group and that 24 (40.7%) patients had complications in the PJ group. When compared to the PG group, there were statistically significant differences in the PJ group in terms of the comprehensive complication index (27.0 ± 2.1 vs 37.0 ± 3.9, $P < 0.05$). In the PG group, three patients (5.9%) had pancreatic fistulas, of which one patient (2.0%) had grade A and two patients (3.9%) had grade B. In the PJ group, eight patients (13.6%) had pancreatic fistulas, of which two patients (3.4%) were grade A, four patients (6.8%) were grade B and two patients (3.4%) were grade C. The PJ group was more likely to have biliary fistula than was the PG group, even though no significant difference was found (11.9% vs 3.9%). However, significant differences in favor of the PG group were investigated regarding intra-abdominal fluid collections (5.9% vs 18.6%, $P < 0.05$) and delayed gastric emptying (3.9% vs 15.3%, $P < 0.05$). The operative time was also significantly different between these two groups (PG, 342.4 ± 11.7 min vs PJ, 390.0 ± 10.8 min, $P < 0.01$), while the time of anastomosis was not significantly different between the PG and PJ groups. The PJ group also had significantly more estimated blood loss than the PG group. All the results are shown in Tables 1 and 3.

Discussion

In this study, the safety and efficacy of mesh-reinforced pancreatojejunostomy and pancreatogastrostomy in patients following pancreatoduodenectomy were compared. We found that patients undergoing pancreatoduodenectomy with the mesh-reinforced technique suffered fewer postoperative complications, especially lower rates of

Table 3 Postoperative outcomes in 110 cases of pancreaticoduodenectomy

Outcome	All (n = 110)	PG group (n = 51)	PJ group (n = 59)	P value
Postoperative complication, n (%)	42 (38.2)	18 (35.3)	24 (40.7)	0.562
Mild complications, n (%)	7 (6.4)	3 (5.9)	4 (6.8)	0.848
Major complications, n (%)	35 (31.8)	15 (29.4)	20 (33.9)	0.614
CCI, mean ± SD	32.7 ± 2.5	27.0 ± 2.1	37.0 ± 3.9	0.045
Pancreatic fistula, n (%)	11 (10.0)	3 (5.9)	8 (13.6)	0.181
Pancreatic fistula grade				0.488
A, n (%)	3 (2.7)	1 (2.0)	2 (3.4)	–
B, n (%)	6 (5.5)	2 (3.9)	4 (6.8)	–
C, n (%)	2 (1.8)	0 (0)	2 (3.4)	–
Biliary fistula, n (%)	9 (8.2)	2 (3.9)	7 (11.9)	0.243
Postoperative stay, mean ± SD	23.2 ± 0.9	23.6 ± 1.6	22.8 ± 1.0	0.674
Abdominal bleeding, n (%)	8 (7.3)	4 (7.8)	4 (6.8)	0.830
Intra-abdominal fluid collection, n (%)	14 (12.7)	3 (5.9)	11 (18.6)	0.045
Delayed gastric empting, n (%)	11 (10.0)	2 (3.9)	9 (15.3)	0.048
Reoperations, n (%)	3 (2.7)	1 (2.0)	2 (3.4)	0.646

PG pancreatogastrostomy, PJ pancreatojejunostomy, CCI comprehensive complication index

pancreatic leakage. This retrospective study also indicated that PG with mesh-reinforced pancreatoduodenectomy resulted in fewer complications and improved the quality and safety of the pancreatic anastomosis more so than did the PJ with mesh-reinforced following PD.

The reported frequency of pancreatic fistula after pancreaticoduodenectomy varied from 10 to 30%, and pancreatic fistula was considered a serious event that even might be life-threatening in almost half of patients [15, 26, 27]. The reasons for pancreatic fistula were primarily its soft parenchyma, making it more likely to develop parenchymal lacerations from shear forces applied during tying of sutures [17]. In addition, the anastomotic technique, the diameter of pancreatic duct, the general condition of the patients and the various definitions of pancreatic fistula could also affect the incidence of postoperative pancreatic fistula [14, 28–30]. It was reported that soft pancreatic parenchyma and the diameter of main pancreatic duct less than 3 mm were risk factors for pancreatic leakage [31, 32]. To prevent these complications, various methods during the preoperative, intraoperative, and postoperative periods have been proposed, especially surgical techniques [33, 34]. For example, it is reported that the application of the novel embeddedness-like pancreaticojejunostomy anastomosis technique in PD was effective and could reduce the incidence of pancreatic fistula [35]. In our hospital, we also introduce a different method of mesh-reinforced technique in PD to reduce postoperative complications.

The rate of pancreatic fistula of 10% in our study was lower than that of other studies. The technique used in our procedure to reduce morbidity and mortality was modified according to the binding pancreaticojejunostomy described by Peng et al. [16]. There exist some advantages of this technique as previously described [36]. First, the safe anchor site was provided by the mesh for sutures, and this resulted in the ability to avoid leakage and bleeding after surgery for soft and fragile pancreatic tissue. Second, it was more convenient to wrap the pancreatic stump with the bowel loop by changing the shape of the pancreas with mesh reinforcement. In addition, the left edge of the mesh was sutured tightening to the posterior wall of the bowel loop, and it facilitated the pancreas sliding into the bowel loop. Fourth, the likelihood of pancreatic leakage and bleeding was diminished by the mesh compression of pancreatic tissue. Finally, the mesh stimulated the growth of fibroblasts and promoted the healing process between the pancreatic capsule and the bowel mucosa [36–38]. In our study, we proposed various mesh-reinforced surgical techniques to prevent complications, and there were lower rates of several surgical complications.

There are two methods for the restoration of pancreatic drainage into the gastrointestinal tract in PD, including PG and PJ [19, 39, 40]. Not all previous studies yielded similar results. Yeo et al. [41] reported that the rate of pancreatic fistula was almost the same for the PG (12.3%) and PJ (11.1%), suggesting that PG was not safer than PJ. However, Bassi et al. [19] found that biliary fistula, postoperative collections and delayed gastric emptying rates were significantly lower in patients with PG than in PJ. Schlitt et al. [20] also suggested that PG was significantly safer than PJ with respect to the incidence of pancreatic fistula. Therefore, there remained a need to compare the two methods following PD. Mesh-reinforced PG and mesh-reinforced PJ were compared with each other in our study. The mesh-reinforced PG showed advantages in PD in that its comprehensive complication index was lower than that of the mesh-reinforced PJ group. We also showed a significant benefit of mesh-reinforced PG reconstruction compared with mesh-reinforced PJ with respect to intra-abdominal fluid collection and delayed gastric emptying. Pancreatic and biliary fistulas also showed lower trends of incidence in mesh-reinforced PG.

There are additional factors supporting our conclusion that mesh-reinforced PG was superior to PJ. First, the blood supply to the stomach is rich, promoting healing between the stomach and the pancreatic stump [42]. Second, in the acidic gastric environment, pancreatic enzymes will not be activated, preventing deleterious tissue digestion around the anastomosis [43]. Third, a nasogastric tube can be used to decompress, and an endoscope can easily access the anastomosis when needed [43, 44]. However, the learning curve of the surgeon and the experience of the center also influence the method we chose. As a result, we suggest that mesh-reinforced PG can be performed in patients following PD to prevent postoperative complications, especially pancreatic fistulas.

There are several limitations in current study. First of all, as this study was a retrospective observational analysis, it could not exclude the impact of residual confounding factors completely, including the fact that patient distribution between groups depended on surgeon's preference. Second, as it is just a single-center study; multicenter studies are needed for further confirmation. Third, the results lacked a control group without a mesh-reinforced technique; a randomized controlled trial would be necessary to conduct to avoid such bias in the future.

Conclusions

The current study confirmed that the mesh-reinforced technique may be beneficial in patients following PD. Although mesh-reinforced PG did not show significant differences in pancreatic fistulas and biliary fistulas, the CCI, intra-abdominal fluid collection, and delayed gastric emptying were significantly lower in patients with the mesh-reinforced PG than in mesh-reinforced PJ. In summary, the mesh-reinforced technique is preferred during pancreaticoduodenectomy, especially mesh-reinforced pancreatogastrostomy.

Abbreviations
BMI: Body mass index; CCI: Comprehensive complication index; PD: Pancreaticoduodenectomy; PG: Pancreatogastrostomy; PJ: Pancreatojejunostomy; POPF: Postoperative pancreatic fistula

Acknowledgements
The authors gratefully acknowledge all of the investigators for their contributions to the trial, as well as Bin Chen, who provided medical writing assistance.

Funding
This study was funded in part by the Zhejiang Provincial Natural Science Foundation (No. 2017C33159 and No. LY18H030006) and Health and Family Planning Commission of Zhejiang Province Grant (No. 2017ZD019).

Authors' contributions
JP and XG contributed to the study conception and design. XG, WZ, XL, and JP contributed to the acquisition of the data. XZ, WQ, and LG contributed to the analysis and interpretation of the data. JP and HZ contributed to the drafting of the manuscript. WZ and XW contributed to the critical revision. All authors read and approved the final manuscript.

Competing interests
The authors declare that they have no competing interests.

References
1. Whipple AO, Parsons WB, Mullins CR. Treatment of carcinoma of the ampulla of vater. Ann Surg. 1935;102(4):763–79.
2. Senda Y, Shimizu Y, Natsume S, Ito S, Komori K, Abe T, et al. Randomized clinical trial of duct-to-mucosa versus invagination pancreaticojejunostomy after pancreatoduodenectomy. Br J Surg. 2018;105(1):48–57.
3. Bannone E, Andrianello S, Marchegiani G, Masini G, Malleo G, Bassi C, et al. Postoperative acute pancreatitis following pancreaticoduodenectomy: a determinant of fistula potentially driven by the intraoperative fluid management. Ann Surg. 2018. https://doi.org/10.1097/SLA.0000000000002900.
4. Wang WG, Babu SR, Wang L, Chen Y, Tian BL, He HB. Use of Clavien-Dindo classification in evaluating complications following pancreaticoduodenectomy in 1,056 cases: a retrospective analysis from one single institution. Oncol Lett. 2018;16(2):2023–9.
5. Kunstman JW, Starker LF, Healy JM, Salem RR. Pancreaticoduodenectomy can be performed safely with rare employment of surgical drains. Am Surg. 2017;83(3):265–73.
6. Hirono S, Kawai M, Okada KI, Miyazawa M, Kitahata Y, Hayami S, et al. Modified Blumgart mattress suture versus conventional interrupted suture in pancreaticojejunostomy during pancreaticoduodenectomy: randomized controlled trial. Ann Surg. 2018. https://doi.org/10.1097/SLA.0000000000002802.
7. De Pastena M, Paiella S, Marchegiani G, Malleo G, Ciprani D, Gasparini C, et al. Postoperative infections represent a major determinant of outcome after pancreaticoduodenectomy: results from a high-volume center. Surgery. 2017;162(4):792–801.
8. Lubrano J, Bachelier P, Paye F, Le Treut YP, Chiche L, Sa-Cunha A, et al. Severe postoperative complications decrease overall and disease free survival in pancreatic ductal adenocarcinoma after pancreaticoduodenectomy. Eur J Surg Oncol. 2018;44(7):1078–82.
9. Qiu J, Du C. Pancreatogastrostomy versus pancreatojejunostomy for RECOnstruction after PANCreatoduodenectomy (RECOPANC, DRKS 00000767): perioperative and long-term results of a multicenter randomized controlled trial. Ann Surg. 2017;266(6):e63–e4.
10. D'Souza MA, Shrikhande SV. Pancreatic resectional surgery: an evidence-based perspective. J Cancer Res Ther. 2008;4(2):77–83.
11. Ball CG, Howard TJ. Does the type of pancreaticojejunostomy after Whipple alter the leak rate? Adv Surg. 2010;44:131–48.
12. Kleeff J, Korc M, Apte M, La Vecchia C, Johnson CD, Biankin AV, et al. Pancreatic cancer. Nat Rev Dis Primers. 2016;2:16022.
13. Buchler MW, Friess H, Wagner M, Kulli C, Wagener V, Z'graggen K. Pancreatic fistula after pancreatic head resection. Brit J Surg. 2000;87(7):883–9.
14. Bassi C, Dervenis C, Butturini G, Fingerhut A, Yeo C, Izbicki J, et al. Postoperative pancreatic fistula: an international study group (ISGPF) definition. Surgery. 2005;138(1):8–13.
15. Trede M, Schwall G. The complications of pancreatectomy. Ann Surg. 1988;207(1):39–47.
16. Peng SY, Mou YP, Liu YB, Su Y, Peng CH, Cai XJ, et al. Binding pancreaticojejunostomy: 150 consecutive cases without leakage. J Gastrointest Surg. 2003;7(7):898–900.
17. Wang XF, Zhou W, Xin Y, Huang DY, Mou YP, Cai XH. A new technique of polypropylene mesh-reinforced pancreaticojejunostomy. Am J Surg. 2007;194(3):413–5.
18. Zhu YP, Zhou W, Zhang NY, Pan JH, Li B, Wang XF. A new technique of mesh-reinforced pancreaticogastrostomy: report of 13 initial cases. J Laparoendosc Adv S. 2013;23(7):617–20.
19. Bassi C, Falconi M, Molinari E, Salvia R, Butturini G, Sartori N, et al. Reconstruction by pancreaticojejunostomy versus pancreaticogastrostomy following pancreatectomy: results of a comparative study. Ann Surg. 2005;242(6):767–71 discussion 71–3.
20. Schlitt HJ, Schmidt U, Simunec D, Jager M, Aselmann H, Neipp M, et al. Morbidity and mortality associated with pancreatogastrostomy and pancreatojejunostomy following partial pancreatoduodenectomy. Br J Surg. 2002;89(10):1245–51.
21. Slankamenac K, Nederlof N, Pessaux P, de Jonge J, Wijnhoven BPL, Breitenstein S, et al. The comprehensive complication index a novel and more sensitive endpoint for assessing outcome and reducing sample size in randomized controlled trials. Ann Surg. 2014;260(5):757–63.
22. Dindo D, Demartines N, Clavien PA. Classification of surgical complications - a new proposal with evaluation in a cohort of 6336 patients and results of a survey. Ann Surg. 2004;240(2):205–13.
23. Slankamenac K, Graf R, Barkun J, Puhan MA, Clavien PA. The comprehensive complication index a novel continuous scale to measure surgical morbidity. Ann Surg. 2013;258(1):1–7.
24. Ge X, Dai X, Ding C, Tian H, Yang J, Gong J, et al. Early postoperative decrease of serum albumin predicts surgical outcome in patients undergoing colorectal resection. Dis Colon Rectum. 2017;60(3):326–34.
25. Shen YF, Jin WY. Reconstruction by pancreaticogastrostomy versus pancreaticojejunostomy following pancreaticoduodenectomy: a meta-analysis of randomized controlled trials. Gastroent Res Pract 2012. 2012:627095. https://doi.org/10.1155/2012/627095.
26. Fabre JM, Arnaud JP, Navarro F, Bergamaschi R, Cervi C, Marrel E, et al. Results of pancreatogastrostomy after pancreatoduodenectomy in 160 consecutive patients. Brit J Surg. 1998;85(6):751–4.
27. vanBergeHenegouwen MI, DeWit LT, VanGulik TM, Obertop H, Gouma DJ. Incidence, risk factors, and treatment of pancreatic leakage after pancreaticoduodenectomy: drainage versus resection of the pancreatic remnant. J Am Coll Surgeons. 1997;185(1):18–24.
28. Poon RTP, Lo SH, Fong D, Fan ST, Wong J. Prevention of pancreatic anastomotic leakage after pancreaticoduodenectomy. Am J Surg. 2002;183(1):42–52.
29. Yang YM, Tian XD, Zhuang Y, Wang WM, Wan YL, Huang YT. Risk factors of pancreatic leakage after pancreaticoduodenectomy. World J Gastroentero. 2005;11(16):2456–61.

30. Azumi Y, Isaji S, Kato H, Nobuoka Y, Kuriyama N, Kishiwada M, et al. A standardized technique for safe pancreaticojejunostomy: pair-watch suturing technique. World J Gastrointest Surg. 2010;2(8):260–4.

31. Bartoli FG, Arnone GB, Ravera G, Bachi V. Pancreatic fistula and relative mortality in malignant disease after pancreaticoduodenectomy. Review and statistical meta-analysis regarding 15 years of literature. Anticancer Res. 1991;11(5):1831–48.

32. Muscari F, Suc B, Kirzin S, Hay JM, Fourtanier G, Fingerhut A, et al. Risk factors for mortality and intra-abdominal complications after pancreatoduodenectomy: multivariate analysis in 300 patients. Surgery. 2006;139(5):591–8.

33. Sakorafas GH, Friess H, Balsiger BM, Buchler MW, Sarr MG. Problems of reconstruction during pancreatoduodenectomy. Dig Surg. 2001;18(5):363–9.

34. Alexakis N, Halloran C, Raraty M, Ghaneh P, Sutton R, Neoptolemos JP. Current standards of surgery for pancreatic cancer. Brit J Surg. 2004;91(11): 1410–27.

35. Xu X, Lv Y, Zhang L, Xin B, Li JA, Wang D, et al. Application of a novel embeddedness-like pancreaticojejunostomy anastomosis technique used in pancreaticoduodenectomy. Oncol Lett. 2018;15(5):8067–71.

36. Zhong X, Wang X, Pan J, Zhu H, Gu L, Shi Z. Mesh-reinforced pancreaticojejunostomy versus conventional pancreaticojejunostomy after pancreaticoduodenectomy: a retrospective study of 126 patients. World J Surg Oncol. 2018;16(1):68.

37. Continenza MA, Vicentini C, Paradiso-Galatioto G, Fileni A, Tchokogoue E. In vitro study of human dermal fibroblasts seeded on two kinds of surgical meshes: monofilamented polypropylene and multifilamented polyestere. Ital J Anat Embryol. 2003;108(4):231–9.

38. Di Vita G, Patti R, D'Agostino P, Ferlazzo V, Angileri M, Sieli G, et al. Modifications in the production of cytokines and growth factors in drainage fluids following mesh implantation after incisional hernia repair. Am J Surg. 2006;191(6):785–90.

39. Marcus SG, Cohen H, Ranson JH. Optimal management of the pancreatic remnant after pancreaticoduodenectomy. Ann Surg. 1995;221(6):635–45 discussion 45-8.

40. Berger AC, Howard TJ, Kennedy EP, Sauter PK, Bower-Cherry M, Dutkevitch S, et al. Does type of pancreaticojejunostomy after pancreaticoduodenectomy decrease rate of pancreatic fistula? A randomized, prospective, dual-institution trial. J Am Coll Surg. 2009;208(5): 738–47 discussion 47–9.

41. Yeo CJ, Cameron JL, Maher MM, Sauter PK, Zahurak ML, Talamini MA, et al. A prospective randomized trial of pancreaticogastrostomy versus pancreaticojejunostomy after pancreaticoduodenectomy. Ann Surg. 1995; 222(4):580–8 discussion 8–92.

42. Sauvanet A, Belghiti J, Panis Y, Gayet B, Camara E, Urrejola G, et al. Pancreaticogastrostomy after pancreatoduodenectomy. HPB Surg. 1992;6(2): 91–5 discussion 5–8.

43. McKay A, Mackenzie S, Sutherland FR, Bathe OF, Doig C, Dort J, et al. Meta-analysis of pancreaticojejunostomy versus pancreaticogastrostomy reconstruction after pancreaticoduodenectomy. Br J Surg. 2006;93(8):929–36.

44. Ricci C, Casadei R, Taffurelli G, Pacilio CA, Beltrami D, Minni F. Is pancreaticogastrostomy safer than pancreaticojejunostomy after pancreaticoduodenectomy? A meta-regression analysis of randomized clinical trials. Pancreatology. 2017;17(5):805–13.

3

The sonographic findings of micropapillary pattern in pure mucinous carcinoma of the breast

Heqing Zhang, Li Qiu and Yulan Peng[*]

Abstract

Background: The aim of this study was to describe the sonographic features of pure mucinous carcinoma with micropapillary pattern (MUMPC) and compare them with conventional pure mucinous breast carcinoma without micropapillary architecture (cPMBC) and mixed mucinous breast carcinoma (MMBC).

Methods: Eighty-eight patients (17 MUMPCs, 43 cPMBCs, and 28 MMBCs) were included in the study. Sonographic features according to the Breast Imaging Reporting and Data System (BI-RADS) lexicon for ultrasound (US) were recorded and analyzed for each patient. The age, sonographic lesion size, menstrual status, mass location, palpation, tenderness, and axillary lymph node metastasis (LNM) were also analyzed.

Results: Most of the MUMPCs showed an irregular shape (82.4%, 14/17), a parallel orientation (94.1%, 16/17), a non-circumscribed margin (88.2%, 15/17), and distal acoustic enhancement (88.2%, 15/17). Furthermore, MUMPC had mixed cystic and solid components (35.3%, 6/17) and hypoechoic (29.4%, 5/17) and isoechoic (35.3%, 6/17) structures, with calcification (29.4%, 5/17) and blood flow (41.2%, 7/17) within the tumor. The differences in sonographic features were not found between the MUMPC and cPMBC and between the MUMPC and MMBC. Moreover, there was no significant difference between the three groups based on age, menstrual status, mass location, palpation, and tenderness ($p > 0.05$). Similar axillary LNMs were observed between MUMPC and cPMBC ($p > 0.05$), but both MUMPC and cPMBC were statistically different from MMBC ($p < 0.05$), so as the lesion size.

Conclusions: At this particular stage, it is challenging to distinguish MUMPC from cPMBC and MMBC on ultrasound according to the BI-RADS-US lexicon.

Keywords: Breast, Mucinous carcinoma, Micropapillary, Ultrasonography

Background

Mucinous breast carcinoma (MBC) is a rare type of breast tumor characterized by large amounts of extracellular mucin. It accounts for about 1–7% of all the breast neoplasms [1–3] and can be divided into two types: pure mucinous breast carcinoma (PMBC) without other malignant components and mixed mucinous breast carcinoma (MMBC) with non-mucinous component. The PMBC is associated with a better prognosis and a lower rate of axillary lymph node metastasis compared with other breast tumors [4–7]. In contrast, invasive micropapillary carcinoma (IMPC), which accounts for approximately 0.7–3% of

invasive breast cancers, is a clinically aggressive variant of invasive ductal cancer with a high frequency of lymph node metastasis [7–9]. The micropapillary formations of IMPC indicate potentially aggressive tumor behavior and influence the choice of therapy [7]. However, the extracellular mucin and micropapillary can coexist within the same tumor. Pure mucinous carcinoma with micropapillary pattern (MUMPC), which was first reported in 2002 by Ng [10], has both architectures with opposite biological behavior [11]. Although, according to WHO Classification of Tumours of the Breast (2012), MUMPC does not classify as one of the breast cancer subtypes [12], MUMPCs are associated with a younger age group and frequent occurrence of nodal metastasis, which warrants special attention [4]. Barbashina et al. [11] have

* Correspondence: zhqpyl2018@163.com
Department of Ultrasound, West China Hospital, Sichuan University, Chengdu, China

demonstrated that MUMPCs constitute a clinically aggressive subset among tumors with mucinous morphology and should be distinguished from conventional pure mucinous carcinomas.

Up to the present time, there are only few studies on MUMPC. To our knowledge, there is no medical literature describing the sonographic findings of MUMPC. Therefore, we used ACR Breast Imaging Reporting and Data System (BI-RADS) lexicon [13] for ultrasound (US) to analyze the sonographic findings of MUMPC; the aim of this study was to characterize the sonographic features of MUMPC and to compare them with those from conventional PMBC without micropapillary architecture (cPMBC) and MMBC. Some clinical characteristics were also compared.

Methods

Patients

A total of 114 patients diagnosed with MBC were recruited at the Department of Ultrasound, West China Hospital, between January 2012 and April 2017. According to the WHO Classification of Tumours of the Breast (2012), PMBC has a mucinous component of more than 90%, while MMBC has a mucinous component of less than 90% [12]. The lower limit of mucinous component in MMBC is still not defined. Nevertheless, the majority of MBC we examined had ≥ 50% of mucinous component. Patients who underwent breast ultrasound and surgical excision at our hospital were included in the research. From 114 patients, 26 patients were excluded from the study; 9 patients who did not have surgery performed at our institute and 17 patients who were excluded from the study due to the loss of sonographic images. At last, a total of 88 lesions in 88 patients (87 women and 1 man) were identified within the study, including 17 patients with MUMPC, 43 with cPMBC, and 28 with MMBC. All the cases were consecutive patients. All patients underwent clinical breast physical exams before the ultrasonography. Furthermore, patients' clinical characteristics were reviewed, including age at diagnosis, menstrual status, mass status (location, palpation, and tenderness), and personal/family history. Our database was password protected, and the study was approved by the Ethics Committee of West China Hospital.

Ultrasonography

Breast ultrasonography was performed in all 88 lesions with the linear array probe (5–15 MHz) supplemented by the 1–5 MHz convex array probe, as needed, to penetrate lager mass (Philips iU22 and HDI 5000, Philips Medical Systems, Bothell, WA, USA; HI VISION Preirus, Hitachi Medical, Tokyo, Japan; Esaote MyLab 90, Esaote, Genova, Italy; GE Logiq E9, General Electric Healthcare,

Milwaukee, WI, USA). The patients were examined by US at supine position with the arms raised over the head. Bilateral breast scan was performed, and both gray-scale and color images of the lesion were acquired. All the US exams had been performed by experienced sonographers. They were familiar with the results of the physical examination, but were blinded to the pathological findings.

The US findings were retrospectively analyzed by one sonographer with more than 8 years of experience based on the criteria from the ACR BI-RADS lexicon for US [13]. The lesion size (maximum dimension), shape (regular, irregular), orientation (parallel, not parallel), margin (circumscribed, non-circumscribed (indistinct, angular, microlobulated, or spiculated)), echogenicity (anechoic, hyperechoic, complex echogenicity (mixed cystic and solid), hypoechoic, isoechoic, or heterogeneous), posterior acoustic features (no features, enhancement, shadowing, or combined pattern), and calcification (present, absent) in tumor mass were all recorded. The vascularity (present, absent) of the breast lesions was also retrospectively reviewed; blood flow was divided into four grades based on Adler et al. [14]: grade 0: no blood flow; grade 1: small amounts of flow (one or two punctate or short rod-like color flow signals); grade 2: medium amounts of flow (three or four punctate color flow signals or a longer blood vessel which may be half of the mass dimension long); grade 3: rich flow (more than four punctate color flow signals or two longer blood vessels). The BI-RADS classification of the tumors was done in the end.

Histopathology

Surgical removal of the breast lesion was performed in all the cases, and the surgical pathologic reports, which were confirmed by experienced pathologists at our hospital, were consequently reviewed. The lymph node metastasis (LNM) of homolateral axillary was also reviewed. Nevertheless, the pathological findings of axillary lymph nodes in eight patients (one MUMPC, five cPMBCs, and two MMBCs) were not acquired.

Statistical analysis

All results were analyzed using the SPSS version 20.0 (Statistical Product and Service Solutions) for Windows (Microsoft). Student's t test was used for comparisons of the age at the time of diagnosis and for the sonographic lesion size between the three groups. χ^2 test (and Fisher's exact test, if necessary) was used to analyze the ultrasound descriptors of the lesion shape, orientation, margin, echogenicity, posterior acoustic features, calcification, vascularity, blood flow grade, and BI-RADS classification, as well as menstrual status (premenopausal, postmenopausal), mass location (right, left), palpation (palpable, nonpalpable), tenderness (positive, negative), and axillary LNM (positive, negative) of the patients, in order to see if there were discrepancies between the three groups. $P < 0.05$ was considered statistically significant.

Results

The non-mucinous component of 28 MMBCs included invasive carcinoma of no special type (17 cases), invasive carcinoma of no special type and invasive micropapillary carcinoma (3 cases), solid papillary carcinoma (2 cases), solid papillary carcinoma and carcinoma with neuroendocrine features (2 cases), invasive carcinoma of no special type and encapsulated papillary carcinoma (1 case), invasive micropapillary carcinoma (1 case), papillary carcinoma (1 case), and other invasive carcinoma (1 case). All patients were Chinese, including 87 women and 1 man; the male patient was diagnosed with MUMPC. Except for one case, patients had no family history of breast cancer. One woman with cPMBC ever suffered from breast cancer before, while another one with cPMBC also had non-mucinous breast carcinoma.

The mean age of patients with MUMPC, cPMBC, and MMBC was 53.7 years (range, 34–85 years; median value, 52 years), 50.9 years (range, 28–83 years; median value, 46 years), and 50.9 years (range, 28–81 years; median value, 48 years), respectively. Nevertheless, no significant difference between MUMPC and cPMBC ($p = 0.47$), between MUMPC and MMBC ($p = 0.55$), and cPMBC and MMBC ($p = 0.99$) was observed.

The clinical characteristics of the histologically proven MUMPC, cPMBC, and MMBC are compared in Table 1. In the present study, the location of MUMPC on the left

or right side was approximately equal. All the tumor masses (100%, 17/17) were palpable, and most of them (88.2%, 15/17) had no tenderness. There were no major differences in the three groups. The differences in lymph node metastasis rates among MUMPC, cPMBC, and MMBC were statistically significant; the axillary LNM was similar between MUMPC and cPMBC ($p = 0.246$); however, both MUMPC and cPMBC were statistically different from MMBC ($p < 0.01$ for both).

All the mucinous carcinomas presented as a mass on ultrasound. The mean values of the maximum dimension (sonographic lesion size) in MUMPC, cPMBC, and MMBC were 26 mm (range 11–51; median value, 23), 26 mm (range 10–50; median value, 23), and 35 mm (range 12–80; median value, 34), respectively. There was no difference between MUMPC and cPMBC ($p = 0.926$). Nevertheless, MUMPC ($p = 0.045$) and cPMBC ($p = 0.006$) were different from MMBC.

The sonographic findings were summarized in Table 2. Most of the MUMPCs had irregular shape (82.4%, 14/17), parallel orientation (94.1%, 16/17), and non-circumscribed margin (88.2%, 15/17) (Figs. 1 and 2). There was no difference between MUMPC, cPMBC, and MMBC. The internal echoes of MUMPCs were mixed cystic and solid (35.3%, 6/17), hypoechoic (29.4%, 5/17), and isoechoic (35.3%, 6/17), and most of the posterior features were enhancement (88.2%, 15/17) (Figs. 1 and 2). Up to 29.4% (5/17) of the MUMPC lesions showed calcification (Fig. 2), while blood flow in the mass was identified in only 7 of 17 (41.2%) lesions with grade 1. Finally,

Table 1 The clinical characteristics of the histologically proven MUMPC, cPMBC, and MMBC

Characteristics	MUMPC	cPMBC	MMBC	Total	Significance
Menopausal status					$\chi^2 = 0.284, p = 0.87$
Premenopausal	9	26	18	87[a]	
Postmenopausal	7	17	10		
Mass location					$\chi^2 = 0.423, p = 0.81$
Right	8	20	11	88	
Left	9	23	17		
Palpation					$F = 1.285, p = 1.00$
Palpable	17	42	28	88	
Nonpalpable	0	1	0		
Tenderness					$\chi^2 = 2.045, p = 0.36$
Positive	2	12	8	87[b]	
Negative	15	30	20		
LNM					$\chi^2 = 25.884, p < 0.001$
Positive	3	3	17	80[c]	
Negative	13	35	9		

F Fisher's exact test

[a]The man patient was excluded

[b]One of the masses was not palpable

[c]The pathological findings of axillary lymph nodes of eight patients were not acquired

Table 2 Sonographic features of MUMPC, cPMBC, and MMBC

Features	MUMPC (n = 17)	cPMBC (n = 43)	MMBC (n = 28)	Significance
Shape				χ^2 = 2.562, p = 0.278
Regular	3	14	5	
Irregular	14	29	23	
Orientation				F = 1.801, p = 0.450
Parallel	16	42	28	
Not parallel	1	1	0	
Margin				χ^2 = 2.421, p = 0.307
Circumscribed	2	13	6	
Non-circumscribed	15	30	22	
Echogenicity				F = 18.418, p = 0.007
Hyperechoic	0	1	1	
Complex echogenicity	6	14	7	
Hypoechoic	5	5	15	
Isoechoic	6	18	5	
Heterogeneous	0	5	0	
Posterior acoustic features				F = 10.588, p = 0.037
No features	2	5	6	
Enhancement	15	38	17	
Shadowing	0	0	3	
Combined pattern	0	0	2	
Calcification				χ^2 = 14.889, p = 0.001
Present	5	6	16	
Absent	12	37	12	
Vascularity				χ^2 = 7.556, p = 0.023
Present	7	17	20	
Absent	10	26	8	
Blood flow grade				F = 10.866, p = 0.045
0	10	26	8	
1	7	15	15	
2	0	0	3	
3	0	2	2	
BI-RADS category				F = 26.427, p < 0.001
3	2	9	0	
4	13	31	12	
5	2	3	16	

F Fisher's exact test

76.5% (13/17) MUMPC masses were assessed as category 4 according to BI-RADS-US. There was no statistically significant difference between MUMPC and cPMBC in BI-RADS category (p = 0.628), but the differences were found between MUMPC and MMBC (p = 0.002), the same as between cPMBC and MMBC (p < 0.001).

Although the margin (circumscribed, non-circumscribed) was not statistically significant among the three groups, the angular and spiculated signs of the masses with non-circumscribed margin were statistically different (p < 0.05). In addition, the ultrasound descriptors with statistically significant differences were also further compared, which included the non-circumscribed margin (angular, spiculated), echogenicity, posterior acoustic features, calcification, vascularity, and blood flow grade. Finally, all the observed differences in the sonographic descriptors were between cPMBC and MMBC (p < 0.05). All the non-circumscribed MUMPCs showed

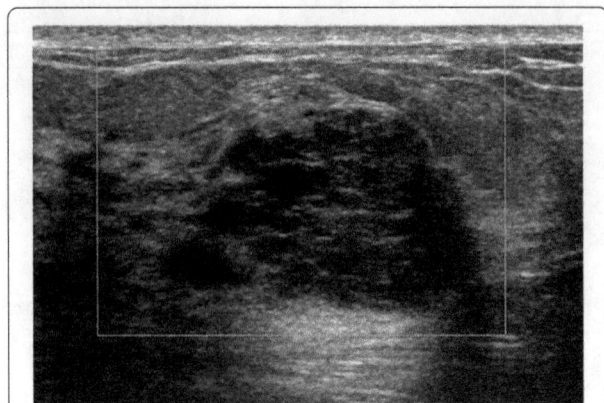

Fig. 1 Ultrasonographic findings of a MUMPC in a 41-year-old patient with a palpable left breast tumor. US shows a 3.0 × 2.2 × 1.9 cm parallel, irregular, and non-circumscribed tumor with mixed solid and cystic components and posterior acoustic accentuation (BI-RADS 4B). No signal of blood flow was found in the mass

an indistinct margin, and most (93.3%, 14/15) showed microlobulated border. Nonetheless, there were less MUMPCs (26.7%, 4/15) with angular border and none of them showed a spiculated margin.

Discussion

In the present study, we showed that there are no significant differences in sonographic features between the MUMPC and cPMBC and between the MUMPC and MMBC. Nevertheless, there is a definite separation between cPMBC and MMBC in echogenicity, posterior acoustic features, calcification, vascularity, and blood flow grade. It seems that MUMPC shows the ultrasonic manifestations in between. Unfortunately, under the present conditions, these features are indistinguishable according to the BI-RADS-US.

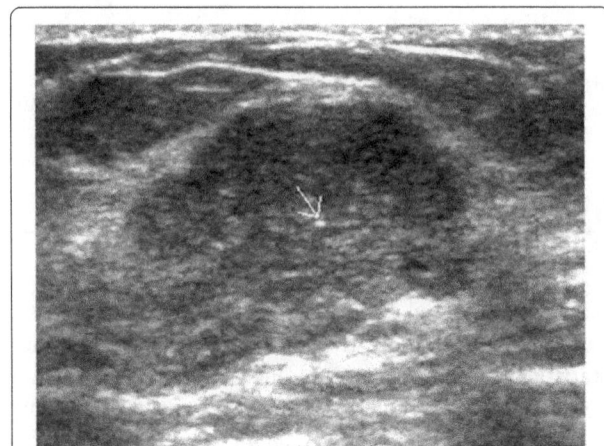

Fig. 2 US image of a MUMPC in a 49-year-old patient with a palpable left breast tumor. A solid, parallel, slightly lobulated, isoechoic tumor with posterior acoustic accentuation and punctate calcification (arrow) (BI-RADS 4B)

Irregular shape can be found in most of the tumors. In the present study, it was identified in 82.4% (14/17) of MUMPC and 67.4% (29/43) of cPMBC. In a different study conducted by Kaoku, irregular shape was found in 90.9% (10/11) of PMBC [15]. Lam et al. [16] have suggested that the irregular shape on sonography is associated with MBC having a less favorable histologic grade.

The nonparallel orientation is characteristic of presumed malignant breast tumors [17]. Nevertheless, in the present study, only one case with MUMPC and one case with cPMBC manifested this feature, while all the MMBC masses were parallel. This feature appears to be related with the size of the mass, as only 20% of malignant nodules > 2.0 cm in maximum diameter are taller than wide [17].

Previous studies have shown that microlobulation, one of the diagnostic features, could be seen in more MBCs [15, 16]. According to Lam et al. [16], the presence of cystic and solid components (37.5%, 12/32) and distal enhancement (43.8%, 14/32) in MBC are important sonographic features for diagnosis. In the present study, MUMPCs were more common with indistinct (88.2%, 15/17) and microlobulated (82.4%, 14/17) margins, while 35.3% (6/17) of MUMPC lesions were mixed cystic and solid, equal to isoechoic (35.3%, 6/17), and slightly above hypoechoic (29.4%, 5/17). 88.2% (15/17) of MUMPCs showed distal acoustic enhancement. The obtained results were higher than those reported by Lam et al. [16], but lower than those reported by (100%, 11/11) Kaoku et al. [15].

Calcification is not a common feature of MBC [18]. Using mammography, Liu et al. have reported that the calcification ratio of MBC is 26.1% (12/46). This was consistent with our results, where ultrasound revealed the calcification in less than one third of MUMPCs (29.4%, 5/17).

MUMPC may have sparse color flow signals. In our study, those signals were observed in 41.2% of MUMPC lesions (7/17), and 39.5% of cPMBC masses (17/43), while blood flow was found in 71.4% of MMBCs (20/28). Thus, the vascularity may be related to the amount of mucin in the MBC masses.

We found that the MUMPC descriptors did not show any significant difference compared to the cPMBCs or MMBCs, except for the rate of nodal involvement, the mean value of the maximum dimension, and BI-RADS category of the tumor, in which the differences were found between MUMPC and MMBC.

Lymph node metastasis is one of the key factors affecting the prognosis in breast cancer patients. Previous studies have reported that the rate of nodal involvement in MUMPC is 20.0–42.9% [4, 7, 10, 11, 19, 20]. It is also considered that the incidence of LNM in MUMPC is higher compared to that in cPMBC [11, 20]. According to Liu et al. [20], this rate is nine times higher compared to the incidence in cPMBC. This suggests that MUMPC is more aggressive than cPMBC. Nonetheless, our results are not consistent with the previous studies. The LNMs in our research were present in 18.8% (3/16) of MUMPC patients, and there was no obvious difference in the rate of LNM between the MUMPCs and cPMBCs ($p > 0.05$). These results were in line with those reported by Kim et al. [7]. In addition, Bal et al. [21] think that the micropapillary pattern is not associated with aggressive or benevolent behavior. Besides, our study revealed that the differences in LNM ratio of MUMPC compared to MMBC were significant ($p < 0.05$). These results suggested that MUMPC and cPMBC were relatively indolent compared with MMBC.

Liu et al. [20] have found that there was no difference in the median tumor size between MUMPC and cPMBC (2.2 vs. 2.0 cm, $p = 0.213$). Likewise, in our study, the median size was 23 mm for both groups (MUMPC and cPMBC), while the average size of MUMPC (26 mm) was smaller compared to MMBC (35 mm), which was higher compared to the mean size of MMBC (25 mm) observed by Ranade et al. [4].

Most of the MUMPCs (76.5%, 13/17) and cPMBCs (72.1%, 31/43) were assessed as category 4, while most of MMBCs (57.1%, 16/28) were categorized as 5. These results show that MMBC is more likely to be malignant.

The physical examination of MUMPC is often unremarkable. In previous study, a palpable mass was identified in 87% MBC cases [18], while the tumor pain was uncommon [22]. Our study was consistent with these previous studies, since it revealed that MUMPC was no different than cPMBC and MMBC.

Shet and Chinoy [19] have suggested that MUMPC generally affects the younger women and that most patients are between 41 and 60 years. According to Kim et al. [7], the mean age is 53.9 years. Our findings (mean age, 53.7 years) were similar to these studies. Nonetheless, Barbashina et al. [11] have found that the median age of the patients with MUMPC is 62 years and that majority of patients are postmenopausal. In the present study, the median age was 52 years and majority of patients were premenopausal (56.3%, 9/16). The observed difference may stem from the difference in the samples or races.

Our study has some limitations. First, this was a retrospective study. Since all the ultrasonic images included were static with one single cross section, some characteristics may not be presented on the image, which in turn could affect the assessment. Second, the sample size was small. MBC is a rare carcinoma, while MUMPC is even more infrequent than MBC. Although, there were 88 patients in the study, there were only 17 persons with MUMPC, and they were all Chinese. Also, 26 patients

were excluded for the loss of information or performing the operations in other institution. These circumstances potentially had causal effect on outcomes. The future study should include a large sample size, especially MUMPC sample. Third, only one sonographer analyzed the images, which can also cause the bias.

Conclusions

In conclusion, MUMPC commonly appears on sonography as an irregular parallel mass with an indistinct and/or microlobulated margin. The tumor may show hypoechoic or isoechoic structure, complex lesion with cystic and solid components, and posterior enhancement with less calcification and inner vascularity. Although the ultrasonic manifestations of MUMPC are in between those of cPMBC and MMBC, there is no statistically significant difference between the MUMPC and cPMBC and between the MUMPC and MMBC. For this reason, it is hard to distinguish MUMPC from the other two subtypes on ultrasound according to the BI-RADS-US lexicon. Larger sample size and experienced sonographers are required for further analysis, as well as additional research means such as contrast-enhanced ultrasonography and ultrasound elastography.

Abbreviations
BI-RADS: Breast Imaging Reporting and Data System; cPMBC: Conventional pure mucinous breast carcinoma without micropapillary architecture; IMPC: Invasive micropapillary carcinoma; LNM: Lymph node metastasis; MBC: Mucinous breast carcinoma; MMBC: Mixed mucinous breast carcinoma; MUMPC: Mucinous carcinoma with micropapillary pattern; PMBC: Pure mucinous breast carcinoma; US: Ultrasound

Funding
This study was supported by the National Natural Science Foundation of China (Grant No. 81571694).

Authors' contributions
HZ carried out the studies, participated in collecting the data, and drafted the manuscript. LQ performed the statistical analysis and participated in its design. YP helped to draft the manuscript. All authors read and approved the final manuscript.

Competing interests
The authors declare that they have no competing interests.

References
1. Di Saverio S, Gutierrez J, Avisar E. A retrospective review with long term follow up of 11,400 cases of pure mucinous breast carcinoma. Breast Cancer Res Treat. 2008;111:541–7.
2. Bae SY, Choi MY, Cho DH, Lee JE, Nam SJ, Yang JH. Mucinous carcinoma of the breast in comparison with invasive ductal carcinoma: clinicopathologic characteristics and prognosis. J Breast Cancer. 2011;14:308–13.
3. Okafuji T, Yabuuchi H, Sakai S, Soeda H, Matsuo Y, Inoue T, et al. MR imaging features of pure mucinous carcinoma of the breast. Eur J Radiol. 2006;60:405–13.

4. Ranade A, Batra R, Sandhu G, Chitale RA, Balderacchi J. Clinicopathological evaluation of 100 cases of mucinous carcinoma of breast with emphasis on axillary staging and special reference to a micropapillary pattern. J Clin Pathol. 2010;63:1043–7.

5. Dumitru A, Procop A, Iliesiu A, Tampa M, Mitrache L, Costache M, et al. Mucinous breast cancer: a review study of 5 year experience from a hospital-based series of cases. Maedica (Buchar). 2015;10:14–8.

6. Barkley CR, Ligibel JA, Wong JS, Lipsitz S, Smith BL, Golshan M. Mucinous breast carcinoma: a large contemporary series. Am J Surg. 2008;196:549–51.

7. Kim HJ, Park K, Kim JY, Kang G, Gwak G, Park I. Prognostic significance of a micropapillary pattern in pure mucinous carcinoma of the breast: comparative analysis with micropapillary carcinoma. J Pathol Transl Med. 2017;51:403–9.

8. Adrada B, Arribas E, Gilcrease M, Yang WT. Invasive micropapillary carcinoma of the breast: mammographic, sonographic, and MRI features. AJR Am J Roentgenol. 2009;193:W58–63.

9. Jones KN, Guimaraes LS, Reynolds CA, Ghosh K, Degnim AC, Glazebrook KN. Invasive micropapillary carcinoma of the breast: imaging features with clinical and pathologic correlation. AJR Am J Roentgenol. 2013;200:689–95.

10. Ng WK. Fine-needle aspiration cytology findings of an uncommon micropapillary variant of pure mucinous carcinoma of the breast: review of patients over an 8-year period. Cancer. 2002;96:280–8.

11. Barbashina V, Corben AD, Akram M, Vallejo C, Tan LK. Mucinous micropapillary carcinoma of the breast: an aggressive counterpart to conventional pure mucinous tumors. Hum Pathol. 2013;44:1577–85.

12. Lakhani SR, Ellis IO, Schnitt SJ. WHO classification of tumours of the breast. World Health Organization classification of tumours, 4th edn. Lyon: IARC press; 2012.

13. Mendelson EB, Böhm-Vélez M, Berg WA. ACR BI-RADS® Ultrasound. In: ACR BI-RADS® Atlas, Breast Imaging Reporting and Data System. Reston: American College of Radiology; 2013.

14. Adler DD, Carson PL, Rubin JM, Quinn-Reid D. Doppler ultrasound color flow imaging in the study of breast cancer: preliminary findings. Ultrasound Med Biol. 1990;16:553–9.

15. Kaoku S, Konishi E, Fujimoto Y, Tohno E, Shiina T, Kondo K, et al. Sonographic and pathologic image analysis of pure mucinous carcinoma of the breast. Ultrasound Med Biol. 2013;39:1158–67.

16. Lam WW, Chu WC, Tse GM, Ma TK. Sonographic appearance of mucinous carcinoma of the breast. AJR Am J Roentgenol. 2004;182:1069–74.

17. Rumack CM, Wilson SR, Charboneau JW, Levine D. Diagnostic Ultrasound. 4th ed., vol. 1. Philadelphia: Elsevier Mosby; 2011.

18. Liu H, Tan H, Cheng Y, Zhang X, Gu Y, Peng W. Imaging findings in mucinous breast carcinoma and correlating factors. Eur J Radiol. 2011;80:706–12.

19. Shet T, Chinoy R. Presence of a micropapillary pattern in mucinous carcinomas of the breast and its impact on the clinical behavior. Breast J. 2008;14:412–20.

20. Liu F, Yang M, Li Z, Guo X, Lin Y, Lang R, et al. Invasive micropapillary mucinous carcinoma of the breast is associated with poor prognosis. Breast Cancer Res Treat. 2015;151:443–51.

21. Bal A, Joshi K, Sharma SC, Das A, Verma A, Wig JD. Prognostic significance of micropapillary pattern in pure mucinous carcinoma of the breast. Int J Surg Pathol. 2008;16:251–6.

22. Hoda SA, Brogi E, Koerner FC, Rosen PP. Rosen's Breast Pathology. 4th ed. Philadelphia: Lippincott Williams & Wilkins; 2014.

4

The mode of progressive disease affects the prognosis of patients with metastatic breast cancer

Ryutaro Mori[*] ⓘ, Manabu Futamura, Kasumi Morimitsu, Yoshimi Asano, Yoshihisa Tokumaru, Mai Kitazawa and Kazuhiro Yoshida

Abstract

Background: According to the Response Evaluation Criteria in Solid Tumors (RECIST), progressive disease (PD) is diagnosed under two conditions: an increase in size of pre-existing lesions (IS) and the appearance of new lesions (NL). We retrospectively investigated the difference in the prognosis between IS and NL.

Methods: Patients receiving drug therapies for metastatic breast cancer between 2004 and 2015 at our institution were reviewed. The survival time after NL and IS was compared and the frequency of NL with each drug calculated.

Results: For the 107 eligible patients, the survival time after NL at second-line chemotherapy was significantly worse than after IS (median survival time 4.3 months vs. 20.3 months, $p = 0.0048$). Maintenance therapy with bevacizumab or trastuzumab had a high frequency of NL (88.9%), and third-line eribulin had a low frequency of NL (16.7%). A multivariate analysis showed that NL at second-line chemotherapy was not an independent risk factor (hazard ratio 1.02, 95%; confidence interval 0.54–1.93, $p = 0.95$) for the total survival time.

Conclusions: Patients with IS had a better survival after PD than those with NL. We may be able to avoid changing drug therapy for patients without NL and allow them to continue drug therapy for longer.

Keywords: Secondary breast neoplasms, Drug therapy, Progressive disease, Prognosis

Background

Patients with metastatic breast cancer (MBC) are treated with drug therapies, such as hormone therapy and chemotherapy. Although MBC is still an incurable disease [1], the survival of such patients has been improved by new therapeutic agents [2, 3]. The efficacy of drug therapies is evaluated by imaging modalities, such as computed tomography (CT), bone scintigraphy, and positron emission tomography (PET), and the therapy is continued as long as it seems to be effective [4]. The efficacy of drug therapies is evaluated based on Response Evaluation Criteria in Solid Tumors (RECIST) especially in clinical trials [5] as well as in daily practice.

Under the RECIST criteria, the efficacy is divided into four categories: complete response (CR), partial response (PR), stable disease (SD), and progressive disease (PD).

Usually, the therapy is changed when the efficacy is evaluated as PD. According to the RECIST criteria, PD is diagnosed under two conditions: an increase in the size of pre-existing lesions and the appearance of new lesions [5]. These situations should be interpreted as indicative of the progress of metastatic disease. However, the precise meanings of these situations seem to differ, as the size of pre-existing lesions may be decreased again by subsequent therapy, while new lesions rarely disappear, regardless of therapy. Thus, the European Medicines Agency (EMA) has recently recommended that the mode of progressive disease (an increase in the size of pre-existing lesions or the appearance of new lesions) should be taken into account when progression-free survival (PFS) is used as the endpoint of a clinical trial [6].

Given the above, we suspected that the prognosis of patients with new metastatic lesions might differ from that of patients whose pre-existing metastatic lesions have only increased in size. Therefore, we retrospectively

* Correspondence: moriry52@gmail.com
Department of Surgical Oncology, Gifu University Graduate School of Medicine, 1-1 Yanagido, Gifu 501-1194, Japan

investigated the prognosis of these patients after PD and the relationship between the mode of PD and drugs.

Methods

The records of breast cancer patients who received drug therapy for locally advanced or metastatic breast cancer at Gifu University Hospital between 2004 and 2015 were reviewed. The therapy in each case was investigated, and the efficacy of drug therapy was evaluated from the viewpoint of the objective response, which was categorized as mentioned above: CR, PR, SD, and PD. This categorization was determined based on the RECIST criteria.

In the present study, PD was further divided into the appearance of new lesions (NL) and an increase in the size of existing lesions (IS). NL indicates that the patient developed new metastatic lesions that had never been detected before, regardless of the size of pre-existing lesions. IS indicates that the target lesions had increased in size, and no new lesions had developed. When judging the mode of PD, the most recent therapies the patients had received were excluded, as the efficacies of these therapies were deemed poor and had not been evaluated sufficiently in most cases. We then compared the survival after PD between the patients with NL and IS using the Kaplan–Meier curves with a log-rank test and calculated the frequency of NL to determine which drugs was most strongly associated with NL. We also analyzed the impact of these factors on the patients' survival using a Cox proportional hazard model. All statistical analyses were carried out using the software EZR software program (version 3.4.1 with R commander 2.4–0).

This study was approved by the ethics committee of Gifu University, Graduate School of Medicine.

Results

Patient characteristics

A total of 127 patients received drug therapy for locally advanced or metastatic breast cancer in our institution. However, 20 patients were excluded because their outcomes were unclear. Thus, we investigated the outcomes of the 107 remaining patients. The patients were a median 58 years of age. Most of the primary tumors exhibited a size of 2–5 cm (T2). Seventy-four patients had N (+) status, 74 had estrogen-receptor (ER)-positive tumors, and 22 had HER2-positive tumors. The metastatic sites included the bones (61 patients), lungs (34 patients), liver (29 patients), lymph nodes (44 patients), pleural (26 patients), local (15 patients), and other organs (17 patients). The details are shown in Table 1.

Selection of drug therapy

The patients received a median of four lines of drug therapy. Among those who received chemotherapies, oral 5-FU

derivatives were administered to 66 cases, taxanes (excluding paclitaxel + bevacizumab therapy) to 47 cases, and anthracyclines to 17 cases. Patients with HER2-positive status also received trastuzumab (33 cases) or trastuzumab + pertuzumab (4 cases), and paclitaxel + bevacizumab was administered to 11 cases. Nine of the cases who had been receiving cytotoxic drugs with targeted drugs, such as trastuzumab, pertuzumab, and bevacizumab, received targeted drugs alone after metastatic lesions were well-controlled. Among the cases who received hormone therapies, non-steroidal aromatase inhibitors (AIs) were administered to 66 cases, steroidal AIs to 36 cases, and selective estrogen receptor modulators (SERMs) to 52 cases. The details are shown in Table 2.

Table 1 Patient characteristics

$n = 107$	No
Age, years	
< 50	20
50–59	38
≥ 60	49
Menopausal status	
Premenopausal	22
Postmenopausal	85
T factor	
T1	15
T2	43
T3	7
T4	20
Unknown	22
Nodal status	
N (−)	19
N (+)	74
Unknown	14
Subtypes	
Luminal A/B	68
Luminal HER2	8
HER2	14
Triple negative	17
Metastatic sites	
Bone	61
Lung	34
Liver	29
Lymph node	44
Pleural	26
Local	15
Brain	9
Others	8

Table 2 Selection of hormone therapy and chemotherapy

	No.
Chemotherapy	
Oral 5FU	62
Taxane	47
Anthracycline	17
Vinorelbine	17
Eribulin	12
Paclitaxel + Bevacizumab	11
Targeted drug alone	9
Others	26
Hormone therapy	
Non-steroidal AI	66
Steroidal AI	36
SERM	52
SERD	9
MPA	6

AI aromatase inhibitor, *SERM* selective estrogen receptor modulator, *SERD* selective estrogen receptor down-regulator, *MPA* medroxyprogesterone 17-Acetate

Comparing the survival time after NL or IS

Among the cases who received chemotherapy, the survival time of the patients with NL tended to be worse than that with IS (Fig. 1a–c). After second-line chemotherapy, in particular, the patients with NL had a shorter survival time than did those with IS (median survival time 4.3 months vs. 20.3 months, $p = 0.0048$) (Fig. 1b). Similarly, among the cases treated with hormone therapy, the survival time of the patients with NL tended to be worse than that of those with IS, albeit not to a statistically significant degree (Fig. 1d–f).

Frequency of NL by drugs

As mentioned above, the patients with NL tended to have poor prognosis after PD. Therefore, we analyzed the frequency of NL for each drug.

All of the drugs used for hormone therapy had similar frequencies of NL (nsAI 48.5%, sAI 50.0%, SERM 42.3%, and SERD 55.6%) (Fig. 2a). The patients treated with oral s and maintenance therapy with targeted drugs alone (such as bevacizumab and trastuzumab) frequently developed NL (oral 5FUs 45.2% and targeted drug alone 88.9%). Anthracycline, vinorelbin, eribulin, taxanes, and paclitaxel with bevacizumab had similar frequencies of NL (Fig. 2b).

We also calculated the frequency of NL among chemotherapy drugs stratified by treatment lines. Paclitaxel with bevacizumab therapy had the highest frequency of NL (58.3%) among first-line therapies (Fig. 3a), and oral 5FUs had the second-highest frequency of NL (41.4%) among first-line therapies and the highest (63.2%) among second-line therapies (Fig. 3b). Eribulin had the lowest frequency of NL (16.7%), even among third-line therapies (Fig. 3c).

A multivariate analysis for the survival after PD with second-line chemotherapy

We analyzed the impact of the factors that seemed to be important for the survival (NL at second-line chemotherapy,

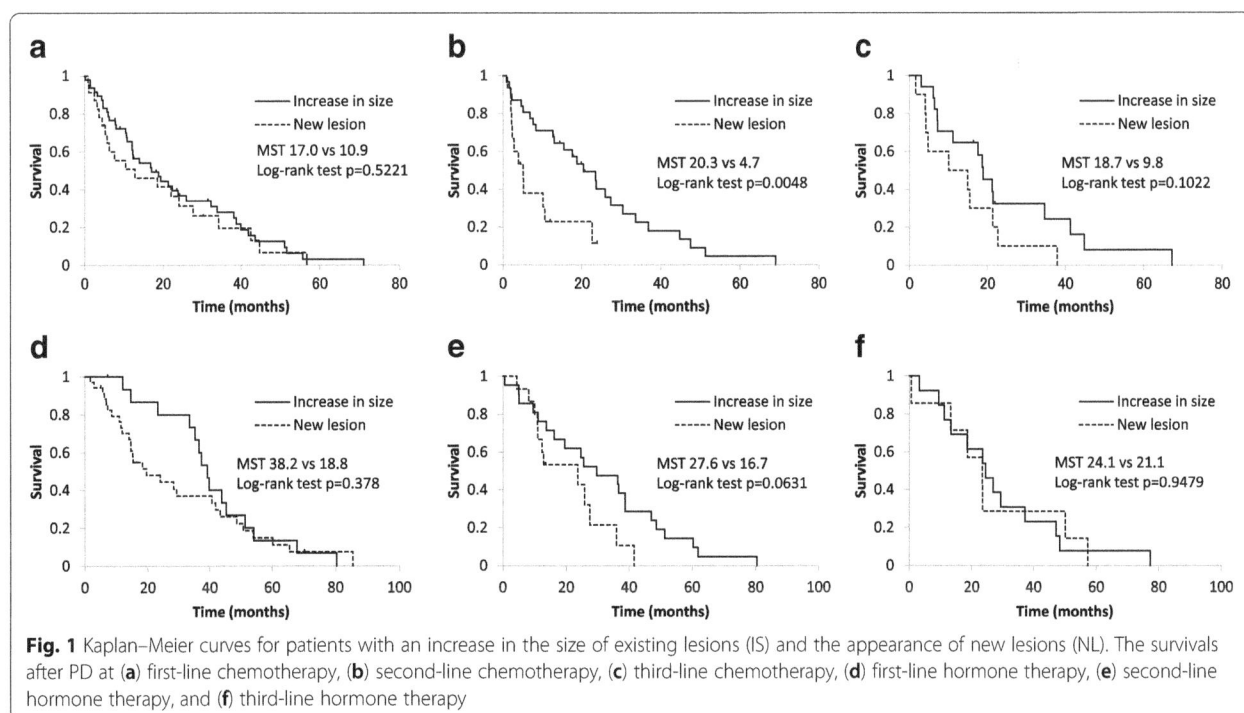

Fig. 1 Kaplan–Meier curves for patients with an increase in the size of existing lesions (IS) and the appearance of new lesions (NL). The survivals after PD at (**a**) first-line chemotherapy, (**b**) second-line chemotherapy, (**c**) third-line chemotherapy, (**d**) first-line hormone therapy, (**e**) second-line hormone therapy, and (**f**) third-line hormone therapy

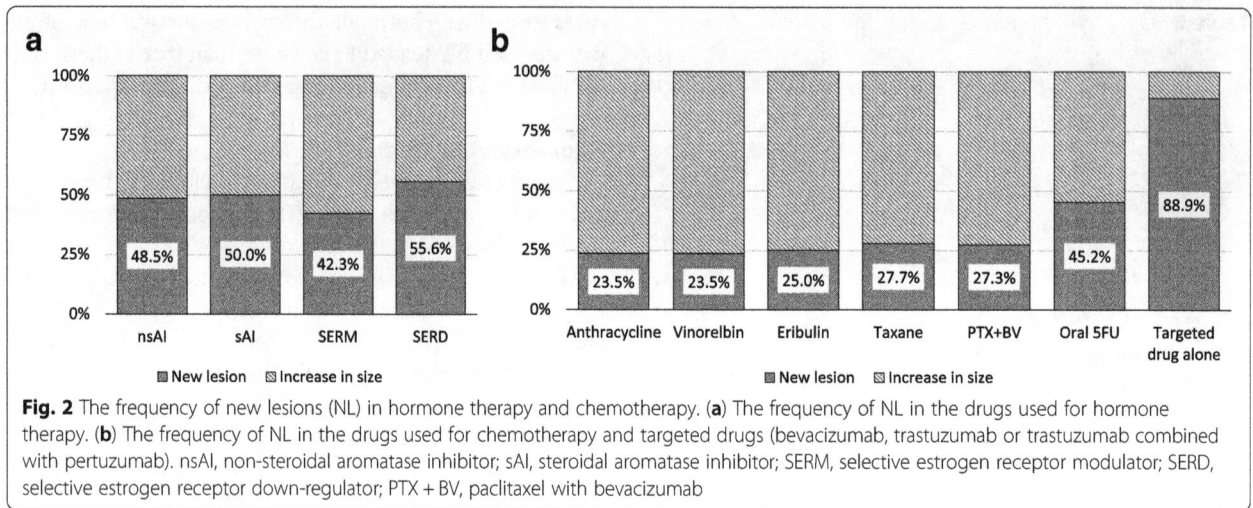

Fig. 2 The frequency of new lesions (NL) in hormone therapy and chemotherapy. (**a**) The frequency of NL in the drugs used for hormone therapy. (**b**) The frequency of NL in the drugs used for chemotherapy and targeted drugs (bevacizumab, trastuzumab or trastuzumab combined with pertuzumab). nsAI, non-steroidal aromatase inhibitor; sAI, steroidal aromatase inhibitor; SERM, selective estrogen receptor modulator; SERD, selective estrogen receptor down-regulator; PTX + BV, paclitaxel with bevacizumab

targeted therapy alone, eribulin administration, ER-positive status, visceral metastasis at first recurrence) on the survival time after the first recurrence using a Cox proportional hazard model.

As shown in Table 3, NL at second-line chemotherapy was not an independent factor for the survival after the first recurrence (hazard ratio [HR] 1.02, 95% confidence interval [CI] 0.54–1.93, $p = 0.95$), although it was related to a poor survival after PD with second-line chemotherapy, as described above. The administration of maintenance therapy with targeted therapy alone was an independent factor for a good prognosis (HR 0.27, 95%

CI 0.12–0.62, $p < 0.01$), although it was related to a high frequency of NL, as described above. The administration of eribulin was also an independent factor for a good prognosis (HR 0.49, 95% CI 0.24–0.99, $p < 0.05$).

Discussion

We analyzed the relationship between the mode of PD and the prognosis and found that the survival time in patients who developed NL at second-line chemotherapy was statistically worse than that in patients with IS.

Some reports have described the relationship between the mode of PD and the prognosis. In the RECORD-1 study

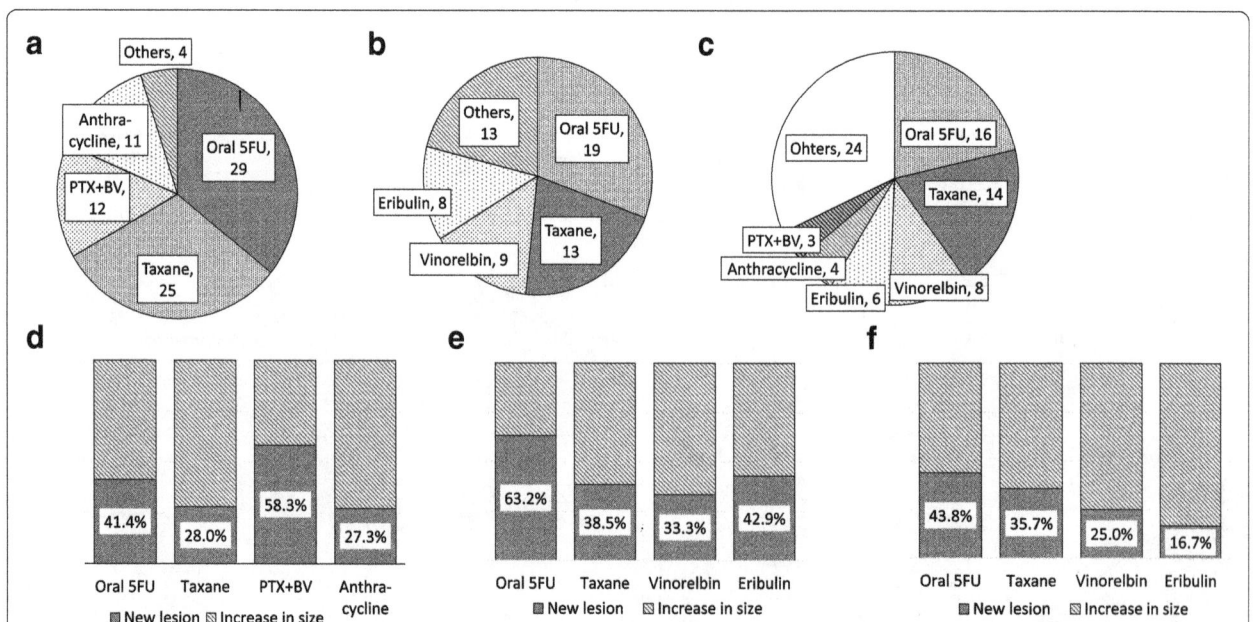

Fig. 3 The distribution of the chemotherapy drugs used in first-, second-, and third-line chemotherapy and the frequency of new lesions (NL) in each drug. The distribution of the chemotherapy drugs at (**a**) first-line chemotherapy, (**b**) second-line chemotherapy, and (**c**) third-line chemotherapy, and the frequency of NL at (**d**) first-line chemotherapy, (**e**) second-line chemotherapy, and (**f**) third-line chemotherapy. PTX + BV, paclitaxel with bevacizumab

Table 3 A multivariate analysis for survival after the first recurrence

Factors	Hazard ratio	95% CI	p value
New lesions at second chemotherapy	1.02	0.54–1.93	0.95
ER (+)	0.28	0.16–0.48	< 0.01
Targeted therapy alone	0.27	0.12–0.62	< 0.01
Eribulin administration	0.49	0.24–0.99	< 0.05
Visceral metastasis at first recurrence	1.10	0.70–1.73	0.68

ER: estrogen receptor

investigating the benefit of everolimus over placebo for metastatic renal cell carcinoma, a multivariate Cox proportional hazard model revealed that the growth of non-target lesions and appearance of new lesions were predictive factors for the overall survival [7]. In the Nordic VI trial comparing FLIRI therapy and Lv5FU2-IR therapy for metastatic colorectal cancer, patients with new lesions or unequivocal progression of non-measurable lesions had a worse prognosis than those with an increase in the size of pre-existing lesions, and a ≥ 10% decrease in the size of pre-existing lesions was a positive prognostic factor [8]. Another report has also described the influence of the mode of PD on the overall survival in MBC. Twelves et al. reported that, in study 301 and study 305, which investigated the efficacy of eribulin for MBC, patients who developed new metastases had a worse prognosis than did those with PD due to the growth of pre-existing lesions [9]. Kotake et al. also reported similar findings based on the data from Japanese patients receiving eribulin [10]. The results of these studies have consistently suggested that new lesions are associated with a worse prognosis than IS after PD, which agrees with the findings of the present study. These present and previous findings suggest that simply observing MBC patients whose lesions have slightly increased in size without changing the therapy may be feasible, as long as new lesions do not appear.

Litiere et al. also reported that an increase in the size of target lesions had a low explanatory value, and the appearance of new lesions and the progression of non-target lesions resulted in a worse overall survival, according to the results of a meta-analysis investigating the explanatory values of the mode of PD based on the RECIST criteria in breast, lung, and colorectal cancer. Therefore, those authors suggested that this information be included in the updated version of RECIST [11]. According to the current consensus, the drug therapy in MBC patients must be changed when PD develops [1]. However, we have limited effective drugs. Therefore, if we were to distinguish the treatment protocol after PD between patients with NL and those with IS, we could continue otherwise effective drug therapies for longer.

Another important finding of our study is that NL at second-line chemotherapy itself was not an independent factor for the total survival. NL at second-line chemotherapy is related to a poor prognosis after PD, and patients receiving maintenance therapy frequently develop NL. However, this does not necessarily mean that the total survival time is shortened. The mode of PD was a factor for predicting not the total survival time but only the survival time after PD.

Despite the small population and retrospective nature of the present study, we believe that our results provide some important evidence to support our hypothesis and that these findings may help prolong the survival of patients using limited drugs for metastatic breast cancer. A larger prospective study investigating the prognoses of patients with NL and IS will be required in the future.

Conclusion

We found that patients with NL had a worse survival after PD than did those with IS. When patients develop NL, their therapy must be changed. However, patients with only IS might be able to be observed without changing their therapy, allowing them to continue otherwise effective drug therapies for longer.

Abbreviations

AI: Aromatase inhibitor; CR: Complete response; CT: Computed tomography; ER: Estrogen receptor; HER2: Human epidermal growth factor receptor 2; IS: Increase in size of pre-existing lesions; MBC: Metastatic breast cancer; MST: Median survival time; NL: Appearance of new lesions; PD: Progressive disease; PET: Positron emission tomography; PR: Partial response; PR: Progesterone receptor; RECIST: Response Evaluation Criteria in Solid Tumors; SD: Stable disease; SERD: Selective estrogen receptor degrader; SERM: Selective estrogen receptor modulator

Authors' contributions

RM wrote the manuscript. RM, MF, KM, YA, YT, and MK participated in the medical treatments for these cases. KY represented our surgical department and supervised the writing of the manuscript. All authors read and approved the final manuscript.

Competing interests

The authors declared that they have no competing interests..

References

1. Greenberg PA, Hortobagyi GN, Smith TL, Ziegler LD, Frye DK, Buzdar AU. Long-term follow-up of patients with complete remission following combination chemotherapy for metastatic breast cancer. J Clin Oncol. 1996; 14:2197–205.
2. Chia SK, Speers CH, D'yachkova Y, Kang A, Malfair-Taylor S, Barnett J, Coldman A, Gelmon KA, O'reilly SE, Olivotto IA. The impact of new chemotherapeutic and hormone agents on survival in a population-based cohort of women with metastatic breast cancer. Cancer. 2007;110:973–9.
3. Dafni U, Grimani I, Xyrafas A, Eleftheraki AG, Fountzilas G. Fifteen-year trends in metastatic breast cancer survival in Greece. Breast Cancer Res Treat. 2010; 119:621–31.
4. Gennari A, Stockler M, Puntoni M, Sormani M, Nanni O, Amadori D, Wilcken N, D'Amico M, DeCensi A, Bruzzi P. Duration of chemotherapy for metastatic breast cancer: a systematic review and meta-analysis of randomized clinical trials. J Clin Oncol. 2011;29:2144–9.
5. Eisenhauer EA, Therasse P, Bogaerts J, Schwartz LH, Sargent D, Ford R, Dancey J, Arbuck S, Gwyther S, Mooney M, Rubinstein L, Shankar L, Dodd L, Kaplan R, Lacombe D, Verweij J. New response evaluation criteria in solid tumours: revised RECIST guideline (version 1.1). Eur J Cancer. 2009;45:228–47.

6.   European Medicines Agency. Appendix 1 to the guidance on the evaluation of anticancer medicinal products in man. 2013. http://www.ema.europa.eu/docs/en_GB/document_library/Scientific_guideline/2013/01/WC500137126.pdf.

7.   Stein A, Bellmunt J, Escudier B, Kim D, Stergiopoulos SG, Mietlowski W, et al. Survival prediction in everolimus-treated patients with metastatic renal cell carcinoma incorporating tumor burden response in the RECORD-1 trial. Eur Urol. 2013;64:994–1002.

8.   Suzuki C, Blomqvist L, Sundin A, Jacobsson H, Byström P, Berglund A, et al. The initial change in tumor size predicts response and survival in patients with metastatic colorectal cancer treated with combination chemotherapy. Ann Oncol. 2012;23:948–54.

9.   Twelves C, Cortes J, Kaufman PA, Yelle L, Awada A, Binder TA, et al. "New" metastases are associated with a poorer prognosis than growth of pre-existing metastases in patients with metastatic breast cancer treated with chemotherapy. Breast Cancer Res. 2015;17:150.

10. Kotake T, Kikawa Y, Takahara S, Tsuyuki S, Yoshibayashi H, Suzuki E, et al. Impact of eribulin monotherapy on post-progression survival in patients with HER2-negative advanced or metastatic breast cancer. Int J Cancer Clin Res. 2017;3:061.

11. Litiere S, de Vries EG, Seymour L, Sargent D, Shankar L, Bogaerts J, et al. The components of progression as explanatory variables for overall survival in the response evaluation criteria in solid tumours 1.1 database. Eur J Cancer. 2014;50:1847–53.

5

Assessment of thyroid cancer risk in more than 334,000 patients with inflammatory bowel disease

Lihong Cao

Abstract

Background: Potential risk of thyroid cancer in patients with inflammatory bowel disease has not been well investigated. The aim of the study was to reveal the relationship between history of inflammatory bowel disease and risk of thyroid cancer.

Methods: First, 1392 patients with inflammatory bowel disease and 1392 controls were included in a case-control study. All patients did not receive immunosuppressive therapy. A multivariate logistic regression analysis was adopted to determine the relationship between history of inflammatory bowel disease and risk of thyroid cancer. Second, a literature search was performed and eight articles were collected. Pooled odds ratios with 95% confidence intervals were reported for relevant risk estimates in fixed or random effect model.

Results: In the case-control study, thyroid cancer was more common in patients with inflammatory bowel disease than in controls ($P = 0.032$). After Bonferroni correction, association of thyroid cancer risk with history of total inflammatory bowel disease or its two subtypes was not found. In the meta-analysis, patients with total inflammatory bowel disease or ulcerative colitis showed an increased risk of thyroid cancer, but patients with Crohn's disease did not. Furthermore, inflammatory bowel disease patients with immunosuppressive therapy showed an increased risk of the cancer, but patients without immunosuppressive therapy did not have this finding.

Conclusions: Risk of thyroid cancer probably elevates in patients with inflammatory bowel disease. Inflammatory bowel disease (particularly ulcerative colitis) itself and use of immunosuppressant might contribute to the development of the cancer.

Keywords: Crohn's disease, Immunosuppressant, Inflammatory bowel diseases, Thyroid neoplasms, Ulcerative colitis

Background

Thyroid cancer (TC) is one kind of endocrine tumors, which originates in the tissue of thyroid gland [1]. Papillary thyroid carcinoma (PTC) is the most common histological subtype and accounts for more than 80% of TC cases. It often occurs at the age of 35–65 years old and usually affects women more than men [2]. In recent years, incidence of TC has significantly increased [3]. Presently, there are more than three million TC patients around the world [3].

Though prognosis of TC is not very poor, it still causes tens of thousands of deaths each year. Family history, radiation exposure, iodine intake abnormality, and obesity are major risk factors [4–7]. Other potential risk factors have not been well investigated.

Inflammatory bowel disease (IBD) including ulcerative colitis (UC) and Crohn's disease (CD) is a precancerous disease of colorectal cancer [8]. Besides, an increased risk of extra-intestinal cancer in IBD patients has been revealed by previous studies [9]. According to these findings, potential relationship between risk of TC and history of IBD has also been explored. Some studies reported that risk of TC was elevated in patients with

Correspondence: caolihong2012@yeah.net
Department of Ear-nose-throat, Tianjin Medical University General Hospital, No. 154, Anshan Road, Heping District, Tianjin 300052, China

IBD [10, 11], but other studies failed to do so [12, 13]. Thus, a firmed conclusion has not been drawn.

Therefore, we conducted a case-control study and a meta-analysis to evaluate the relationship between the risk of TC and the history of IBD and to further explore the mechanism involved.

Methods

Case-control study

Outpatients in Tianjin Binjiang Hospital between 1991 and 2000 enrolled in a health system database, which contained the huge data of these patients from baseline to 2015. All these outpatients signed the written informed consents and agreed to participate in a series of clinical studies including this study. A total of 1392 IBD patients (1022 UC patients, 370 CD patients) were identified in this database according to ICD-9 codes (codes of CD: 555, 550.0, 555.1 and 555.9; codes of UC: 556, 556.0, 556.1, 556.2, 556.3, 556.5, 556.6, 556.8, and 556.9) and served as the IBD group. All these patients did not have any kind of cancer on admission. And, 1392 age- and gender-matched patients with diverticulitis (codes of diverticulitis 62.11 and 562.13) were randomly collected from the database and served as control group.

Research data such as demographic information, personal history, medical history, treatment history, and other useful information from baseline to 2015 were collected from the database. Major endpoint was the development of PTC, and all the patients with PTC should be confirmed pathologically. Total follow-up period of these IBD patients were 27,448 person-years.

Most of the IBD patients received 5-ASA treatment and other supportive treatment. They did not receive any kind of biologics or immunosuppressant. They did not receive any surgical therapy.

History of smoking was defined as smoking (≥ 7 cigarettes per week) for more than 6 months in one's life. History of drinking was defined as drinking alcohol (≥ 3 times per week) for more than 6 months in one's life. History of iodized salt intaking was defined as having iodized salt for more than 6 months in one's life. History of radiation exposure was defined as having radiation exposure (≥ 1 time per month) for more than 6 months in one's life.

Difference of continuous variables was determined using independent sample t test, and difference of categorical variables was determined using chi-square test. If a P value was less than 0.05, it was considered to be statistically significant. Relationship between the history of IBD and the risk of PTC was determined using multivariate logistic regression analysis. Odds ratios (ORs), 95% confidence intervals (CIs), and P values were reported. Bonferroni correction was adopted for multiple analyses, and Bonferroni corrected P

value was 0.004 (0.05/12 variables). If a P value was less than 0.004, it was statistically significant. These analyses were conducted using SPSS 17.0 (SPSS Inc., Chicago, IL, USA).

The study was separately approved by the ethics committee of Tianjin Medical University General Hospital (TMUGH-2016-0657) and Tianjin People's Hospital (Tianjin Binjiang Hospital) (TJRMYY-2016-087).

Meta-analysis

A structured literature search in MEDLINE/PubMed, EMBASE, Web of Science, and Cochrane Database of Systematic Reviews was conducted between January 1998 and December 2017. Search parameters were "Thyroid Cancer" [Title/Abstract], "Thyroid Neoplasms" [MeSH Terms], "Inflammatory Bowel Disease" [Title/Abstract], "Inflammatory Bowel Diseases" [MeSH Terms], "Ulcerative Colitis" [Title/Abstract], "Colitis, Ulcerative" [MeSH Terms], "Crohn's Disease" [Title/Abstract], "Crohn Disease" [MeSH Terms] and their combinations.

Inclusion criteria were listed as follows: (1) There were IBD group and control group in each study. (2) Number of TC patients in each group was reported. Only English articles were included. Subsequently, references in the included articles were searched. If any reference met the inclusion criteria, it was also adopted.

Two trained reviewers independently performed the data selection according to a predefined survey form, which had several contents: first author, year of publication, country, study design, age at diagnosis, gender, period of follow-up, use of immunosuppressant, size of study, and so on. All data were double entered.

Our meta-analysis was conducted according to the recommendations from the Cochrane Collaboration and the Quality of Reporting of Meta-analyses guidelines [14, 15]. The fourfold table data (events/total in group one, events/total in group two) of each included study were input to a data matrix in Review Manager Version 5.2 (The Cochrane Collaboration, Software Update, Oxford). If P values for heterogeneity > 0.05, the results were performed by fixed effects method. If not, the random effects model was adopted. Then, OR and 95%CI were reported. It was statistically significant, if the 95% CI did not include the value one.

The study adopted three strategies to ensure the research quality. (1) Funnel plot obtained by Review Manager Software was used to evaluate the publication bias [16, 17]. (2) Sensitivity analysis was performed. In this process, each included study was sequentially removed from the meta-analysis to measure its contribution to the overall effect size. (3) All studies in the meta-analysis were scored by the Newcastle-Ottawa Scale to assess their overall quality [18].

Results

Case-control study

In Table 1, there were 1392 patients with IBD and 1392 controls with diverticulitis in the case-control study. Compared with the controls, body mass index was higher in the IBD patients ($P < 0.001$). More IBD patients had history of smoking, radiation exposure, or benign thyroid nodule ($P < 0.001$, $P < 0.001$, $P < 0.001$). More IBD patients had family history of TC ($P < 0.001$). Furthermore, the development of PTC was more common in the IBD patients than in the controls ($P = 0.032$).

In Table 2, after adjusted for several confounding factors (i.e., age, gender, body mass index, smoking, drinking alcohol, iodized salt intaking, radiation exposure, benign thyroid nodule and family history of thyroid cancer), a multivariate logistic regression analysis reported that the history of smoking, radiation exposure, benign thyroid nodule, inflammatory bowel disease, or ulcerative colitis was associated with the increased risk of PTC (OR 3.81, 95%CI 1.27~11.37, $P = 0.016$; OR 5.37, 95%CI 1.78~16.13, $P = 0.003$; OR 9.22, 95%CI 1.21~70.54, $P = 0.031$; OR 3.70, 95%CI 1.04~13.26, $P = 0.044$; OR 4.12, 95%CI 1.12~15.24, $P = 0.033$). Family history of TC was also related to the elevated risk of the cancer (OR 13.02, 95%CI 4.47~37.97, $P < 0.001$). After Bonferroni correction, only history of radiation exposure and

Table 1 Characteristics of inflammatory bowel disease patients and controls in the case-control study

	IBD	Control	P value
Total (n)[b]	1392	1392	–
Male (n)	634	658	0.362
Age (years)[b]	37.0 ± 5.8	36.7 ± 5.8	0.454
BMI (kg/m^2)[a]	23.2 ± 4.3	22.4 ± 4.3	< 0.001
History of smoking (n)	604	296	< 0.001
History of drinking (n)	410	395	0.531
History of iodized salt intaking (n)	754	708	0.081
History of radiation exposure (n)	251	14	< 0.001
History of benign thyroid nodule (n)	1064	570	< 0.001
Family history of TC (n)[a]	135	22	< 0.001
Age at diagnosis of IBD (years)[a]	26.9 ± 6.3	–	–
Duration of IBD on admission (years)	10.1 ± 2.8	–	–
Extraintestinal manifestations (n)	708	–	–
5-ASA treatment (n)[a]	1334	–	–
PTC development (n)[a]	11	3	0.032

[a]BMI Body mass index, IBD inflammatory bowel disease, 5-ASA 5-aminosalicylic acid, PTC papillary thyroid carcinoma, TC thyroid cancer
[b]Categorical and continuous variables were separately showed by frequency and mean ± standard deviation

family history of TC reached the Bonferroni-corrected level of statistical significance.

Meta-analysis

As shown in Fig. 1, during the literature search using the parameters described above, 411 potential articles were found. Their abstracts were carefully reviewed, and 339 articles were directly excluded from the meta-analysis. Major reasons were that they were clinical studies with other topic (205), reviews (53), case reports (34), articles in other languages (27), or basic studies (20). Full texts of the remaining 72 articles were collected and reviewed. Among them, six articles focusing on this topic without required data, seven duplicate articles, and 52 articles focusing on other topics were excluded from the meta-analysis. Then, seven articles were included [11, 13, 19–23]. Their references were researched, and no suitable article was found. Meanwhile, our case-control study was also adopted. Thus, a total of eight studies were included in the meta-analysis.

Major characteristics of the included studies are presented in Table 3. There were 334,015 patients with IBD in the meta-analysis. The study with the largest sample size had 289,935 IBD patients, and the study with the smallest sample size had 374 patients. During the follow-up of more than 339,558 person-years, 244 patients had suffered from TC. Though time range of the literature search was 1998–2017, most of the included articles were published in the last 5 years. Improved detection for TC in the recent years was believed to be one of the possible reasons to explain this phenomenon. Five studies had normal controls, and the other three studies had patient controls with diverticulitis.

In Fig. 2, eight studies focused on the relationship between the history of IBD and the risk of TC in the patients. The fixed-effect pooled OR was 1.75 (95%CI 1.48~2.07, P for heterogeneity = 0.31). After excluding our study, the fixed-effect pooled OR was 1.72 (95%CI 1.45~2.04, P for heterogeneity = 0.33).

Five studies explored the possible association between the history of UC and the risk of TC, and the fixed-effect pooled OR was 1.62 (95%CI 1.26~2.09, P for heterogeneity = 0.25) (Fig. 2). After excluding our study, the fixed-effect pooled OR was 1.54 (95%CI 1.19~2.00, P for heterogeneity = 0.32).

Six studies showed the relationship between the history of CD and the risk of TC. The fixed-effect pooled OR was 1.41 (95%CI 0.91~2.18, P for heterogeneity = 0.65) (Fig. 2). After excluding our study, the fixed-effect pooled OR was 1.36 (95%CI 0.86~2.14, P for heterogeneity = 0.57).

In the subgroup analysis, the data were separately stratified by several factors, such as gender, race, case type, control type, use of immunosuppressant, and

Table 2 Association of several variables with risk of papillary thyroid carcinoma in the case-control study

Group	Subgroup	PTC[a]	Total	Univariate OR (95%CI)[a,b]	Univariate P value [c]	Multivariate OR (95%CI)[b]	Multivariate P value[c]
Gender	Female	9	1492	Reference		Reference	
	Male	5	1292	0.64 (0.20~1.92)	0.425	0.65 (0.21~1.93)	0.424
Age (years)	< 36.9 years	6	1428	Reference		Reference	
	≥ 36.9 years	8	1356	1.41 (0.49~4.06)	0.529	1.42 (0.49~4.07)	0.528
BMI (kg/m²)[a]	< 22.8 kg/m²	5	1408	Reference		Reference	
	≥ 22.8 kg/m²	9	1376	1.85 (0.61~5.54)	0.272	1.86 (0.62~5.54)	0.271
History of smoking	Absent	5	1884	Reference		Reference	
	Present	9	900	3.80 (1.27~11.36)	0.017	3.81 (1.27~11.37)	0.016
History of drinking	Absent	7	1979	Reference		Reference	
	Present	7	805	2.47 (0.86~7.07)	0.092	2.48 (0.87~7.08)	0.092
History of ISI[a]	Absent	4	1322	Reference		Reference	
	Present	10	1462	2.26 (0.72~7.24)	0.167	2.27 (0.72~7.25)	0.166
History of RE[a]	Absent	9	2519	Reference		Reference	
	Present	5	265	5.36 (1.78~16.12)	0.003	5.37 (1.78~16.13)	0.003
History of BTN[a]	Absent	1	1150	Reference		Reference	
	Present	13	1634	9.21 (1.20~70.53)	0.032	9.22 (1.21~70.54)	0.031
Family history of TC[a]	Absent	8	2627	Reference		Reference	
	Present	6	157	13.01 (4.47~37.96)	< 0.001	13.02 (4.47~37.97)	< 0.001
History of IBD[a]	Control	3	1392	Reference		Reference	
	IBD	11	1392	3.69 (1.04~13.25)	0.045	3.70 (1.04~13.26)	0.044
History of CD[a]	Control	3	1392	Reference		Reference	
	CD	2	370	2.52 (0.43~15.12)	0.313	2.53 (0.43~15.13)	0.313
History of UC[a]	Control	3	1392	Reference		Reference	
	UC	9	1022	4.11 (1.12~15.23)	0.034	4.12 (1.12~15.24)	0.033

[a]*BMI* body mass index, *ISI* iodized salt intaking, *RE* radiation exposure, *BTN* benign thyroid nodule, *IBD* inflammatory bowel disease, *UC* ulcerative colitis, *CD* Crohn's disease, *TC* thyroid cancer, *PTC* papillary thyroid carcinoma, *OR* odds ratio, *CI* confidence interval

[b]Univariate analysis was not adjusted by potential confounding factor. Multivariate analysis was adjusted by age, gender, body mass index, smoking, drinking alcohol, iodized salt intaking, radiation exposure, benign thyroid nodule, and family history of thyroid cancer

[c]Bonferroni correction was adopted for multiple analyses, and Bonferroni corrected P value was 0.004 (0.05/12 variables). If a P value was less than 0.004, it was statistically significant

number of IBD patients. The results were showed in Table 4. The meta-analysis with hospital-based or small sample size (less than 10,000 cases) studies did not report any statistically significant results, revealing that study design had great influence on the result.

Jung et al. and So et al. reported that 35.3% and 40.0% of the IBD patients separately in their studies received the immunosuppressant, and these two studies were defined as "ever use" studies [13, 19]. Sonu et al. in their study and our case-control study reported that the IBD patients did not adopt any kind of immunosuppressant before the development of TC, and these studies were defined as "never use" study [22]. Then, a subgroup analysis was done (Table 4). The IBD patients who ever received the immunosuppressant showed the increased the risk of TC, but the patients who never received these drugs did not show any change of the TC risk compared with the controls.

Discussion

At present, only a few clinical and epidemiological studies focused on the risk of TC in IBD patients around the world. Most of the studies were based on their national health or medical insurance databases and had a huge sample size [11, 13, 19, 20, 23]. Because many potential confounding factors were not taken into account, these studies actually conducted an unadjusted analysis. In addition, there were two hospital-based studies. One was from Yano et al. and examined all kinds of cancers in CD patients [21]. Another one came from Sonu et al., and their results were only adjusted by age and gender [22]. Both the studies did not have a well-adjusted design. Therefore, we carried out this case-control study, which had taken into account many confounding factors, such as family history, radiation exposure, iodine intake

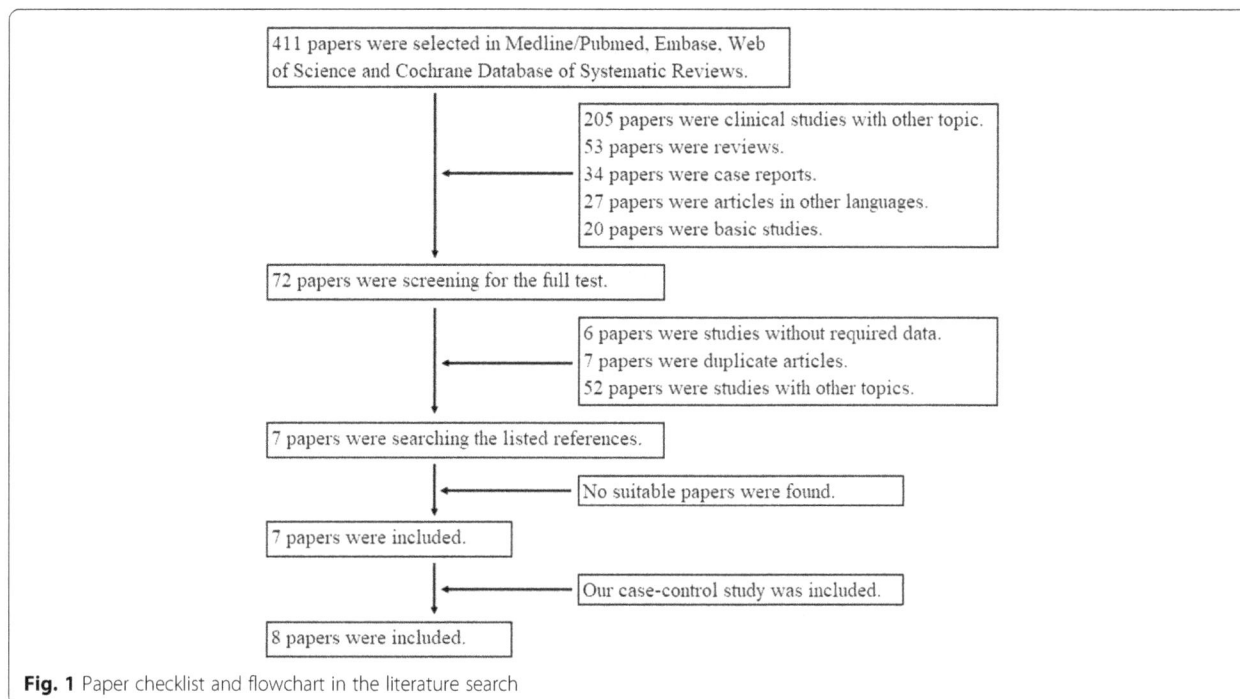

411 papers were selected in Medline/Pubmed, Embase, Web of Science and Cochrane Database of Systematic Reviews.

205 papers were clinical studies with other topic.
53 papers were reviews.
34 papers were case reports.
27 papers were articles in other languages.
20 papers were basic studies.

72 papers were screening for the full test.

6 papers were studies without required data.
7 papers were duplicate articles.
52 papers were studies with other topics.

7 papers were searching the listed references.

No suitable papers were found.

7 papers were included.

Our case-control study was included.

8 papers were included.

Fig. 1 Paper checklist and flowchart in the literature search

abnormality, and obesity. We believed that our study might supplement the shortcomings of the previous studies.

Incidence of TC in the case-control study seemed to be higher than many previous studies [19, 20]. Possible reasons were listed as follows: First, TC was a relatively quiet tumor, and could be asymptomatic for a long time. Second, due to the improvement of health consciousness, many local people began to receive regular physical examination. Third, great progress had been made in diagnostic technology for TC. So, many cases of TC were found in recent years. The incidence of the cancer might be underestimated in the previous studies [19, 20].

Based on the adjusted analysis, the case-control study reported that the patients with IBD or its subtype UC had a more than 2-time or 3-time increased risk of PTC compared with the controls. However, these results did not reach the Bonferroni-corrected statistical significance.

In the meta-analysis, there were eight case-control studies with a total of 334,015 IBD patients. All the eligible studies had been included. Based on the pooled results, the patients with IBD showed a 45–100% increased risk of TC and the patients with its subtype UC showed a 20–100% increased risk of TC compared with the controls. The pooled results demonstrated the significant increase of the cancer risk in patients with IBD

Table 3 Characteristics of included studies in the meta-analysis

First author	Year	Country	No. of IBD (n)[a]	IBD male (n)	IBD age at diagnosis (years)	IBD type	No. of controls (n)	Control type	Quality score
This study	2018	China	1392	634	Mean 26.9	Single center	1392	Patient	7
Jung	2017	Korea	15,291	9743	Mean 38.6	Population	1,529,100	Normal	7
So	2017	China	1603	893	Median CD 40/UC 53 [a]	Population	160,300	Normal	7
Wadhwa	2016	USA	289,935	125,635	Mean 50.1	Population	315,145	Patient	7
Jussila	2013	Finland	21,964	11,810	NM	Population	2,196,400	Normal	7
Yano	2013	Japan	770	531	Mean 23.1	Single center	77,000	Normal	6
Sonu	2013	USA	2686	913	Mean 47.5	Single center	1638	Patient	6
Jess	2004	Denmark	374	157	NM	Population	37,400	Normal	7

[a]*IBD* inflammatory bowel disease, *NM* not mentioned, *CD* Crohn's disease, *UC* ulcerative colitis

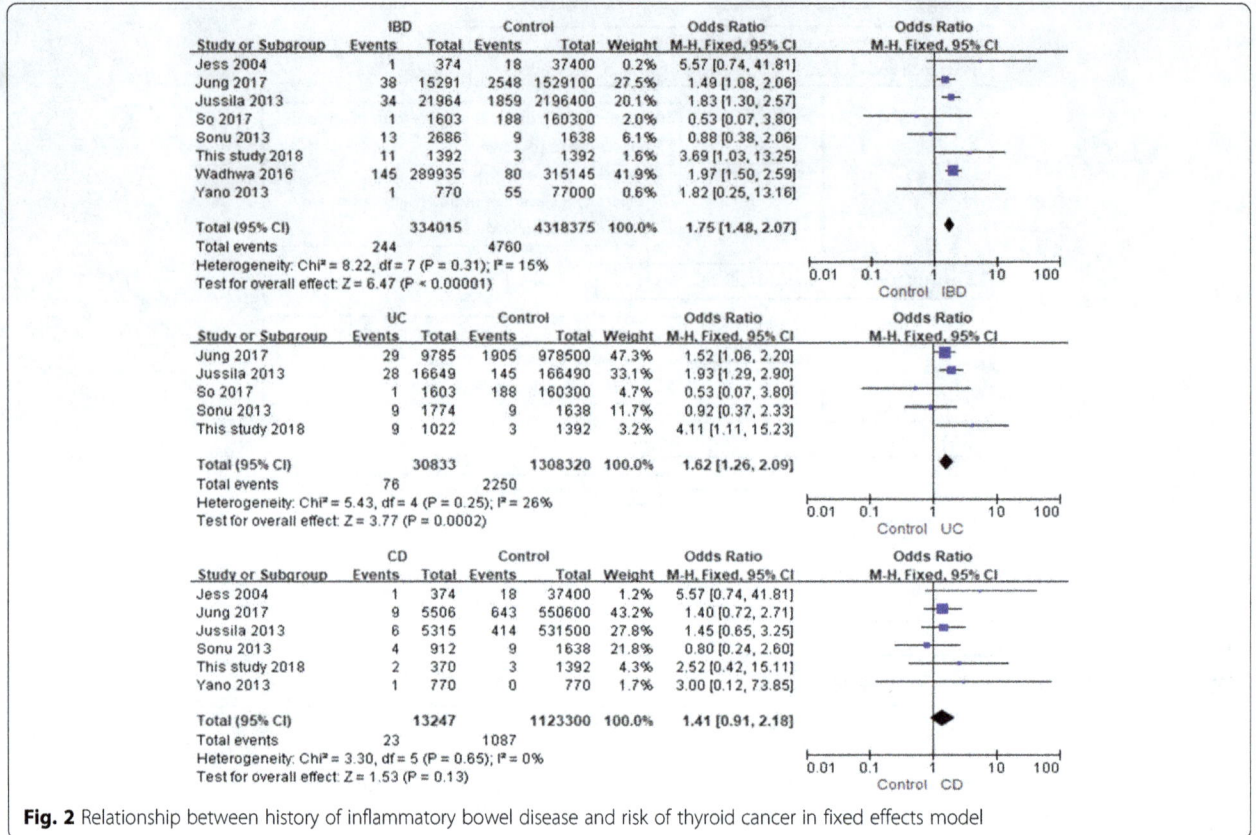

Fig. 2 Relationship between history of inflammatory bowel disease and risk of thyroid cancer in fixed effects model

Table 4 Results of meta-analysis in the subgroup

Subgroup	No. of studies (n)	No. of IBD (n)[a]	OR (95%CI)[a]	P value for heterogeneity
Gender				
Male	2	21,553	2.05 (1.38~3.05)	0.26
Female	2	15,702	1.48 (1.11~1.97)	0.79
Race				
Asian	4	19,056	1.55 (1.15~2.08)	0.39
Caucasian	2	22,338	1.87 (1.34~2.61)	0.29
Case type				
Population	5	329,167	1.77 (1.49~2.11)	0.36
Hospital	3	4848	1.50 (0.78~2.88)	0.18
Control type				
Normal	5	40,002	1.61 (1.28~2.02)	0.48
Patient	3	292,621	1.89 (1.47~2.44)	0.12
Immunosuppressant				
Ever use	2	16,894	1.43 (1.04~1.96)	0.31
Never use	2	4078	1.47 (0.74~2.92)	0.07
No. of IBD patients				
≥ 10,000	3	327,190	1.79 (1.50~2.14)	0.42
< 10,000	5	5433	1.39 (0.78~2.48)	0.19

[a]*IBD* inflammatory bowel disease, *OR* odds ratio, *CI* confidence interval

or its subtype UC. In the subgroup analysis, the relationship between the history of IBD and the risk of TC always existed in men, women, Asians, and Caucasians, suggesting that the increased risk of TC in IBD might not be a single race or gender problem.

To our knowledge, it was the first meta-analysis exploring the relationship between the history of IBD and the risk of TC. Pedersen et al. obtained an estimate of the risk of extra-intestinal cancer in CD and UC by performing a meta-analysis of population-based cohort studies and reported that the risk of upper gastrointestinal tract cancer, lung cancer, urinary bladder cancer, or skin cancer was significantly increased among patients with CD, and the risk of liver-biliary cancer or leukemia was significantly increased in patients with UC [9]. However, only two cohort studies with not enough subjects focused on TC, and their pooled results did not demonstrate a relationship between the history of IBD and the risk of TC [9]. Another meta-analysis from Huai et al. explored the impact of IBD on cholangiocarcinoma, and suggested the risk of cholangiocarcinoma was significantly increased among IBD patients, especially in intra-hepatic cholangiocarcinoma cases [24]. Though there were no positive or available results on TC, both meta-analyses demonstrated the relationship between the history of IBD and the risk of extra-intestinal cancer.

In addition, the results of the case-control study were basically the same as those of the meta-analysis, though the Bonferroni-corrected results in the case-control study were not statistically significant. A possible explanation for the negative results after Bonferroni-correction was the lack of sample size. This explanation had been confirmed in the subgroup meta-analysis. The population-based studies in the subgroup meta-analysis reported a 50–110% increased risk of TC in the IBD patients. But, the studies with small sample size failed to do so.

At present, immunosuppressant became one common therapeutic drug for IBD. Some previous studies reported that the use of immunosuppressant increased the risk of cancer [25, 26]. In particular, immunosuppressant caused lymphoproliferative disorder, which was related to the development of TC [26]. In the case-control study, the patients did not receive the immunosuppressant and provided a negative result. In the meta-analysis, the patients who ever use immunosuppressant showed an increased risk of TC, but the patients who never used the drug did not. So, the strategy of immunosuppressive therapy might be a possible carcinogenic factor for TC.

Radiation exposure was another important confounding factor. A previous study reported that the IBD patients frequently received X-ray or computed tomography examination, which was a potential hazard to the human body [27]. In the case-control study,

the history of radiation exposure was related to the increased risk of the cancer. Therefore, excessive exposure to radiation in IBD patients probably contributed to the development of TC.

Potential role of IBD in the development of TC could not be completely negated. The meta-analysis found that the risk of TC was higher in the UC patients than in the CD patients. The case-control study supported it, though the results did not reach Bonferroni-corrected statistical significance. This finding apparently could not be explained by the use of immunosuppressant and excessive exposure to radiation, but could be partly explained by chronic inflammation in IBD. It was well known that the pathogenesis of UC and CD was not exactly the same. CD was clearly identified as a Th1 inflammation [28], and Th2 mainly improved the development of UC [29]. Interleukin-13 (IL-13) was the key Th2 cytokine, and affected epithelial tight junctions, apoptosis and cell restitution in UC [30]. IL-5 was another Th2 cytokine, which could attract eosinophils to intestinal tissue and caused tissue damage and intestinal inflammation in UC [31]. Furthermore, Th2 cytokines (IL-4, IL-5 and IL-13), but not Th1 cytokines, were implicated in the pathogenesis of TC. Simonovic et al. suggested that peripheral blood cells of differentiated TC patients produced significantly higher concentrations of Th2 cytokines (IL-5 and IL-13) than control subjects, and radioactive 131-I therapy led to reduced secretion of these Th2 cytokines [32]. Joshi et al. demonstrated that IL-4 receptor-α (IL-4Rα) was over-expressed in anaplastic TC and might represent a novel therapeutic target in this cancer [33]. Taken together, there was no enough evidence that IBD was an independent risk factor for TC, but IBD might provide an appropriate inflammatory environment and promote the development of the cancer.

Quality evaluation of the meta-analysis was conducted and mainly involved three aspects: participant selection, group comparability, and outcome assessment. All included studies received satisfactory scores (Table 3). Major results were based on the fixed effects model (P values for heterogeneity were > 0.05). So, included studies showed good homogeneity. Publication bias was an important problem and could not be ignored. As shown in Fig. 3, the studies created roughly funnel-shaped distributions and formed symmetric graphs. So, significant publication bias had not been detected.

"Reverse causality" might be a potential limitation in case-control study. But, the studies in our meta-analysis were nested case-control studies with follow-ups of 6000–236,000 person-years. "Recall bias" was another potential problem in retrospective study. But, all included studies obtained their research data from medical

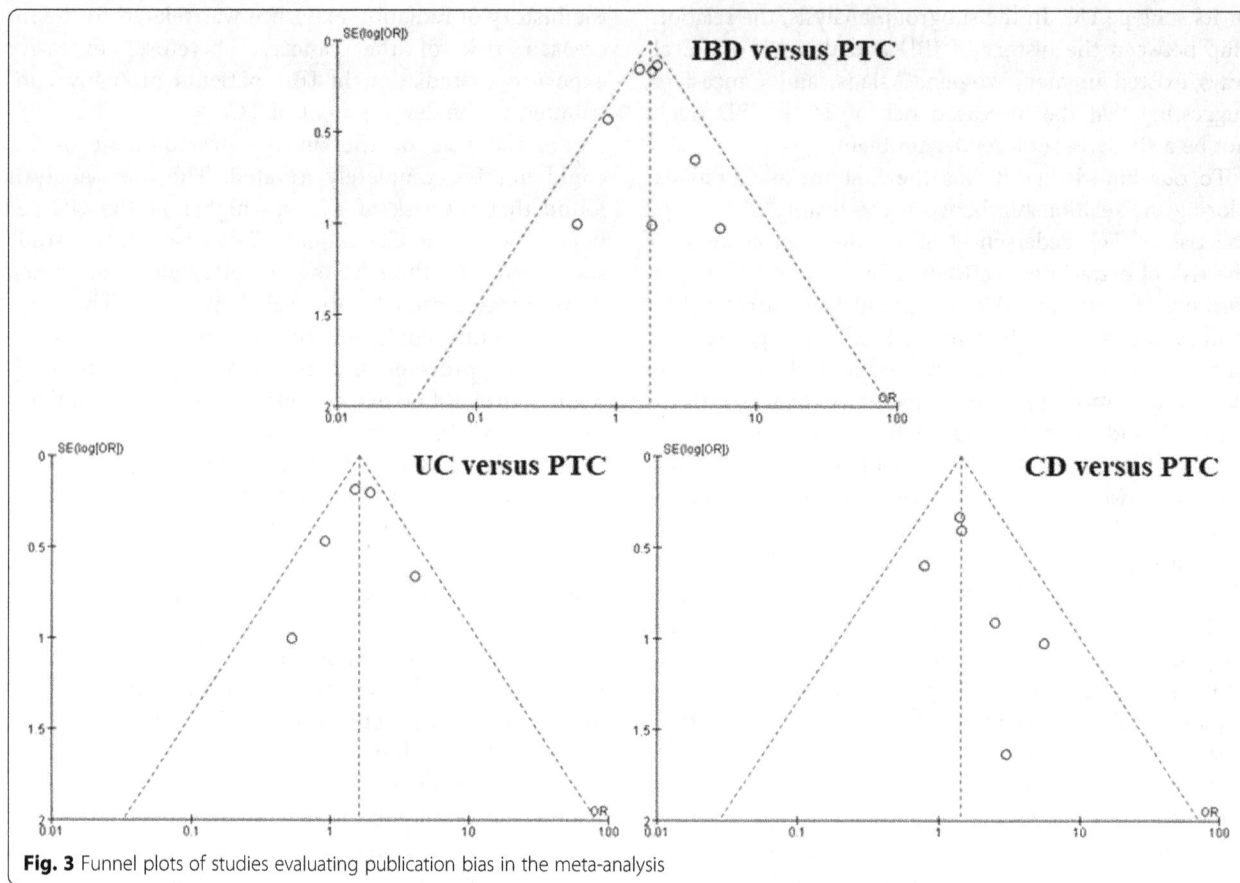

Fig. 3 Funnel plots of studies evaluating publication bias in the meta-analysis

records or health data system. The cases of IBD and TC were collected according to ICD-10 system. So, we did not think these issues affected our results.

TC was classified into medullary cancer, follicular cancer, undifferentiated cancer, and PTC. The case-control study focused on the PTC patients. But, most of the included studies in the meta-analysis explored the association of IBD with total TC. This limitation might cause bias, though PTC was the most common tissue subtype and accounted for more than 80% of total TC cases. More research should be conducted in different tissue types of TC.

Conclusions

In conclusion, there were some defects in the current studies, but their achievements could be the basis for future research. Based on the results of our case-control study and meta-analysis, we suggested that the risk of TC probably elevated in patients with IBD, and this increase was more significant in its subtype UC. Inflammatory response of IBD itself, use of immunosuppressant and other undefined factors contributed to the development of TC. Well-adjusted and population-based studies should be conducted to verify our conclusion.

Abbreviations
CD: Crohn's disease; CI: Confidence interval; IBD: Inflammatory bowel disease; >OR: Odds ratio; PTC: Papillary thyroid carcinoma; TC: Thyroid cancer; UC: Ulcerative colitis

Acknowledgements
I want to take this chance to thank to Dr. LQ (Tianjin Binjiang Hospital, Tianjin People's Hospital). In the process of data collection, he gives me many academic and constructive advices and helps me to correct my paper.

Author's contribution
CL collected, analyzed, and interpreted the data. Then, she wrote and approved the final manuscript.

Competing interests
The author declares that she has no competing interests.

References
1. Burns WR, Zeiger MA. Differentiated thyroid cancer. Semin Oncol. 2010;37: 557–66.
2. Jonklaas J, Nogueras-Gonzalez G, Munsell M, Litofsky D, Ain KB, Bigos ST, et al. The impact of age and gender on papillary thyroid cancer survival. J Clin Endocrinol Metab. 2012;97:878–87.
3. Davies L, Morris L, Hankey B. Increases in thyroid cancer incidence and mortality. JAMA. 2017;318:389–90.
4. Leux C, Truong T, Petit C, Baron-Dubourdieu D, Guénel P. Family history of malignant and benign thyroid diseases and risk of thyroid cancer: a population-based case-control study in New Caledonia. Cancer Causes Control. 2012;23:745–55.
5. Takamura N, Orita M, Saenko V, Yamashita S, Nagataki S, Demidchik Y. Radiation and risk of thyroid cancer: Fukushima and Chernobyl. Lancet Diabetes Endocrinol. 2016;4:647.

6. Zimmermann MB, Galetti V. Iodine intake as a risk factor for thyroid cancer: a comprehensive review of animal and human studies. Thyroid Res. 2015;8:8.

7. Oberman B, Khaku A, Camacho F, Goldenberg D. Relationship between obesity, diabetes and the risk of thyroid cancer. Am J Otolaryngol. 2015;36:535–41.

8. Harpaz N, Ward SC, Mescoli C, Itzkowitz SH, Polydorides AD. Precancerous lesions in inflammatory bowel disease. Best Pract Res Clin Gastroenterol. 2013;27:257–67.

9. Pedersen N, Duricova D, Elkjaer M, Gamborg M, Munkholm P, Jess T. Risk of extra-intestinal cancer in inflammatory bowel disease: meta-analysis of population-based cohort studies. Am J Gastroenterol. 2010;105:1480–7.

10. Biancone L, Armuzzi A, Scribano ML, D'Inca R, Castiglione F, Papi C. Inflammatory bowel disease phenotype as risk factor for cancer in a prospective multicentre nested case-control IG-IBD study. J Crohns Colitis. 2016;10:913–24.

11. Jussila A, Virta LJ, Pukkala E, Färkkilä MA. Malignancies in patients with inflammatory bowel disease: a nationwide register study in Finland. Scand J Gastroenterol. 2013;48:1405–13.

12. Biancone L, Zuzzi S, Ranieri M, Petruzziello C, Calabrese E, Onali S, et al. Fistulizing pattern in Crohn's disease and pancolitis in ulcerative colitis are independent risk factors for cancer: a single-center cohort study. Crohns Colitis. 2012;6:578–87.

13. So J, Tang W, Leung WK, Li M, Lo FH, Wong MTL, et al. Cancer risk in 2621 Chinese patients with inflammatory bowel disease: a population-based cohort study. Inflamm Bowel Dis. 2017;23:2061–8.

14. Clarke M, Horton R. Bringing it all together: Lancet – Cochrane collaborate on systematic reviews. Lancet. 2001;357:1728.

15. Stroup DF, Berlin JA, Morton SC, Olkin I, Williamson GD, Rennie D, et al. Meta-analysis of observational studies in epidemiology: a proposal for reporting. Meta-analysis Of Observational Studies in Epidemiology (MOOSE) group. JAMA. 2000;283:2008–12.

16. Egger M, Davey Smith G, Schneider M, Minder C. Bias in meta-analysis detected by a simple, graphical test. BMJ. 1997;315:629–34.

17. Egger M, Smith GD. Misleading meta-analysis. BMJ. 1995;311:753–4.

18. Athanasiou T, Al-Ruzzeh S, Kumar P, Crossman MC, Amrani M, Pepper JR, et al. Off-pump myocardial revascularization is associated with less incidence of stroke in elderly patients. Ann Thorac Surg. 2004;77:745–53.

19. Jung YS, Han M, Park S, Kim WH, Cheon JH. Cancer risk in the early stages of inflammatory bowel disease in Korean patients: a nationwide population-based study. J Crohns Colitis. 2017;11:954–62.

20. Wadhwa V, Lopez R, Shen B. Crohn's disease is associated with the risk for thyroid Cancer. Inflamm Bowel Dis. 2016;22:2902–6.

21. Yano Y, Matsui T, Hirai F, Okado Y, Sato Y, Tsurumi K, et al. Cancer risk in Japanese Crohn's disease patients: investigation of the standardized incidence ratio. J Gastroenterol Hepatol. 2013;28:1300–5.

22. Sonu IS, Blonski W, Lin MV, Lewis J, Aberra F, Lichtenstein GR. Papillary thyroid cancer and inflammatory bowel disease: is there a relationship? World J Gastroenterol. 2013;19:1079–84.

23. Jess T, Winther KV, Munkholm P, Langholz E, Binder V. Intestinal and extra-intestinal cancer in Crohn's disease: follow-up of a population-based cohort in Copenhagen County, Denmark. Aliment Pharmacol Ther. 2004;19:287–93.

24. Huai JP, Ding J, Ye XH, Chen YP. Inflammatory bowel disease and risk of cholangiocarcinoma: evidence from a meta-analysis of population-based studies. Asian Pac J Cancer Prev. 2014;15:3477–82.

25. Jiyad Z, Olsen CM, Burke MT, Isbel NM, Green AC. Azathioprine and risk of skin cancer in organ transplant recipients: systematic review and meta-analysis. Am J Transplant. 2016;16:3490–503.

26. Kandiel A, Fraser AG, Korelitz BI, Brensinger C, Lewis JD. Increased risk of lymphoma among inflammatory bowel disease patients treated with azathioprine and 6-mercaptopurine. Gut. 2005;54:1121–5.

27. Peloquin JM, Pardi DS, Sandborn WJ, Fletcher JG, McCollough CH, Schueler BA, et al. Diagnostic ionizing radiation exposure in a population-based cohort of patients with inflammatory bowel disease. Am J Gastroenterol. 2008;103:2015–22.

28. Brand S. Crohn's disease: Th1, Th17 or both? The change of a paradigm: new immunological and genetic insights implicate Th17 cells in the pathogenesis of Crohn's disease. Gut. 2009 Aug;58(8):1152 67.

29. Bamias G, Kaltsa G, Ladas SD. Cytokines in the pathogenesis of ulcerative colitis. Discov Med. 2011 May;11(60):459–67.

30. Heller F, Florian P, Bojarski C, Richter J, Christ M, Hillenbrand B, Mankertz J, Gitter AH, Bürgel N, Fromm M, Zeitz M, Fuss I, Strober W, Schulzke JD. Interleukin-13 is the key effector Th2 cytokine in ulcerative colitis that affects epithelial tight junctions, apoptosis, and cell restitution. Gastroenterology. 2005 Aug;129(2):550–64.

31. Lampinen M, Carlson M, Sangfelt P, Taha Y, Thörn M, Lööf L, Raab Y, Venge P. IL-5 and TNF-alpha participate in recruitment of eosinophils to intestinal mucosa in ulcerative colitis. Dig Dis Sci. 2001 Sep;46(9):2004–9.

32. Simonovic SZ, Mihaljevic O, Majstorovic I, Djurdjevic P, Kostic I, Djordjevic OM, Teodorovic LM. Cytokine production in peripheral blood cells of patients with differentiated thyroid cancer: elevated Th2/Th9 cytokine production before and reduced Th2 cytokine production after radioactive iodine therapy. Cancer Immunol Immunother. 2015 Jan;64(1):75–82.

33. Joshi BH, Suzuki A, Fujisawa T, Leland P, Varrichio F, Lababidi S, Lloyd R, Kasperbauer J, Puri RK. Identification, characterization, and targeting of IL-4 receptor by IL-4-pseudomonas exotoxin in mouse models of anaplastic thyroid cancer. Discov Med. 2015 Nov;20(111):273–84.

6

Current practice patterns of preoperative bowel preparation in colorectal surgery

Zheng Liu[†], Ming Yang[†], Zhi-xun Zhao[†], Xu Guan, Zheng Jiang, Hai-peng Chen, Song Wang, Ji-chuan Quan, Run-kun Yang and Xi-shan Wang[*]

Abstract

Background: The optimal preoperative bowel preparation for colorectal surgery remains controversial. However, recent studies have established that bowel preparation varies significantly among countries and even surgeons at the same institution. This survey aimed to obtain information on the current practice patterns of bowel preparation for colorectal surgery in China.

Methods: A paper-based survey was circulated to the members of the Chinese Society of Colorectal Cancer (CSCC). The survey responses were collected and analyzed. Statistical analysis was performed for all the categorical variables according to the responses to individual questions.

Results: Three hundred forty-one members completed the questionnaire. Regarding surgical practice, 203 (59.5%) performed > 50% of the colorectal operations laparoscopically or robotically; the use of mechanical bowel preparation (MBP) alone was significantly higher (63.5 vs 31.9%; $P < 0.001$). The respondents who performed > 200 colonic or rectal resections provided significantly more MBP alone (79.6 vs 39.1%, $P < 0.001$; 76.6 vs 43.2%, $P < 0.001$; respectively). Among hospitals with fewer than 500 beds, 52.4% of the respondents used MBP + oral antibiotics preparation (OAP) + enema, a significantly higher percentage than the respondents of hospitals with more than 500 beds ($P < 0.001$). Nearly 40% of the respondents prescribed OAP in regimens; meanwhile, 74.8% prescribed preoperative intravenous antibiotics.

Conclusions: The study demonstrates considerable variation among members from the CSCC. These findings should be considered when developing multicenter trials and to provide more definitive answers.

Keywords: Bowel preparation, Mechanical bowel preparation, Colorectal surgery, Survey

Background

Although preoperative bowel preparation is a standard practice for the most elective colorectal surgical procedures and is routinely used, the method and practice still vary widely [1–3]. In the past few decades, various regimens of mechanical bowel preparation (MBP) and oral antibiotics preparation (OAP) have been widely debated

* Correspondence: wxshan1208@126.com
[†]Zheng Liu, Ming Yang and Zhi-xun Zhao contributed equally to this work.
Department of Colorectal Surgery, National Cancer Center/National Clinical Research Center for Cancer/Cancer Hospital, Chinese Academy of Medical Sciences and Peking Union Medical College, Beijing, China

[4–7]. Previous investigators have suggested that MBP or OAP reduces the risk of anastomotic leaks and infectious complications [8, 9]. It is widely accepted that MBP/OAP could help to reduce the stool burden and further reduce the bacterial counts [10, 11].

A recent study has added fuel to this debate. The analysis of the American College of Surgeons National Surgical Quality Improvement Program (ACS-NSQIP) indicated that the combined use of MBP/OAP was associated with significantly lower rates of postoperative complications compared with the use of other bowel preparation strategies [12]. However, a multicenter randomized trial of 1354 patients found that performing colorectal surgery safely without MBP was justified [13]. This is in keeping with common belief that clinical practice is not always evidence-based but is based on tradition and an individual's opinion and previous experiences [14].

Although optimal bowel preparation remains elusive, understanding these differences in practice can help continually improve the clinical practices and implement multicenter trials. To the best of our knowledge, no such survey of preoperative bowel preparation has been previously undertaken in China. The purpose of this study was to describe the current practice patterns of preoperative bowel preparation in colorectal surgery among members of the Chinese Society of Colorectal Cancer (CSCC).

Methods

A 19-question paper-based survey was developed (see Additional file 1). The permission to conduct the survey was obtained from the CSCC. The anonymous survey was announced by posters to the active members who attended the Annual Meeting of the CSCC on August 18–20, 2017. The participants could complete the questionnaire immediately before, during, or after the meeting, depending on their individual needs and predilections. Participation was encouraged by the program coordinators but was not mandatory.

Key demographic information was collected, including gender, age, experience time, medical specialty, affiliations, position, and volume. Specific questions were aimed at the methods and practices used for preoperative bowel preparation in colorectal surgery in the respondent's practice. The survey consisted of questions

Table 1 General characteristics

	Number	Percent
Gender		
Male	318	93.3
Female	23	6.7
Age		
< 40 years	197	57.8
40–50 years	121	35.5
> 50 years	23	6.7
Working experience		
< 10 years	98	28.7
10–20 years	155	45.5
> 20 years	88	25.8
Medical specialty		
General surgery	169	49.6
Gastrointestinal surgery	81	23.8
Colorectal surgery	50	14.7
Other	41	12.0
Hospital setting		
General	295	86.5
Specialized	46	13.5
Hospital volume		
< 500 beds	63	18.5
500–1000 beds	87	25.5
1000–1500 beds	60	17.6
> 1500 beds	131	38.4
Colonic resections per year		
< 100	181	53.1
100–200	62	18.2
> 200	98	28.7
Rectal resections per year		
< 100	194	56.9
100–200	70	20.5
> 200	77	22.6
Resection performed laparoscopically or robotically		
< 30%	76	22.3
30–50%	62	18.2
> 50%	203	59.5

Table 2 Answers according to bowel preparation

	Number	Percent
Bowel preparation regimens		
MBP alone	173	50.7
MBP + OAP + enema	81	23.8
MBP + OAP	55	16.1
Enema alone	20	5.9
Other	12	3.5
Indication for bowel preparation		
Colonic resection only	9	2.6
Rectal resection only	35	10.3
Colonic resection + rectal resection	297	87.1
Bowel preparation for intestinal obstruction		
Yes	243	71.3
No	98	28.7
Preoperative intravenous antibiotic		
Yes	255	74.8
No	86	25.2
Postoperative intravenous antibiotic		
Yes	307	90.0
No	34	10.0
Length of postoperative intravenous antibiotic usage		
< 1 days	14	4.6
1–3 days	125	40.7
> 3 days	168	54.7

MBP mechanical bowel preparation, *OAP* oral antibiotics preparation

regarding the use of MBP, OAP, and perioperative intravenous antibiotics for colorectal surgery. We also asked for information on whether the respondents had used bowel preparation in incomplete bowel obstruction.

Based on the responses obtained, the response rates of respondents were calculated; Fisher's exact test analysis was used to compare groups using SPSS (version 19.0; IBM Corporation, Armonk, NY).

Results

Demographics

Overall, 341 members finally completed the questionnaire, representing 31 provincial administrative regions. Table 1 shows the demographic characteristics of the respondents. There were 318 (93.3%) male respondents and 23 (6.7%) female respondents. Most of the

respondents had more than 10 years of working experience (71.3%), and working in general hospitals (86.5%), and were under the age of 40 (57.8%). The most common specialty for the respondents was general surgery (49.6%), and 38.4% reported working in hospitals with more than 1500 beds. Regarding the surgical volume, 28.7% performed > 200 colonic resections per year and 56.9% performed < 100 rectal resections per year. Among the respondents, 59.5% performed > 50% of colorectal operations laparoscopically or robotically.

Bowel preparation strategies

For colorectal surgery, all the respondents routinely used preoperative bowel preparation. Approximately half of the respondents used MBP alone; MBP + OAP was used by 16.1%, and MBP + OAP combined with an enema

Table 3 Subgroup analysis of preoperative bowel preparation use

	MBP alone	Enema alone	MBP + OAP	MBP + OAP + enema	Other	P value
Age						
< 40 years	101	16	22	51	7	0.032
40–50 years	60	2	27	27	5	
> 50 years	12	2	6	3	0	
Working experience						
< 10 years	55	8	8	24	3	0.128
10–20 years	76	9	26	36	8	
> 20 years	42	3	21	21	1	
Hospital setting						
General	148	16	49	72	10	0.738
Specialized	25	4	6	9	2	
Hospital volume						
< 500 beds	10	6	13	33	1	< 0.001
500–1000 beds	35	2	20	28	2	
1000–1500 beds	35	3	7	10	5	
> 1500 beds	93	9	15	10	4	
Colonic resections per year						
< 100	61	11	40	62	7	< 0.001
100–200	34	4	6	15	3	
> 200	78	5	9	4	2	
Rectal resections per year						
< 100	70	11	41	64	8	< 0.001
100–200	44	3	6	15	2	
> 200	59	6	8	2	2	
Resection performed laparoscopically or robotically						
< 30%	20	3	16	35	2	< 0.001
30–50%	24	5	12	17	4	
> 50%	129	12	27	29	6	

MBP mechanical bowel preparation, *OAP* oral antibiotics preparation

(MBP + OAP +enema) was used by 23.8% (Table 2). No respondent used OAP alone. Enema alone and other regimens were prescribed preoperatively by 5.9 and 3.5%, respectively. The percentage of the respondents performing preoperative bowel preparation for colonic resection only or rectal resection only was 2.6 and 10.3%, respectively. Moreover, 71.3% of the respondents reported using bowel preparation for intestinal obstruction patients.

The respondent's age, hospital volume, volume of resections per year, and percentage of resections performed laparoscopically or robotically showed significant differences in the use of preoperative bowel preparation (Table 3). In the cohort performing > 50% of colorectal operations laparoscopically or robotically ($n = 203$), the use of MBP alone was significantly higher (63.5 vs 31.9%; $P < 0.001$) (Fig. 1). The respondents who performed > 200 colonic or rectal resections gave significantly more MBP alone (79.6 vs 39.1%, $P < 0.001$; 76.6 vs 43.2%, $P < 0.001$; respectively) (Figs. 2 and 3). Of hospitals with less than 500 beds, 52.4% of the respondents used MBP + OAP + enema, which is significantly higher than the respondents of hospitals with more than 500 beds ($P < 0.001$) (Fig. 4). The respondent's working experience and hospital setting did not significantly affect the use of bowel preparation.

OAP and intravenous antibiotics
Preoperative oral antibiotics were administered by 39.9% of the respondents. The most common specified antibiotic drug used was metronidazole (83.9%). Preoperative or postoperative intravenous antibiotics were administered by most respondents (74.8 vs 90.0%, respectively). The length of postoperative usage was < 1 day in 4.6%, 1–3 days in 40.7%, and > 3 days in 54.7% of the respondents.

Discussion
For several decades, surgeons have utilized bowel preparation to reduce infectious complications, but the value has remained controversial. The current survey is the first nation-wide attempt to document the current trends of preoperative bowel preparation in China. Among the respondents who were older, were working in a large volume hospital, and were performing a higher percentage of minimally invasive surgeries, a significantly higher use of MBP alone was noted. This study observed variations in bowel preparation across respondents from CSCC.

The use of MBP in elective colorectal surgery is supported by emerging evidence, although several published randomized controlled trials have shown that preoperative MBP should be omitted before colon surgery [13, 15, 16]. There is ongoing debate on the role of bowel preparation in colorectal surgery, MBP is still used in routine clinical practice before both colon and rectal surgery in China, with a similar picture in the USA and Japan [17–19]. Unlike European practice, American-enhanced recovery guidelines often include MBP [20]. Why is this discrepancy evident between American and European guidelines? One possible reason may be that the European recommendation is not to be revisited at present [1].

The 2017 clinical practice guidelines from the American Society of Colon and Rectal Surgeons (ASCRS) and Society of American Gastrointestinal and Endoscopic Surgeons (SAGES) recommend MBP + OAP before colorectal surgery as preferred preparation to reduce complication rates [21]. Surveys have shown a change in the use of laparoscopic procedures compared with open procedures depending on the type of preparation used. A survey from the European Society of Coloproctology (ESCP) found that the routine use of MBP prescribed by laparoscopic surgeons was significantly lower (19.7 vs 51.5%,

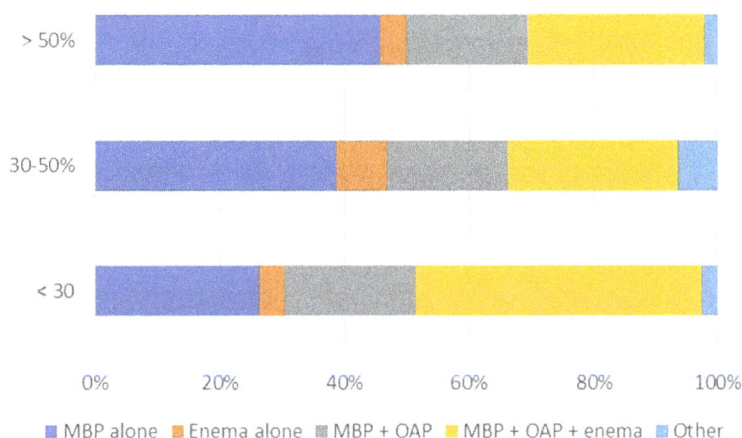

Fig. 1 Association between percentages of resections performed laparoscopically or robotically and bowel preparation. MBP mechanical bowel preparation; OAP oral antibiotics preparation

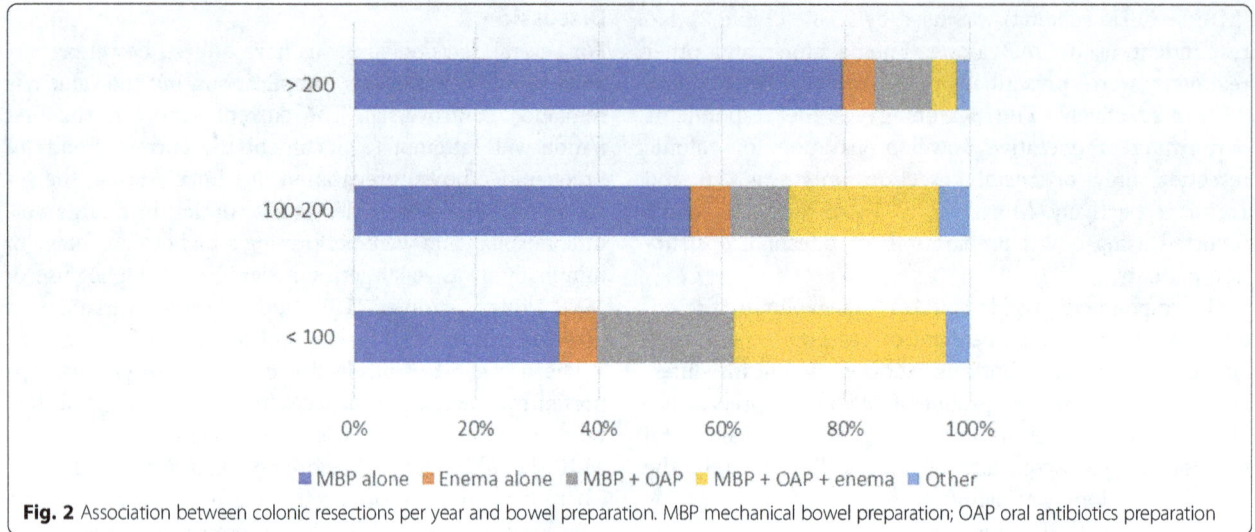

Fig. 2 Association between colonic resections per year and bowel preparation. MBP mechanical bowel preparation; OAP oral antibiotics preparation

$P < 0.01$) [22]. By contrary, a survey from the UK showed that a higher proportion of laparoscopic right-sided procedures was performed with MBP compared with open procedures (16.8 vs 9.5%; $P = 0.08$); however, the need for MBP for a left-sided procedure remains controversial [23]. Despite the survey limitation of unclear procedure classification in the questionnaire, this study showed a similar picture of the high use of MBP in laparoscopic or robotic surgery. Although previous studies have suggested that MBP did not improve postoperative outcomes in laparoscopic colorectal resections [24], there is an inconsistency between opinion and practice, with individual surgeons often using different regimens for their open and laparoscopic resections [23].

OAP is generally believed to help protect against infectious complication in elective colorectal resections [25]. Currently, it is becoming increasingly clear that MBP + OAP combined with intravenous antibiotics is the most

effective method. Previous surveys from the USA, Europe, and Japan have shown a low rate of oral antibiotic usage [17–19, 22]. This obviously contrasts with the patterns of practice in China, because nearly 40% of the respondents prescribed OAP in regimens, meanwhile 49.3% prescribed a longer duration (> 3 days) of postoperative intravenous antibiotics. Our results showed that, despite the clear recommendations from the literature and the guidelines, there remains some concern about the overuse of antibiotics in China.

Moreover, in our subgroup analysis, different bowel preparation strategies are associated with hospital volume. Our results may reflect the surgeon's bias or limitations inherent in this type of survey. Regarding the lower use of OAP, our results showed that, despite the disparity among hospitals, high-volume hospitals tend to follow guidelines more closely. The other interesting finding in our study is that bowel preparation (enema)

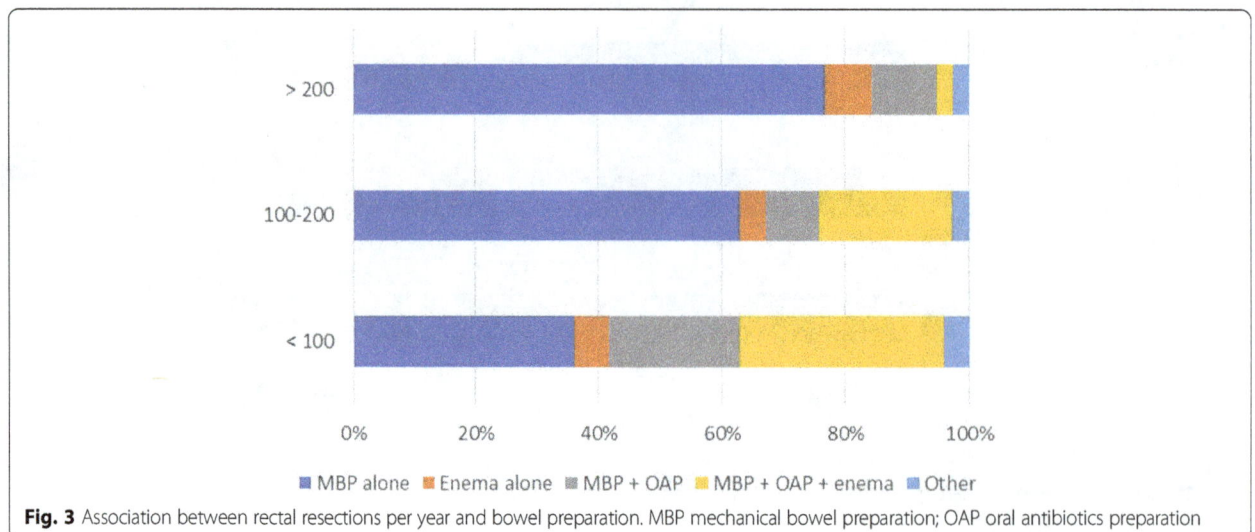

Fig. 3 Association between rectal resections per year and bowel preparation. MBP mechanical bowel preparation; OAP oral antibiotics preparation

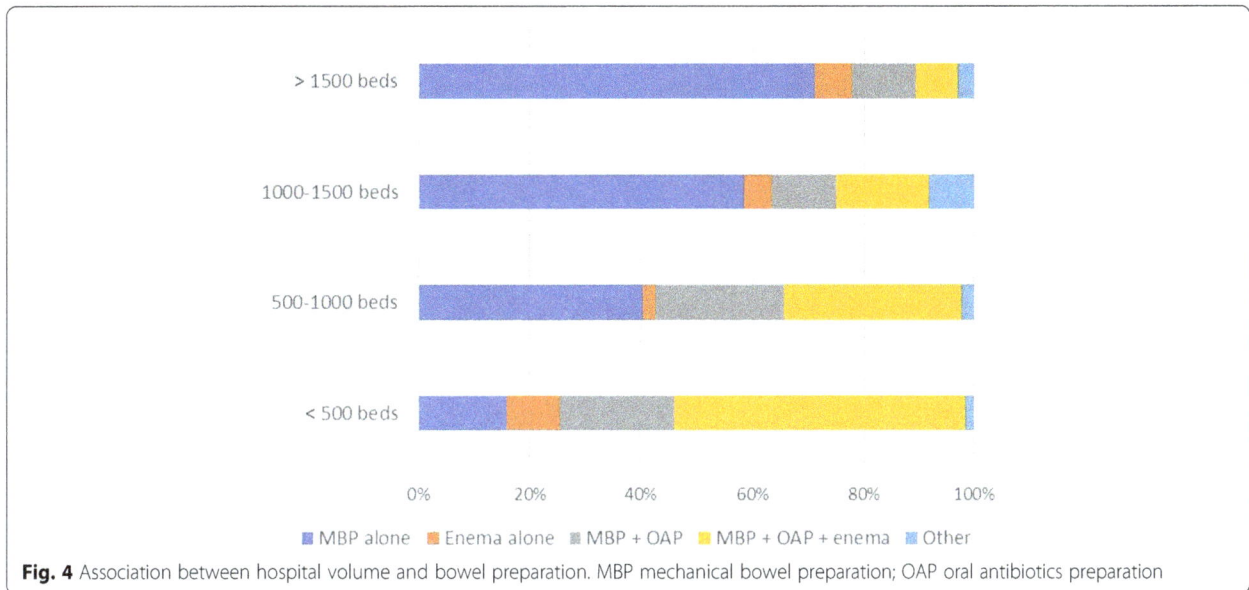

Fig. 4 Association between hospital volume and bowel preparation. MBP mechanical bowel preparation; OAP oral antibiotics preparation

for intestinal obstruction is common (71.3%). Although enema could stimulate the colon to contract and eliminate stool, it may cause serious adverse events, such as perforation or metabolic derangement [26]. Our findings should lead to a careful consideration of appropriate bowel preparation to intestinal obstruction.

Conclusions

In conclusion, this survey provides an adequate response from the CSCC members, describing the preoperative bowel preparation in current practices. Regarding the respondent's age, hospital, and resection volume, as well as the percentage of minimally invasive resections, the study shows that there is no current standardization of preoperative bowel preparation among colorectal surgeons in China, especially concerning the use of oral or intravenous antibiotic prophylaxis. Therefore, we recommend the CSCC should use these results to develop new protocols for multicenter trials and provide more definitive answers.

Abbreviations
ACS-NSQIP: American College of Surgeons National Surgical Quality Improvement Program; ASCRS: American Society of Colon and Rectal Surgeons; CSCC: Chinese Society of Colorectal Cancer; ESCP: European Society of Coloproctology (ESCP); MBP: Mechanical bowel preparation; OAP: Oral antibiotics preparation; SAGES: Society of American Gastrointestinal and Endoscopic Surgeons

Funding
This study was supported by the Beijing Municipal Science & Technology Commission (No. Z161100000116090); the National Key Research and Development Program of the Ministry of Science and Technology of China (No. 2016YFC0905303); the CAMS Innovation Fund for Medical Sciences (CIFMS) (No.2016-I2M-1-001); and the Beijing Science and Technology Program (No. D17110002617004).

Authors' contributions
ZL, MY, ZZ, and XW are responsible for the design, acquisition of data, analysis and interpretation of data, drafting of the manuscript, critical revision, and final approval. GX and ZJ are responsible for the acquisition of data, critical revision, and final approval. HC, SW, and JQ are responsible for the critical revision and final approval. All authors read and approved the final manuscript.

Competing interests
The authors declare that they have no competing interests.

References
1. Slim K, Kartheuser A. Mechanical bowel preparation before colorectal surgery in enhanced recovery programs: discrepancy between the American and European guidelines. Dis Colon Rectum. 2018;61:e13–4.
2. Parthasarathy M, Greensmith M, Bowers D, Groot-Wassink T. Risk factors for anastomotic leakage after colorectal resection: a retrospective analysis of 17 518 patients. Color Dis. 2017;19:288–98.
3. Midura EF, Jung AD, Hanseman DJ, Dhar V, Shah SA, Rafferty JF, Davis BR, Paquette IM. Combination oral and mechanical bowel preparations decreases complications in both right and left colectomy. Surgery. 2018;163:528–34.
4. Mik M, Berut M, Trzcinski R, Dziki L, Buczynski J, Dziki A. Preoperative oral antibiotics reduce infections after colorectal cancer surgery. Langenbeck's Arch Surg. 2016;401:1153–62.
5. Anjum N, Ren J, Wang G, Li G, Wu X, Dong H, Wu Q, Li J. A randomized control trial of preoperative oral antibiotics as adjunct therapy to systemic antibiotics for preventing surgical site infection in clean contaminated, contaminated, and dirty type of colorectal surgeries. Dis Colon Rectum. 2017;60:1291–8.
6. Vo E, Massarweh NN, Chai CY, Tran Cao HS, Zamani N, Abraham S, Adigun K, Awad SS. Association of the addition of oral antibiotics to mechanical bowel preparation for left colon and rectal cancer resections with reduction of surgical site infections. JAMA Surg. 2018;153:114–21.
7. Ohman KA, Wan L, Guthrie T, Johnston B, Leinicke JA, Glasgow SC, Hunt SR, Mutch MG, Wise PE, Silviera ML. Combination of oral antibiotics and mechanical bowel preparation reduces surgical site infection in colorectal surgery. J Am Coll Surg. 2017;225:465–71.
8. Garfinkle R, Abou-Khalil J, Morin N, Ghitulescu G, Vasilevsky CA, Gordon P, Demian M, Boutros M. Is there a role for oral antibiotic preparation alone before colorectal surgery? ACS-NSQIP analysis by coarsened exact matching. Dis Colon Rectum. 2017;60:729–37.

9. Klinger AL, Green H, Monlezun DJ, Beck D, Kann B, Vargas HD, Whitlow C, Margolin D. The role of bowel preparation in colorectal surgery: results of the 2012-2015 ACS-NSQIP data. Ann Surg. 2017; https://doi.org/10.1097/SLA.0000000000002568.

10. Nichols RL, Smith JW, Garcia RY, Waterman RS, Holmes JW. Current practices of preoperative bowel preparation among North American colorectal surgeons. Clin Infect Dis. 1997;24:609–19.

11. Cannon JA, Altom LK, Deierhoi RJ, Morris M, Richman JS, Vick CC, Itani KM, Hawn MT. Preoperative oral antibiotics reduce surgical site infection following elective colorectal resections. Dis Colon Rectum. 2012;55:1160–6.

12. Scarborough JE, Mantyh CR, Sun Z, Migaly J. Combined mechanical and oral antibiotic bowel preparation reduces incisional surgical site infection and anastomotic leak rates after elective colorectal resection: an analysis of Colectomy-Targeted ACS NSQIP. Ann Surg. 2015;262:331–7.

13. Contant CM, Hop WC, van't Sant HP, Oostvogel HJ, Smeets HJ, Stassen LP, Neijenhuis PA, Idenburg FJ, Dijkhuis CM, Heres P, van Tets WF, Gerritsen JJ, Weidema WF. Mechanical bowel preparation for elective colorectal surgery: a multicentre randomised trial. Lancet. 2007;370:2112–7.

14. McCoubrey AS. The use of mechanical bowel preparation in elective colorectal surgery. Ulster Med J. 2007;76:127–30.

15. Bucher P, Gervaz P, Soravia C, Mermillod B, Erne M, Morel P. Randomized clinical trial of mechanical bowel preparation versus no preparation before elective left-sided colorectal surgery. Br J Surg. 2005;92:409–14.

16. Jung B, Påhlman L, Nyström PO, Nilsson E; Mechanical Bowel Preparation Study Group. Multicentre randomized clinical trial of mechanical bowel preparation in elective colonic resection. Br J Surg 2007;94:689–695.

17. Zmora O, Wexner SD, Hajjar L, Park T, Efron JE, Nogueras JJ, Weiss EG. Trends in preparation for colorectal surgery: survey of the members of the American Society of Colon and Rectal Surgeons. Am Surg. 2003;69:150–4.

18. Solla JA, Rothenberger DA. Preoperative bowel preparation. A survey of colon and rectal surgeons. Dis Colon Rectum. 1990;33:154–9.

19. Watanabe M, Murakami M, Aoki T, Takahashi K, Yasuno M, Masaki T, Itabashi M, Yoshimatsu K, Saida Y, Funahashi K, Kan H, Ota M. The current perioperative care in elective colorectal surgery in Japan: a questionnaire survey of members of the Tokyo Colon Seminar Committee. Nihon Daicho Komonbyo Gakkai Zasshi. 2015;68:391–402.

20. Slim K, Martin G. Mechanical bowel preparation before colorectal surgery. Where do we stand? J Visc Surg. 2016;153(2):85–7.

21. Carmichael JC, Keller DS, Baldini G, Bordeianou L, Weiss E, Lee L, Boutros M, McClane J, Feldman LS, Steele SR. Clinical practice guidelines for enhanced recovery after colon and rectal surgery from the American Society of Colon and Rectal Surgeons and Society of American Gastrointestinal and Endoscopic Surgeons. Dis Colon Rectum. 2017;60:761–84.

22. Devane LA, Proud D, O'Connell PR, Panis Y. A European survey of bowel preparation in colorectal surgery. Color Dis. 2017;19:O402–6.

23. Drummond RJ, McKenna RM, Wright DM. Current practice in bowel preparation for colorectal surgery: a survey of the members of the Association of Coloproctology of GB & Ireland. Color Dis. 2011;13:708–10.

24. Chan MY, Foo CC, Poon JT, Law WL. Laparoscopic colorectal resections with and without routine mechanical bowel preparation: A comparative study. Ann Med Surg (Lond). 2016;9:72–6.

25. Koller SE, Bauer KW, Egleston BL, Smith R, Philp MM, Ross HM, Esnaola NF. Comparative effectiveness and risks of bowel preparation before elective colorectal surgery. Ann Surg. 2018;267:734–42.

26. Niv G, Grinberg T, Dickman R, Wasserberg N, Niv Y. Perforation and mortality after cleansing enema for acute constipation are not rare but are preventable. Int J Gen Med. 2013;6:323–8.

7

Radiofrequency ablation versus resection for technically resectable colorectal liver metastasis

Li-Jun Wang[1], Zhong-Yi Zhang[2], Xiao-Luan Yan[1], Wei Yang[2], Kun Yan[2*] and Bao-Cai Xing[1*]

Abstract

Background: Liver resection is the first-line treatment for patients with resectable colorectal liver metastasis (CRLM), while radiofrequency ablation (RFA) can be used for small unresectable CRLM because of disease extent, poor anatomical location, or comorbidities. However, the long-term outcomes are unclear for RFA treatment in resectable CRLM. This study aimed to compare the recurrence rates and prognosis between resectable CRLM patients receiving either liver resection or RFA.

Methods: Consecutive patients who underwent RFA or hepatic resection from November 2010 to December 2015 were assigned in this retrospective study. Propensity score analysis was used to eliminate baseline differences between groups. Survival and recurrence rates were compared between patients receiving liver resection and RFA.

Results: With 1:2 ratio of propensity scoring, 46 patients in the RFA group and 92 in the resection group were successfully matched. Overall survival was similar between the two groups, but the resection group had a higher disease-free survival (median, 22 months vs. 14 months). Whereas among patients with a tumor size of ≤ 3 cm, disease-free survival was similar in the two groups (median, 24 months vs. 21 months). Compared to the resection group, the RFA group had a higher rate of intrahepatic recurrence (34.8% vs. 12.0%) and a shorter recurrence free period. The local and systemic recurrence rate and recurrence-free period for the same were insignificant in the two groups. Poor disease-free survival was associated with RFA, T4, tumor diameter > 3 cm, and lymph node positivity.

Conclusion: Among patients with technically resectable CRLM, resection provided greater disease-free survival, although both treatment modalities provided similar overall survival.

Keywords: Radiofrequency ablation, Resection, Liver metastasis, Colorectal cancer, Survival

Background

Liver metastasis is the leading cause of cancer-related mortality in patients with colorectal cancer [1, 2]. Approximately 50% of patients with colorectal cancer develop liver metastases, with 15–25% have it at their diagnosis [3, 4], with 35% at stage IV disease at presentation, and 20 to 50% with stage II or III disease progress to stage IV [5]. Surgical resection remains the gold standard for treating colorectal

liver metastases (CRLM) and can cure some patients or substantially prolong their survival. Recent 5-year survival rates are 30–50% as reported [6–9]. However, most patients are not initially candidates for resection because of disease extent, anatomical location, or comorbidities [10–13]. In addition, concerns regarding complications and mortality have limited the use of resection.

Radiofrequency ablation (RFA) is a widely used minimally invasive modality that provides acceptable local control for small tumors [14, 15] and may be an alternative for treating unresectable CRLM. The European Society for Medical Oncology guidelines for metastatic colorectal cancer recommends RFA with surgery to achieve R0 resection or as a liver-preserving alternative to resection in cases of poor anatomical localization [16]. An international panel of

* Correspondence: ydbz@vip.sina.com; xingbaocai88@sina.com
[2]Key laboratory of Carcinogenesis and Translational Research (Ministry of Education/Beijing), Department of Ultrasound, Peking University Cancer Hospital and Institute, 52 Fucheng Road, Haidian District, Beijing 100142, China
[1]Key laboratory of Carcinogenesis and Translational Research (Ministry of Education/Beijing), Department of Hepatopancreatobiliary Surgery Unit I, Peking University Cancer Hospital and Institute, 52 Fucheng Road, Haidian District, Beijing 100142, China

ablation experts has also reached a consensus regarding the use of thermal ablation for CRLM [17].

Previous research indicate RFA as inferior to resection in treating liver metastases > 3-cm tumor size [18, 19]. However, improvements in RFA have facilitated the ablation of a spherical zone with a diameter of > 5 cm [20, 21], which has enhanced its applicability. Nevertheless, it remains unclear whether the long-term outcomes of RFA are comparable to those of hepatic resection for resectable CRLM, and so far, no randomized controlled trial has been published. Furthermore, retrospective studies may be limited by patient selection bias and publication bias, although propensity score matching analysis has been successfully used to minimize bias in retrospective studies [22, 23]. Therefore, the present study compared the recurrence and survival rates for RFA and hepatic resection among patients with technically resectable CRLM using propensity score analysis.

Methods
Study design, selection of patients, and grouping
This retrospective study evaluated collected data from 428 consecutive patients who underwent RFA or resection for CRLM at the Peking University Cancer Hospital between November 2010 and December 2015. The study was approved by the Clinical Research Ethics Committee of the same hospital and was performed in compliance with the Helsinki Declaration. Written informed consent was obtained from all patients.

Inclusion criteria was patients with ≤ 3 tumors, well-located tumor size of ≤ 5 cm, and absence of uncontrolled extrahepatic disease. The exclusion criteria were patients with recurrent CRLM after previous resection or RFA, or who underwent both RFA and resection in one session, and those who received palliative treatment. The patients' preoperative images were retrospectively viewed to confirm the technically resectable disease CRLM which was feasibility of complete macroscopic resection to maintain at least 30% future liver remnant [24]. Based on these criteria, we included 50 patients who received RFA and 160 patients who underwent resection with curative intent.

Study outcomes
Baseline data included sex, age, timing of metastasis, location of primary cancer, T stage and N stage, number and diameter of hepatic metastases, carcinoembryonic antigen (CEA) level, and neoadjuvant chemotherapy in the two groups. Disease-free survival and overall survival was determined in both the groups. Variables between the two groups and those included in clinical risk score that could have impacted on survival were identified.

The propensity scores were estimated using a logistic regression model that included the following five covariates primary lymph node status, synchronicity, number of metastases, size of the largest metastasis, and preoperative

CEA levels. A 1:2 "nearest neighbor" match paradigm was used. Patients were matched using a caliper of 0.15 in each group (Fig. 1).

Hepatic resection
The liver was examined, and intraoperative ultrasonography was performed to identify the number and locations of metastases. The extent of hepatic resection was determined by the number, diameter, and locations of the tumors, and lobectomy, segmentectomy, or limited resection was adopted. Parenchymal dissections were performed using the clamp method with Peng's multifunctional operative dissector (Hangzhou Shuyou Medical Instrument Co., Ltd., PR China; FDA 510[K] number K040780). An intermittent Pringle's maneuver with clamping of the hepatoduodenal ligament was occasionally performed during parenchymal transection for vascular occlusion. The preserved margin during parenchymal dissection was ≥ 5 mm.

Radiofrequency ablation
The indications for RFA were complete necrosis achieved based on the tumor size and its position, patients' comorbidities that precluded general anesthesia or surgery, and patient choice. RFA was more often used in deeply situated tumors that would have required excessive sacrifice of the normal parenchyma in resection. Ablation of tumors next to major bile ducts (common bile duct, common hepatic, right and left hepatic ducts) within 1 cm, in contact with larger blood vessels (portal vein and hepatic vein), or in close proximity to vulnerable structures (colon, gallbladder etc.) were relatively restricted. All RFA procedures were performed using the Celon system (Teltow, Germany) by radiologists with > 5 years of interventional experience. The bipolar electrode needles were 16G, and scanning/guidance ultrasonography was performed using the Aloka α-10 (Tokyo, Japan) and GE Logiq E9 (Connecticut, USA) devices. Electrodes were inserted into the tumor under ultrasonographic guidance, and overlapping ablations were used for > 3-cm tumors. The ablation end-point was determined based on the impendence and output power, as well as coverage of the safety margins. Track ablation was performed after the treatment. The ablative area appeared hyperechoic on ultrasound during RFA procedure, which should cover the tumor area. For cases of difficult to assess, contrast-enhanced ultrasound was performed immediately after RFA. If tumor residual occurred, additional RFA session was performed.

Follow-up and definition of recurrence
Patients were evaluated by contrast-enhanced computed tomography (CECT) or magnetic resonance imaging (MRI) at 1 month after resection or RFA procedure. Then, CEA test, MRI of the abdomen, CT of the chest, and MRI or CT of the pelvis were repeated every 3 months for

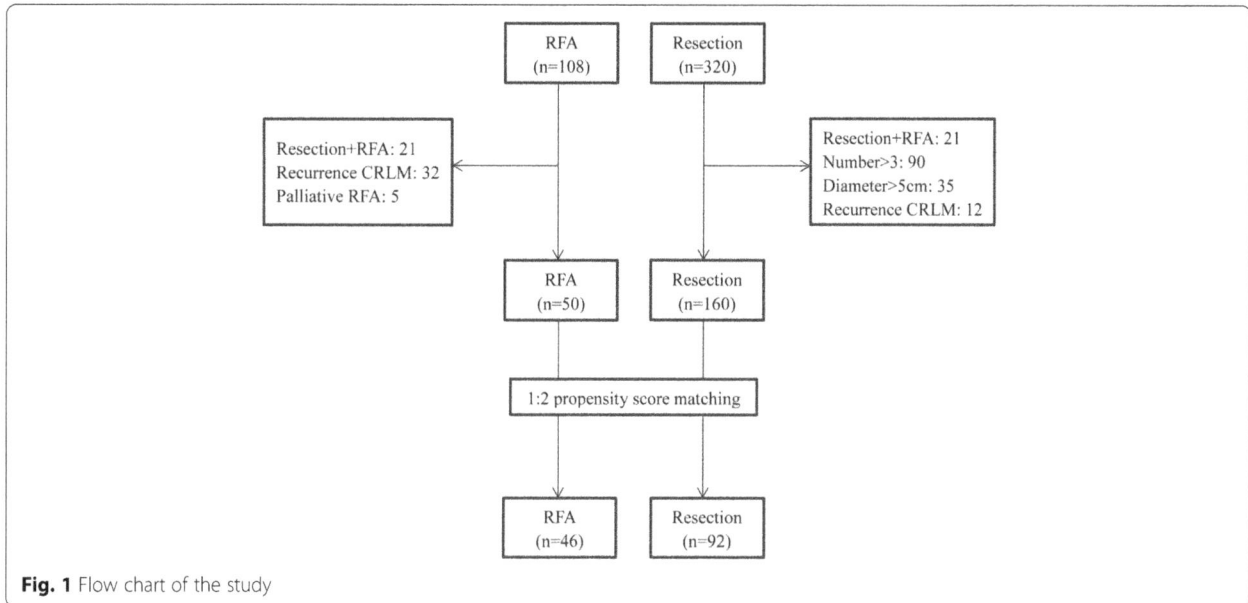

Fig. 1 Flow chart of the study

2 years and every 6 months thereafter. Recurrences were typically identified radiologically.

Local recurrence was defined as tumor growth at the treatment site. Intrahepatic recurrence was defined as new liver lesions emerging at a non-treatment site. Systemic recurrence was defined as tumors at both hepatic and extrahepatic sites, including recurrence at the site of the primary tumor.

Statistical analysis

Continuous variables were reported as median and inter-quartile range. Inter-group differences were analyzed using the chi-square test, Fisher's exact test, or Student's t test, as appropriate. Survival data were analyzed using the Kaplan-Meier method and the log-rank test. Variables with a univariate p value of < 0.1 were entered into the Cox regression model for multivariate analysis. A p value of < 0.05 was considered statistically significant.

Results

Clinicopathological characteristics

The resection group included 92 patients (58 males, 34 females) with a median age of 63 years (interquartile range 51.0–65.8), and the RFA group included 46 patients (29 males, 17 females) with a median age of 63 years (inter-quartile range 50.8–67.0). The patients' clinicopathological characteristics are shown in Table 1. After matching ac-cording to the propensity score, there was no significant difference between the two groups although differences were originally observed for preoperative CEA levels and the number, size, and location of the liver metastases. The 46 patients in the RFA group underwent treatment for 55 lesions (1.2 ± 0.5 lesions/patient), and the 92 patients in the resection group underwent treatment for 114 lesions (1.2 ±

0.4 lesions/patient). The median diameter in the RFA group was 2.3 cm (range, 1.7–3.6 cm), compared to 3 cm (range, 1.9–3.6 cm) in the resection group. Thirty-four patients (37.0%) in resection group and 22 patients (47.8%) in the RFA group received neoadjuvant chemotherapy. Patients in the two groups received regular systemic chemotherapy regimens, such as FOLFOX, CAPEOX, or FOLFIRI, combining biologic-targeted agents (bevacizumab or cetuximab) which were selectively used in high risk of recurrence patients only. After treatment, 45 (48.9%) patients in the resection group and 16 (34.8%) patients in the RFA group received adjuvant chemotherapy according to preoperative chemother-apy response, Fong's score, and postoperative recov-ery condition, and the difference was not statistically significant ($P = 0.115$).

Survival analysis

All follow-ups ended in July 2018, and the median follow-up was 44 months (range, 6–96 months). The over-all survival (OS) rates were similar in the resection and RFA groups at 1 year (97.8% vs. 95.7%), 2 years (83.6% vs. 91.3%), and 3 years (66.8% vs. 71.6%). Based on the Kaplan-Meier analyses, the median OS was 74 months in the resection group and was 59 months in the RFA group ($P = 0.484$, Fig. 2a). The median disease-free survivals (DFS) were 22 months after resection and 14 months after RFA ($P = 0.032$, Fig. 2b). However, the DFS for resection and RFA were similar among patients with a tumor size of ≤ 3 cm (24 months vs. 21 months, $P = 0.41$).

Recurrence and treatment

The first sites of disease progression after treatment are shown in Table 2. Intrahepatic recurrence was

Table 1 The patients' demographic and clinical characteristics

Characteristics	Surgery (n = 92)	RFA (n = 46)	P value
Sex			1.000
Male/female	58/34	29/17	
Age (years)	58.0 (51.0–65.8)	58.5 (50.8–67.0)	0.492
Preoperative CEA (ng/mL)	6.7 (2.9–22.3)	5.4 (3.2–12.9)	0.731
Location of primary cancer			0.802
Colon/rectum	58/34	30/16	
Timing of metastasis			0.277
Synchronous/ metachronous	70/22	31/15	
T stage			0.798
T4/T1–3	30/62	16/30	
N stage			0.899
N0/N+	31/61	16/30	
Median diameter (mm)	30.0 (18.5–35.8)	22.5 (16.8–36.3)	0.249
No. of tumors			0.878
1/2–3	75/17	37/9	
Location of liver metastasis			0.076
Unilobar/bilobar	73/19	42/4	
Neoadjuvant chemotherapy			0.220
Yes/no	34/58	22/24	
Extrahepatic disease			0.160
Yes/no	4/88	5/41	
Comorbidities			0.232
Hypertension	14	5	
Diabetes	8	1	
Cardiac	5	3	
Cerebrovascular	5	2	
Pulmonary or others	2	4	

CEA carcinoembryonic antigen, *RFA* radiofrequency ablation

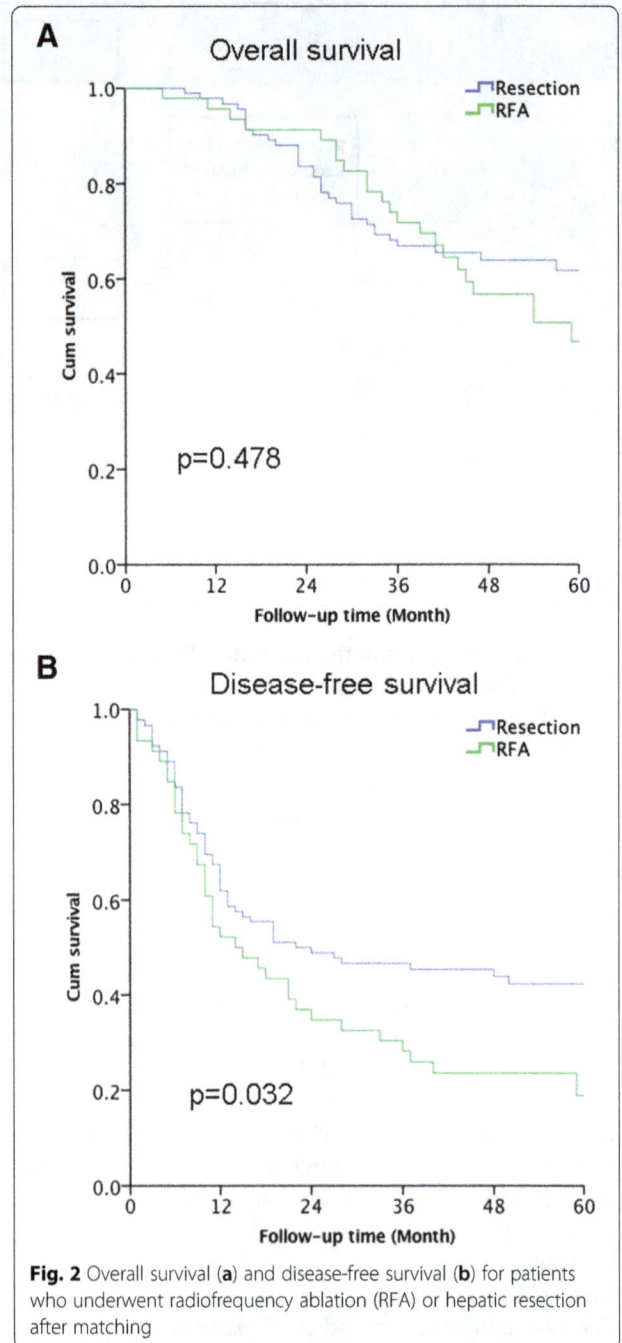

Fig. 2 Overall survival (**a**) and disease-free survival (**b**) for patients who underwent radiofrequency ablation (RFA) or hepatic resection after matching

significantly common (36.9% vs. 11.9%, *P* = 0.001), and local recurrence was more common in the RFA group (15.2% vs. 6.5%, *P* = 0.099) (Table 2). The systemic recurrence rates were similar in both groups (26.1% vs. 39.1%, *P* = 0.129). Hepatic recurrence was more common after RFA compared to resection (69.6% vs. 32.6%, *P* < 0.001) (Table 2).

The time to local, intrahepatic, and systemic recurrences are shown in Fig. 3. The RFA group had a significantly shorter time to intrahepatic recurrence, compared to the resection group (*P* < 0.001). No significant differences were observed between the two groups for the times to local recurrence (*P* = 0.083) or systemic recurrence (*P* = 0.478). Additional treatments with curative intent (resection, RFA, radiotherapy, or combination therapy) were performed after recurrence

for 18 patients (50.0%) in the RFA group and 17 patients (37.0%) in the resection group (*P* = 0.089).

Multivariate analyses of DFS and OS

Cox multivariate analyses were used to evaluate DFS, and the results revealed that poorer DFS was independently associated with RFA, T4 status, lymph node positivity, and tumor diameter > 3 cm (Table 3). OS was independently associated with tumor diameter > 3 cm and T4 stage, but was not significantly associated with RFA or resection as first-line treatment.

Table 2 Recurrence after treatment using RFA or surgery and the subsequent treatment

Recurrence	Surgery (n = 92)	RFA (n = 46)	P value
First recurrence pattern	53	36	
Local recurrence	6	7	0.099
Intrahepatic recurrence (de novo)	11	17	< 0.001
Systemic recurrence	36	12	0.129
Hepatic recurrence			0.001
Yes	30	32	
No	62	14	
Treatment for first recurrence			0.089
Curative treatment	17	18	
Resection		5	
RFA	2	11	
Resection + RFA	1	1	
Radiotherapy	3	1	
Resection + radiotherapy	2	0	
Palliative treatment	36	18	
Chemotherapy	27	15	
Best supportive care	9	3	

RFA radiofrequency ablation

Discussion

Hepatic resection is the first-line treatment for patients with resectable disease and may provide a cure or survival benefit [6, 10]. However, RFA has emerged as a less invasive alternative that has a lower complication rate and shorter hospital stays [25, 26]. RFA is effective for unresectable CRLM among patients with comorbidities and recurrent liver disease and may be added to surgery to increase the chance of curative resection and improve survival rates [14, 16, 27].Nevertheless, design challenges have prevented researchers from performing randomized controlled trials to compare RFA and resection among patients with resectable CRLM. Furthermore, the retrospective studies of RFA versus resection for resectable CRLM have been limited by imbalances in the lesion and patient characteristics [28, 29], although propensity score analysis can be used to address these issues in retrospective studies. Previous studies have suggested that tumor diameter and number are the most important factors that influence the effect of RFA, although primary lymph node status, timing of metastasis, and CEA levels can also influence patient survival and recurrence [30–33]. To prevent selection bias towards RFA, we analyzed multiple clinicopathological characteristics to identify inter-group differences and were able to create propensity score-matched groups of patients who underwent RFA or resection for CRLM.

The Kaplan-Meier analysis revealed that the RFA group had shorter DFS and more patients who experienced hepatic recurrence, compared to the resection group. Thus, it is important to understand if patients were harmed by including them in the RFA treatment protocol. DFS outcomes were similar in both the groups for tumor diameter of ≤ 3 cm, demonstrating that the best indication for RFA were patients with resectable CRLM having ≤ 3-cm tumor diameter.

Recent studies have reported local disease progression rates of 9–48% for percutaneous RFA, compared to 2–9% for resection [34–36]. Evaluation of local recurrence patterns and time to recurrence demonstrated the treatment efficacy of resection over RFA. This relatively high local failure rate in the RFA group could be related to incomplete ablation of larger lesions, the heat sink effect, and/or treatment modality-specific limitations. Interestingly, the de novo intrahepatic recurrence was significantly shorter for the RFA group. This finding may have several explanations. Firstly, previous studies have demonstrated that additional unidentified liver metastases may be revealed during surgical exploration, which would not be treated using percutaneous RFA [37–39]. In the present study, 5.4% of patients

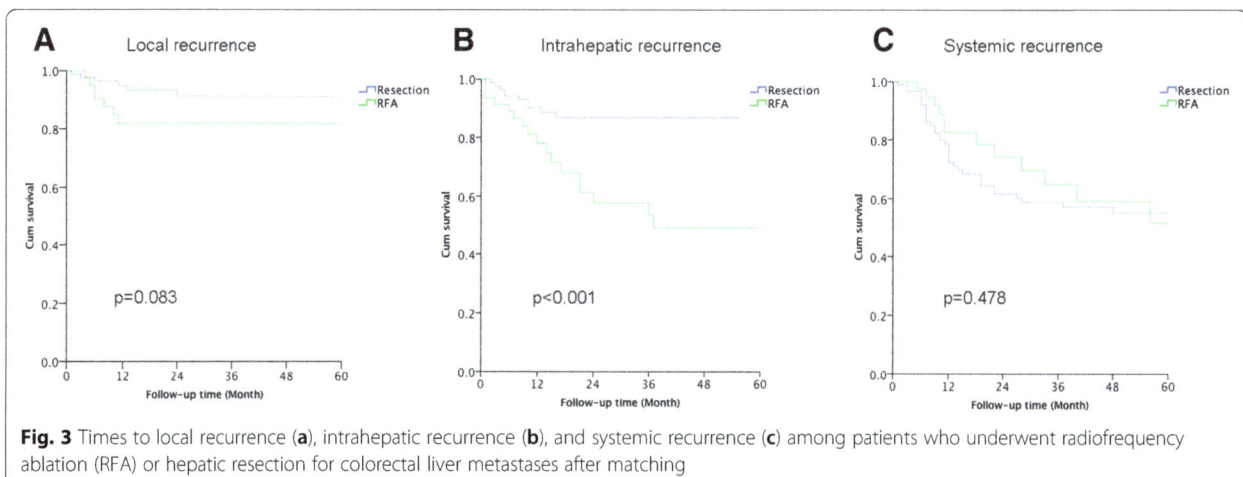

Fig. 3 Times to local recurrence (**a**), intrahepatic recurrence (**b**), and systemic recurrence (**c**) among patients who underwent radiofrequency ablation (RFA) or hepatic resection for colorectal liver metastases after matching

Table 3 Multivariable analyses of disease-free survival and overall survival

Characteristics	Number	Risk ratio	95% CI	P value
Disease-free survival				
Sex (male/female)	87/51	1.338	0.859–2.085	0.197
RFA/resection	46/92	1.661	1.085–2.543	0.020
T stage (T4/T1–3)	46/92	1.652	1.059–2.579	0.027
N stage (N+/N0)	91/47	1.872	1.163–3.014	0.010
Diameter (> 3 cm/≤ 3 cm)	52/86	2.315	1.504–3.564	< 0.001
Overall survival				
RFA/resection	46/92	1.198	0.453–1.778	0.494
T stage (T4/T1–3)	46/92	2.152	1.293–3.583	0.003
Diameter (> 3 cm/≤ 3 cm)	52/86	1.925	1.156–3.206	0.012
Adjuvant chemotherapy (no/yes)	77/61	1.460	0.523–1.460	0.608

RFA radiofrequency ablation, *CI* confidence interval

had initially undetected liver metastases that were identified during the surgery. Secondly, the RFA group had a relative lower proportion of patients who received adjuvant chemotherapy, compared to the resection group, which was related to their comorbidities, unwillingness to receive adjuvant chemotherapy, and other reasons. Thirdly, RFA may contribute to the dissemination of tumor cells and may induce immunological processes that favor tumor growth [34, 40], although we cannot exclude the possibility of resection accelerating the growth of new lesions [29, 41]. Similar to the findings of previous studies, we observed that both groups had similar rates of systemic metastases.

The prolonged survival that we observed in the present study may be related to treatment selectivity, as approximately 25% of patients experience locoregional recurrence after RFA or resection for CRLM [41]. In addition, repeated hepatic resection and RFA are associated with long-term survival and possible cure [21, 42], although resection should be performed if the extrahepatic metastases can be completely removed [43]. In the present study, patients with recurrence underwent a comprehensive assessment and then received curative or palliative chemotherapy according to the recurrence pattern. Survival analysis revealed that repeated curative treatment increases the likelihood of long-term survival among patients with recurrent colorectal metastases.

Several studies have reported conflicting results regarding whether RFA is inferior or equivalent to resection among patients with resectable colorectal disease [34, 44, 45]. However, these studies were limited by selection bias, as the groups were not equivalent. Previous studies have also reported varying 3-year survival rates in both treatment groups. For example, Oshowo et al. [25] reported 3-year OS rates of 55.4% for hepatic resection and 52.6% for RFA, while Otto et al. [46] reported 3-year OS rates of 67% for

hepatic resection and 60% for RFA. The 3-year survival rates in the present study were similar for both treatment groups (66.8% for resection vs. 71.7% for RFA). OS rates in this study are higher than the rates from previous studies, which may be related to our patient selection criteria based on the European Society for Medical Oncology consensus (oligometastatic disease with relatively less invasive behavior). Although RFA provided inferior DFS in the present study, the multivariate analysis did not reveal any significant difference in OS. This finding is partially related to the frequency of curative therapy after recurrence in the RFA group (50% vs. 37%). Another reason is that the follow-up period is short (median 44 months) and it is likely that OS superiority is not reached in the resection group. Thus, larger studies are needed to provide more reliable evidence regarding this association.

The present study has several limitations. First, we used a retrospective design and the patients could not be randomized, as the two groups had different burdens of disease and oncological statuses, although a propensity score-based analysis cannot account for the effects of variables that were not analyzed. Second, the sample size was relatively small because we only considered patients with resectable disease. Third, the RFA group had a smaller proportion of patients who received perioperative chemotherapy, which is likely related to the RFA group including patients with more severe comorbidities, patients who were unwilling to receive chemotherapy, and/or patients with treatment selection bias. Thus, the association of perioperative chemotherapy with poorer DFS in the RFA group should not be ignored.

The strength of the study lies in the propensity score-based analysis used to overcome the effects of potential confounders, the Cox multivariable analysis for DFS, and OS; all these performed for the small sample size to arrive at a conclusion for RFA and resection as treatment options for colorectal metastases.

Conclusions

In conclusion, hepatic resection provided superior DFS, compared to RFA, among patients with technically resectable CRLM. However, multivariate analysis did not reveal any significant treatment-related differences in OS between the RFA and resection groups.

Abbreviations

CEA: Carcinoembryonic antigen; CI: Confidence interval; CRLM: Colorectal liver metastasis; DFS: Disease-free survivals; OS: Overall survival; RFA: Radiofrequency ablation

Acknowledgements

The authors are grateful to Ying-Jian He, a statistician at the Peking University Cancer Hospital and Institute, Beijing, People's Republic of China. This project was supported by the National Natural Science Foundation of China (No. 81371868) and the Beijing Municipal Science & Technology Commission (Z151100004015186).

Funding

This study was supported by a grant (No. 81371868) from the National Nature Science Foundation of China and the Beijing Municipal Science & Technology Commission (Z151100004015186).

Authors' contributions

LJW and ZYZ contributed equally to the work. KY and BCX contributed to the conception and design. XLY and WY are responsible for the provision of the study materials and data collection. LJW and ZYZ contributed to the data analysis and interpretation. All authors contributed to the manuscript writing. All authors read and approved the final manuscript.

Competing interests

The authors declare that they have no competing interests.

References

1. Ferlay J, Soerjomataram I, Dikshit R, Eser S, Mathers C, Rebelo M, Parkin DM, Forman D, Bray F. Cancer incidence and mortality worldwide: sources, methods and major patterns in GLOBOCAN 2012. Int J Cancer. 2015;136: E359–86.
2. Ferlay J, Steliarova-Foucher E, Lortet-Tieulent J, Rosso S, Coebergh JWW, Comber H, Forman D, Bray F. Cancer incidence and mortality patterns in Europe: estimates for 40 countries in 2012. Eur J Cancer Oxf Engl 1990. 2013;49:1374–403.
3. Fong Y, Cohen AM, Fortner JG, Enker WE, Turnbull AD, Coit DG, Marrero AM, Prasad M, Blumgart LH, Brennan MF. Liver resection for colorectal metastases. J Clin Oncol Off J Am Soc Clin Oncol. 1997;15:938–46.
4. Hayashi M, Inoue Y, Komeda K, Shimizu T, Asakuma M, Hirokawa F, Miyamoto Y, Okuda J, Takeshita K, Shibayama Y, Tanigawa N. Clinicopathological analysis of recurrence patterns and prognostic factors for survival after hepatectomy for colorectal liver metastasis. BMC Surg. 2010;10:27.
5. Field K, Lipton L. Metastatic colorectal cancer-past, progress and future. World J Gastroenterol. 2007;13:3806–15.
6. Kanas GP, Taylor A, Primrose JN, Langeberg WJ, Kelsh MA, Mowat FS, Alexander DD, Choti MA, Poston G. Survival after liver resection in metastatic colorectal cancer: review and meta-analysis of prognostic factors. Clin Epidemiol. 2012;4:283–301.
7. Hur H, Ko YT, Min BS, Kim KS, Choi JS, Sohn SK, Cho CH, Ko HK, Lee JT, Kim NK. Comparative study of resection and radiofrequency ablation in the treatment of solitary colorectal liver metastases. Am J Surg. 2009;197:728–36.
8. Abdalla EK, Adam R, Bilchik AJ, Jaeck D, Vauthey J-N, Mahvi D. Improving resectability of hepatic colorectal metastases: expert consensus statement. Ann Surg Oncol. 2006;13:1271–80.
9. Nordlinger B, Sorbye H, Glimelius B, Poston GJ, Schlag PM, Rougier P, Bechstein WO, Primrose JN, Walpole ET, Finch-Jones M, Jaeck D, Mirza D, Parks RW, Mauer M, Tanis E, Van Cutsem E, Scheithauer W, Gruenberger T, EORTC Gastro-Intestinal Tract Cancer Group, Cancer Research UK, Arbeitsgruppe Lebermetastasen und—tumoren in der Chirurgischen Arbeitsgemeinschaft Onkologie (ALM-CAO), Australasian Gastro-Intestinal Trials Group (AGITG), Fédération Francophone de Cancérologie Digestive (FFCD). Perioperative FOLFOX4 chemotherapy and surgery versus surgery alone for resectable liver metastases from colorectal cancer (EORTC 40983): long-term results of a randomised, controlled, phase 3 trial. Lancet Oncol. 2013;14:1208–15.
10. Adam R, Hoti E, Folprecht G, Benson AB. Accomplishments in 2008 in the management of curable metastatic colorectal cancer. Gastrointest Cancer Res GCR. 2009;3:S15–22.
11. Adams RB, Aloia TA, Loyer E, Pawlik TM, Taouli B, Vauthey J-N, Americas Hepato-Pancreato-Biliary Association, Society of Surgical Oncology, Society for Surgery of the Alimentary Tract. Selection for hepatic resection of colorectal liver metastases: expert consensus statement. HPB. 2013;15:91–103.
12. McKay A, Dixon E, Taylor M. Current role of radiofrequency ablation for the treatment of colorectal liver metastases. Br J Surg. 2006;93:1192–201.
13. Siperstein AE, Berber E, Ballem N, Parikh RT. Survival after radiofrequency ablation of colorectal liver metastases: 10-year experience. Ann Surg. 2007; 246:559–65 discussion 565-567.
14. Solbiati L, Livraghi T, Goldberg SN, Ierace T, Meloni F, Dellanoce M, Cova L, Halpern EF, Gazelle GS. Percutaneous radio-frequency ablation of hepatic metastases from colorectal cancer: long-term results in 117 patients. Radiology. 2001;221:159–66.
15. Ruers T, Punt C, Van Coevorden F, JPEN P, Borel-Rinkes I, Ledermann JA, Poston G, Bechstein W, Lentz MA, Mauer M, Van Cutsem E, Lutz MP, Nordlinger B, EORTC Gastro-Intestinal Tract Cancer Group, Arbeitsgruppe Lebermetastasen und—tumoren in der Chirurgischen Arbeitsgemeinschaft Onkologie (ALM-CAO) and the National Cancer Research Institute Colorectal Clinical Study Group (NCRI CCSG). Radiofrequency ablation combined with systemic treatment versus systemic treatment alone in patients with non-resectable colorectal liver metastases: a randomized EORTC Intergroup phase II study (EORTC 40004). Ann Oncol Off J Eur Soc Med Oncol. 2012;23:2619–26.
16. Van Cutsem E, Cervantes A, Adam R, Sobrero A, Van Krieken JH, Aderka D, Aranda Aguilar E, Bardelli A, Benson A, Bodoky G, Ciardiello F, D'Hoore A, Diaz-Rubio E, Douillard J-Y, Ducreux M, Falcone A, Grothey A, Gruenberger T, Haustermans K, Heinemann V, Hoff P, Köhne C-H, Labianca R, Laurent-Puig P, Ma B, Maughan T, Muro K, Normanno N, Österlund P, Oyen WJG, Papamichael D, Pentheroudakis G, Pfeiffer P, Price TJ, Punt C, Ricke J, Roth A, Salazar R, Scheithauer W, Schmoll HJ, Tabernero J, Taïeb J, Tejpar S, Wasan H, Yoshino T, Zaanan A, Arnold D. ESMO consensus guidelines for the management of patients with metastatic colorectal cancer. Ann Oncol Off J Eur Soc Med Oncol. 2016;27:1386–422.
17. Gillams A, Goldberg N, Ahmed M, Bale R, Breen D, Callstrom M, Chen MH, Choi BI, de Baere T, Dupuy D, Gangi A, Gervais D, Helmberger T, Jung E-M, Lee F, Lencioni R, Liang P, Livraghi T, Lu D, Meloni F, Pereira P, Piscaglia F, Rhim H, Salem R, Sofocleous C, Solomon SB, Soulen M, Tanaka M, Vogl T, Wood B, Solbiati L. Thermal ablation of colorectal liver metastases: a position paper by an international panel of ablation experts, The Interventional Oncology Sans Frontières meeting 2013. Eur Radiol. 2015;25:3438–54.
18. Tanis E, Nordlinger B, Mauer M, Sorbye H, van Coevorden F, Gruenberger T, Schlag PM, Punt CJA, Ledermann J, Ruers TJM. Local recurrence rates after radiofrequency ablation or resection of colorectal liver metastases. Analysis of the European Organisation for Research and Treatment of Cancer #40004 and #40983. Eur J Cancer Oxf Engl 1990. 2014;50:912–9.
19. McKay A, Fradette K, Lipschitz J. Long-term outcomes following hepatic resection and radiofrequency ablation of colorectal liver metastases. HPB Surg World J Hepatic Pancreat Biliary Surg. 2009;2009:346863.
20. Hammill CW, Billingsley KG, Cassera MA, Wolf RF, Ujiki MB, Hansen PD. Outcome after laparoscopic radiofrequency ablation of technically resectable colorectal liver metastases. Ann Surg Oncol. 2011;18:1947–54.
21. Nielsen K, van Tilborg AAJM, Meijerink MR, Macintosh MO, Zonderhuis BM, de Lange ESM, Comans EFI, Meijer S, van den Tol MP. Incidence and treatment of local site recurrences following RFA of colorectal liver metastases. World J Surg. 2013;37:1340–7.
22. Lim C, Doussot A, Osseis M, Salloum C, Gomez Gavara C, Compagnon P, Brunetti F, Calderaro J, Azoulay D. Primary tumor versus liver-first strategy in patients with stage IVA colorectal cancer: a propensity score analysis of long-term outcomes and recurrence pattern. Ann Surg Oncol. 2016;23:3024–32.
23. Lee Y-H, Hsu C-Y, Chu C-W, Liu P-H, Hsia C-Y, Huang Y-H, Su C-W, Chiou Y-Y, Lin H-C, Huo T-I. Radiofrequency ablation is better than surgical resection in patients with hepatocellular carcinoma within the Milan criteria and preserved liver function: a retrospective study using propensity score analyses. J Clin Gastroenterol. 2015;49:242–9.
24. Clavien P-A, Petrowsky H, DeOliveira ML, Graf R. Strategies for safer liver surgery and partial liver transplantation. N Engl J Med. 2007;356:1545–59.
25. Oshowo A, Gillams AR, Lees WR, Taylor I. Radiofrequency ablation extends the scope of surgery in colorectal liver metastases. Eur J Surg Oncol J Eur Soc Surg Oncol Br Assoc Surg Oncol. 2003;29:244–7.
26. Evrard S, Becouarn Y, Fonck M, Brunet R, Mathoulin-Pelissier S, Picot V. Surgical treatment of liver metastases by radiofrequency ablation, resection, or in combination. Eur J Surg Oncol J Eur Soc Surg Oncol Br Assoc Surg Oncol. 2004;30:399–406.
27. Wong SL, Edwards MJ, Chao C, Simpson D, McMasters KM. Radiofrequency ablation for unresectable hepatic tumors. Am J Surg. 2001;182:552–7.
28. Stang A, Fischbach R, Teichmann W, Bokemeyer C, Braumann D. A systematic review on the clinical benefit and role of radiofrequency ablation as treatment of colorectal liver metastases. Eur J Cancer Oxf Engl 1990. 2009;45:1748–56.

29. Mulier S, Ruers T, Jamart J, Michel L, Marchal G, Ni Y. Radiofrequency ablation versus resection for resectable colorectal liver metastases: time for a randomized trial? An update. Dig Surg. 2008;25:445–60.

30. Solbiati L, Ahmed M, Cova L, Ierace T, Brioschi M, Goldberg SN. Small liver colorectal metastases treated with percutaneous radiofrequency ablation: local response rate and long-term survival with up to 10-year follow-up. Radiology. 2012;265:958–68.

31. Veltri A, Sacchetto P, Tosetti I, Pagano E, Fava C, Gandini G. Radiofrequency ablation of colorectal liver metastases: small size favorably predicts technique effectiveness and survival. Cardiovasc Intervent Radiol. 2008;31: 948–56.

32. Hamada A, Yamakado K, Nakatsuka A, Uraki J, Kashima M, Takaki H, Yamanaka T, Inoue Y, Kusunoki M, Takeda K. Radiofrequency ablation for colorectal liver metastases: prognostic factors in non-surgical candidates. Jpn J Radiol. 2012;30:567–74.

33. Gillams AR, Lees WR. Radio-frequency ablation of colorectal liver metastases in 167 patients. Eur Radiol. 2004;14:2261–7.

34. Abdalla EK, Vauthey J-N, Ellis LM, Ellis V, Pollock R, Broglio KR, Hess K, Curley SA. Recurrence and outcomes following hepatic resection, radiofrequency ablation, and combined resection/ablation for colorectal liver metastases. Ann Surg. 2004;239:818–25 discussion 825-827.

35. de Baere T, Elias D, Dromain C, Din MG, Kuoch V, Ducreux M, Boige V, Lassau N, Marteau V, Lasser P, Roche A. Radiofrequency ablation of 100 hepatic metastases with a mean follow-up of more than 1 year. AJR Am J Roentgenol. 2000;175:1619–25.

36. Wang X, Sofocleous CT, Erinjeri JP, Petre EN, Gonen M, Do KG, Brown KT, Covey AM, Brody LA, Alago W, Thornton RH, Kemeny NE, Solomon SB. Margin size is an independent predictor of local tumor progression after ablation of colon cancer liver metastases. Cardiovasc Intervent Radiol. 2013; 36:166–75.

37. Grobmyer SR, Fong Y, D'Angelica M, Dematteo RP, Blumgart LH, Jarnagin WR. Diagnostic laparoscopy prior to planned hepatic resection for colorectal metastases. Arch Surg Chic Ill 1960. 2004;139:1326–30.

38. Elias D, Sideris L, Pocard M, de Baere T, Dromain C, Lassau N, Lasser P. Incidence of unsuspected and treatable metastatic disease associated with operable colorectal liver metastases discovered only at laparotomy (and not treated when performing percutaneous radiofrequency ablation). Ann Surg Oncol. 2005;12:298–302.

39. Chung MH, Wood TF, Tsioulias GJ, Rose DM, Bilchik AJ. Laparoscopic radiofrequency ablation of unresectable hepatic malignancies. A phase 2 trial. Surg Endosc. 2001;15:1020–6.

40. Mulier S, Ni Y, Jamart J, Michel L, Marchal G, Ruers T. Radiofrequency ablation versus resection for resectable colorectal liver metastases: time for a randomized trial? Ann Surg Oncol. 2008;15:144–57.

41. Meredith K, Haemmerich D, Qi C, Mahvi D. Hepatic resection but not radiofrequency ablation results in tumor growth and increased growth factor expression. Ann Surg. 2007;245:771–6.

42. Butte JM, Gönen M, Allen PJ, Peter Kingham T, Sofocleous CT, DeMatteo RP, Fong Y, Kemeny NE, Jarnagin WR, D'Angelica MI. Recurrence after partial hepatectomy for metastatic colorectal cancer: potentially curative role of salvage repeat resection. Ann Surg Oncol. 2015;22:2761–71.

43. Warwick R, Page R. Resection of pulmonary metastases from colorectal carcinoma. Eur J Surg Oncol J Eur Soc Surg Oncol Br Assoc Surg Oncol. 2007;33(Suppl 2):S59–63.

44. Majeed AW. Comparison of resection and radiofrequency ablation for treatment of solitary colorectal liver metastases. Br J Surg. 2003; 90:1611.

45. Aloia TA, Vauthey J-N, Loyer EM, Ribero D, Pawlik TM, Wei SH, Curley SA, Zorzi D, Abdalla EK. Solitary colorectal liver metastasis: resection determines outcome. Arch Surg Chic Ill 1960. 2006;141:460–6 discussion 466-467.

46. Otto G, Düber C, Hoppe-Lotichius M, König J, Heise M, Pitton MB. Radiofrequency ablation as first-line treatment in patients with early colorectal liver metastases amenable to surgery. Ann Surg. 2010;251: 796–803.

8

A pancreatic zone at higher risk of fistula after enucleation

Pauline Duconseil[1], Ugo Marchese[1], Jacques Ewald[1], Marc Giovannini[2], Djamel Mokart[3], Jean-Robert Delpero[1] and Olivier Turrini[4]* ⓘ

Abstract

Background: To determine predictive factors of postoperative pancreatic fistula (POPF) in patients undergoing enucleation (EN).

Methods: From 2005 to 2017, 47 patients underwent EN and had magnetic resonance imaging available for precise analysis of tumor location. Three pancreatic zones were delimited by the right side of the portal vein and the main pancreatic head duct (zone #3 comprising the lower head parenchyma and the uncinate process).

Results: The mortality and morbidity rates were 0% and 62%, respectively. POPF occurred in 23 patients (49%) and was graded as B or C (severe) in 15 patients (32%). Four patients (8.5%) developed a postoperative hemorrhage, and 5 patients (11%) needed a reintervention. In univariate and multivariate analyses, the pancreatic zone was the unique predictive factor of overall ($P = .048$) or severe POPF ($P = .05$). We did not observe any difference in postoperative courses when comparing the EN achieved in zones #1 and #2. We noted a longer operative duration ($P = .016$), higher overall ($P = .017$) and severe POPF ($P = .01$) rates, and longer hospital stays ($P = .04$) when comparing the EN achieved in zone #3 versus that in zones #1 and #2. Patients who underwent EN in zone #3 had a relative risk of developing a severe POPF of 3.22 compared with patients who underwent EN in the two other pancreatic zones.

Conclusion: Our study identifies the lower head parenchyma and the uncinate process as a high-risk zone of severe POPF after EN. Patients with planned EN in this zone could be selected and benefit from preoperative and/or intraoperative techniques to reduce the severe POPF rate.

Keywords: Enucleation, Pancreatic fistula, Magnetic resonance imaging

Background

Parenchyma-sparing pancreatectomies were proposed as an alternative to standard pancreatectomy for noninvasive tumors to avoid pancreatic endocrine and exocrine insufficiencies [1–4]. In this manner, enucleation (EN) was first performed in the 1960s [5]; currently, neuroendocrine tumors (particularly insulinoma) and branch-duct intraductal papillary mucinous neoplasms (IPMNs) are the more frequent tumors resected by EN [6–15]. As EN induces parenchyma incision and, occasionally, deep pancreas opening, it exposes patients to postoperative pancreatic fistula (POPF) by unknown main pancreatic duct injury or weakening, especially if thermo-coagulation

has been used too closely. Consequently, several reports have shown that EN leads to the same or a higher rate of POPF than does standard pancreatectomy, but with a "toward zero" mortality [4, 7, 10, 12, 15–17]. Predictive factors of POPF after EN have already been reported, such as age [6], body mass index [10], distance from the main pancreatic duct (≤ 2 mm) [17], cystic morphology [6], history of acute pancreatitis [6], and New York Heart Association class [14] (Table 1). These factors are not a contraindication for EN but could help pancreatic surgeons inform patients about possible prolonged postoperative courses, counterbalanced by the very low risk of developing diabetes mellitus and/or steatorrhea [1–4]. The pancreatic location of the EN (i.e., the head/uncinate process versus body/tail) seemed to be a relevant factor of POPF [9, 10, 13] (Table 1), but the head and uncinate

* Correspondence: oturrini@yahoo.fr
[4]Department of Surgery, Aix-Marseille University, Institut Paoli-Calmettes, CNRS, Inserm, CRCM, Marseille, France
Full list of author information is available at the end of the article

Table 1 Reported risk factors of POPF after enucleation

	n	Head and uncinate together	POPF	Severe POPF	Risk factors
Turrini et al. [16]	7	Yes	43%	14%	–
Brient et al. [17]	52	Yes	27%	14%	Distance to MPD ≤ 2 mm
Jilesen et al. [10]	60	Yes	–	31%	Head/uncinate BMI
Kaiser et al. [8]	74	Yes	46%	27%	–
Faitot et al. [13]	126	Yes	57%	41%	Head/uncinate
Song et al. [9]	65	Separated	20%	9%	Head/uncinate
Strobel et al. [11]	166	Yes	41%	21%	Cystic morphology
Wang et al. [6]	142	Yes	53%	16%	Age Acute pancreatitis Cystic morphology
Zhang et al. [14]	119	Yes	40%	28%	NYHA class
Present series	47	Separated	49%	32%	Lower head + uncinate

BMI body mass index, *POPF* postoperative pancreatic fistula, *NYHA* New York Heart Association

process are usually considered a single location. Indeed, the uncinate process is defined by a portion of the head of the pancreas that hooks around posterior to the superior mesenteric vessels but is actually difficult to delimit from the proper head parenchyma on preoperative imaging and during surgery.

The present study, based on a precise tumor location on pancreatic magnetic resonance imaging (MRI), seeks to determine predictive factors of POPF in patients who underwent EN.

Methods

Initial population

From January 1, 2005, to December 31, 2017, 95 patients were eligible for EN at Institut Paoli-Calmettes (Marseille, France). All patient data were entered into a clinical database (CHIRPAN database: N°Sy50955016U) approved by both the Institut Paoli Calmettes Institutional Review/Ethical and the CNIL ("Commission Nationale de l'Informatique et des Libertés" the French national board for databases) boards. Eligibility criteria for EN were (a) neuroendocrine or cystic tumor (side branch IPMN without worrying features, mucinous cystadenoma), (b) absence of main pancreatic duct dilatation, (c) absence of mural nodule or thickness of cyst wall, and (c) ability to preserve the main pancreatic duct.

Initial staging and final selected population (Fig. 1)

All patients were staged by physical examination, endoscopic ultrasound, and thin-section contrast-enhanced helical dual-phase scanning. As we supported that MRI was the most relevant imaging exam to assess pancreatic tumors [18], only patients who had a recent preoperative (within the month before surgery) MRI available on our picture archiving and communication system were

included in the present study (n = 56) (Fig. 1). Consequently, for each EN, we could precisely determine the tumor location based on (a) the center of the tumor, for a spherical tumor, and (b) the crossing point between length and width, for a non-spherical tumor, as well as the tumor size (mm), and the distance to the main pancreatic duct (mm). Three pancreatic zones were arbitrarily delimited by the right side of the portal vein and the main pancreatic head duct; consequently, the pancreatic head was divided into two easily identifiable zones: zone #2, corresponding to the upper head parenchyma, and zone #3, comprising the lower head parenchyma and the uncinate process (Fig. 2). Zone #1 grouped the body and tail of the pancreas from the right side of the mesenteric vessels to the left parenchyma. Patients whose postoperative courses were not precisely known (within 90 postoperative days) were also excluded (n = 2) (Fig. 1).

Surgery

EN was achieved through laparotomy or laparoscopy according to surgeon preference and tumor location. Direct intraoperative ultrasound exploration was routinely performed to identify the main pancreatic duct and its distance to the tumor. Seven patients (5 in zone #2, 1 in zone #1, and 1 in zone #3) did not undergo EN because the tumor directly contacted the main pancreatic duct on intraoperative ultrasound; consequently, these patients with tumor located in zones #2 and #3 underwent pancreaticoduodenectomy and the patient with tumor located in zone #1 underwent distal pancreatectomy. Finally, 47 patients underwent EN and formed our population for the present study (Fig. 1); their tumor locations are

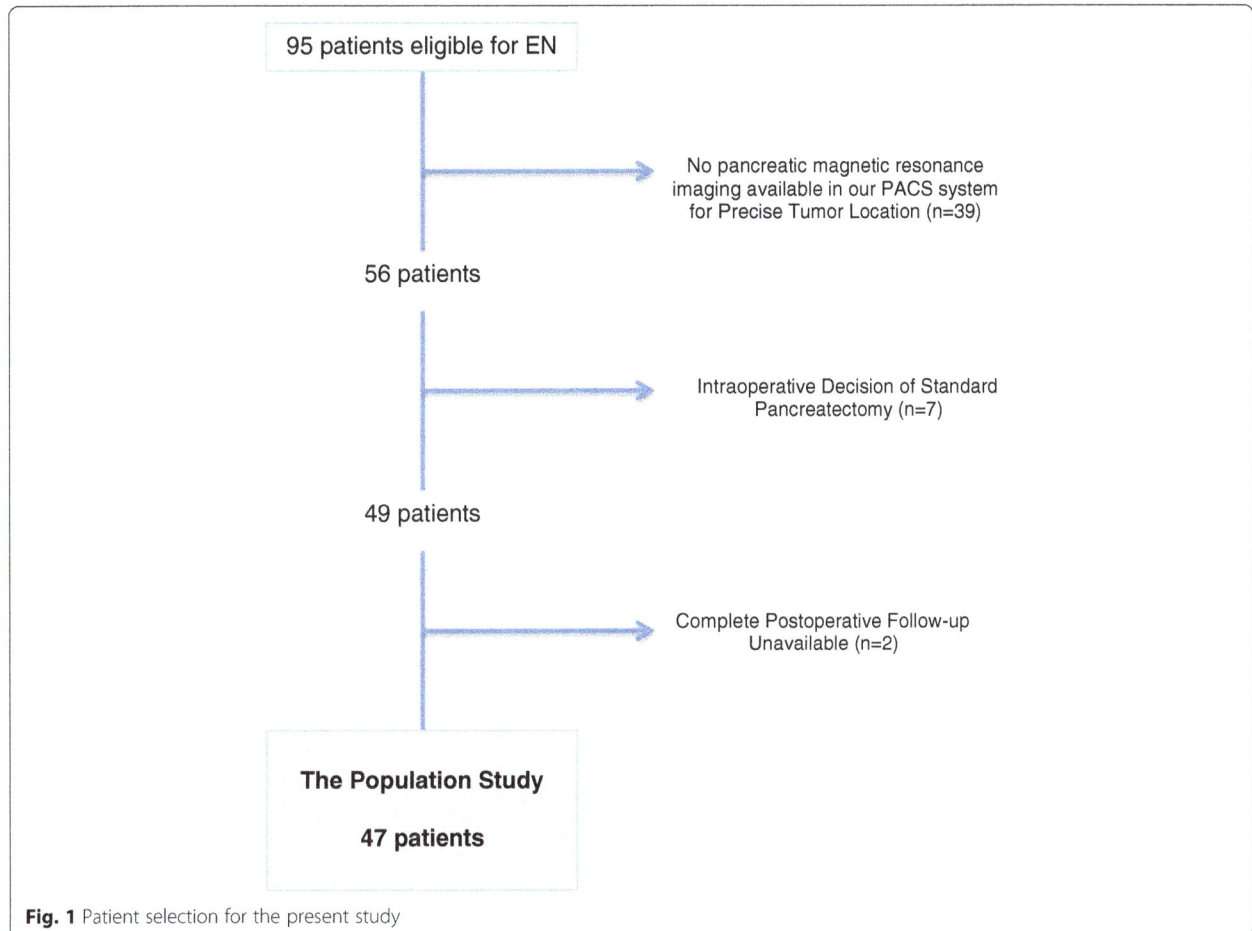

Fig. 1 Patient selection for the present study

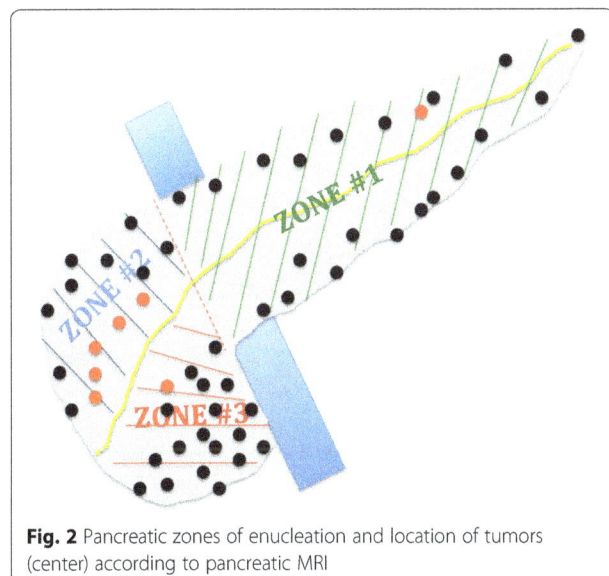

Fig. 2 Pancreatic zones of enucleation and location of tumors (center) according to pancreatic MRI

presented in Fig. 2. The operative technique has already been described for pancreatic head IPMNs [16], and the global technical approach was not different for the body/tail or other cystic/solid tumors; coagulation was avoided to the greatest extent possible to avoid exposing the main pancreatic duct to thermal injury (Additional file 1: Figure S1). In cases of EN in zones #2 and #3, an intraoperative cholangiography with retrograde contrast back filling of the pancreatic duct was achieved to assess the integrity of both the biliary and pancreatic ducts. If the tumor was located in the "posterior" zone #3 (i.e., on the posterior face of the head of the pancreas), a larger Kocher maneuver was achieved to optimally expose the EN area. A non-aspirating drain was left in contact with the EN area, and the drain amylase level was measured on postoperative days 1 and 3. No patient had had a preventive preoperative stent inserted in the main pancreatic duct. Octreotide was not routinely used in prevention or with curative intent in the case of a POPF diagnosis.

End-points studied

The variables evaluated included age, sex, body mass index, location of the tumor (i.e., zone #1, #2, or #3), laparoscopic or open approaches, operative duration (minutes), POPF according to ISGPF grading [19] (grade A fistula was defined by a drain amylase level threefold higher than the serum amylase level; grades B and C defined severe POPF), and the overall morbidity [20] rate, including postoperative bleeding, reoperation, and perioperative red cell transfusion rates; endoscopic or radiologic drainage of a deep collection was noted, as was interventional embolization. The length of hospital stay (days) and the readmission rate were also recorded. The need of a standard pancreatectomy (salvage pancreatectomy) due to unresolved POPF was noted. Tumor morphology (i.e., cystic or solid (mixed tumors were considered as cystic type)) and exact histologic denomination (i.e., neuroendocrine tumor, IPMN, and others) were the recorded histological criteria.

Statistical analyses

The categorical factors were compared using Fisher's exact test, and the continuous variables were compared using Student's t test. Significance was set after a two-sided $P \leq .05$. Prognostic factors with a $P < .1$ in univariate analysis or that were known to be relevant to predicting POPF were entered into a multivariable regression model to determine the independent predictors. Data analyses were performed using Graph-Pad Prism software, version 5.0d (GraphPad Software Inc., La Jolla, CA, USA) and SAS statistical software version 9.1 (SAS Institute, Inc., Cary, NC, USA).

Results

Patient characteristics (Table 2)

Patients were mainly women (74%), with a median age of 55 years (range, 19–78) and a median BMI of 22.7 (range, 18–35). Tumors were located in zone #1 in 20 patients (43%), in zone #2 in 9 patients (19%), and in zone #3 in 18 patients (38%) (Fig. 2); the most common morphology was cystic (53%), and the median size was 20 mm (range, 4–61). Twenty-one patients (45%) had a tumor distance from the main pancreatic duct ≤ 2 mm. Among patients who underwent EN in zone #3, 6 (33%) had an uncinectomy.

Surgery and postoperative course (Table 2)

The median operative duration was 180 min (range, 90–400). We detected one (2.1%) main pancreatic duct injury (in zone #3) according to intraoperative cholangiography: main pancreatic duct was electively closed with interrupted stich (Prolen 7/0) controlled by another cholangiography; a large drainage was positioned close to the suture. The mortality and overall morbidity rates were 0% and 62%, respectively. Dindo grade 3–4 complications were diagnosed in 16 patients (34%). POPF occurred in 23 patients (49%) and was severe in 15

Table 2 Patients and tumor characteristics. Intraoperative data and postoperative courses

	n or median	% or range
Male gender	12	26%
Age (years old)	55	19–78
BMI (kg/m²)	22.7	18–35.1
Pancreatic zones		
1	20	43%
2	9	19%
3	18	38%
Distance to main duct (mm)		
≤ 2 mm	21	45%
> 2 mm	26	55%
Indication		
Neuroendocrine tumors	20	43%
Branch-duct IPMN	17	36%
Others	18	21%
Tumor morphology		
Cystic	25	53%
Solid	22	47%
Tumor size (mm)	20	4–61
Operative duration (min)	180	90–400
POPF		
Grade A	8	17%
Grades B and C	15	33%
Total	23	50%
Delay surgery—POPF	7	4–26
Hemorrhage	4	8.5%
Reintervention	5	11%
Dindo morbidity		
Grades 3–4	16	34%
Overall	29	62%
Perioperative transfusion	4	8.5%
Length of hospital stay (days)	15	6–90
Readmission	3	6.4%

BMI body mass index, *IPMN* intraductal papillary mucinous neoplasm, *POPF* postoperative pancreatic fistula)

patients (32%). The median delay between EN and POPF diagnosis was 7 days (range, 4–26). Four patients (8.5%) developed a postoperative hemorrhage in the EN zone, who all required red blood cell transfusion (range, 2–6 units). Five patients (11%) needed a reintervention for hemorrhage ($n = 4$) or duodenal fistula ($n = 1$) (cf infra). No patient required a salvage pancreatectomy. The length of hospital stay was 19 days (range, 6–90). Three patients (6.4%) needed a readmission for medical complications (urinary infection ($n = 2$), benign pulmonary embolism ($n = 1$)).

Table 3 Univariate and multivariate analysis of risk factor for (a) all grade of postoperative pancreatic fistula and (b) grades B to C of postoperative pancreatic fistula

a)	POPF (n = 23)%	No POPF (n = 24)%	Univariate P value	Odd ratio [95% CI]	Multivariate P value
Gender				–	–
Male	8 (35)	4 (17)	.19		
Female	15 (65)	20 (83)			
Age (years old)	52	56	.39	–	–
BMI (kg/m^2)	24.6	22 .7	.17	–	–
Pancreatic zones			.03	2.03 [1.01–4.07]	.048
1	8 (35)	12 (50)			
2	2 (9)	7 (29)			
3	13 (56)	5 (21)			
Distance to main duct (mm)				–	–
≤ 2 mm	10 (44)	11 (46)	1		
> 2 mm	13 (46)	13 (54)			
Tumor morphology			1	–	–
Cystic	13 (47)	12 (50)			
Solid	10 (44)	12 (50)			
Tumor size (mm)	24	22	.55	–	–
Laparoscopic approach	5 (22)	6 (25)	1	–	–
Operative duration (min)	205	180	.26	–	–
b)	POPF B/C (n = 15)%	No POPF B/C (n = 32)%	Univariate P value	Odd ratio [95% CI]	Multivariate P value
Gender			.16	–	–
Male	6 (40)	6 (19)			
Female	9 (60)	26 (81)			
Age (years old)	54	53	.85	–	–
BMI (kg/m^2)	24.6	23.1	.32	–	–
Pancreatic zones			.02	2.06 [1.01–4.3]	.05
1	3 (20)	17 (53)			
2	2 (13)	7 (22)			
3	10 (67)	8 (25)			
Distance to main duct (mm)			.15		
≤ 2 mm	9 (60)	12 (38)		–	–
> 2 mm	6 (40)	20 (62)			
Tumor morphology			.99		
Cystic	8 (53)	17 (53)		–	–
Solid	7 (47)	15 (47)		–	–
Tumor size (mm)	22	22	.98	–	–
Laparoscopic approach	2 (13)	9 (28)	.27	–	–
Operative duration (min)	200	190	.53	–	–

BMI body mass index, *POPF* postoperative pancreatic fistula, *CI* confidence interval

Pancreatic fistula and risk factors (Table 3a and b)

All patients (*n* = 8) with grade A POPF (of whom three patients with main pancreatic duct direct leakage (all after EN in zone #3) including the patient with main pancreatic duct injury detected intraoperatively) were managed with continuous normal alimentation and progressive drain withdrawal; the median POPF resolution delay (i.e., from POPF diagnosis) was

9 days (range, 4–16). Among the 15 patients with severe POPF, 12 (80%) required an endoscopic or radiologic drainage of a deep collection, 4 patients (27%) required a reintervention for hemorrhage, and one patient (6.7%) developed a duodenal fistula treated by conservative surgery (i.e., direct suture and drainage with progressive fistula spontaneous closure). Two patients who developed a hemorrhage needed a reintervention after an attempt at interventional embolization because the responsible artery could not be reached; another two patients underwent direct reintervention due to bleeding of the gastric wall after a transgastric drainage of a deep collection (Additional file 2: Figure S2a–e).

In the univariate and multivariate analyses, the pancreatic zone was the unique predictive factor of overall ($P = .048$) or severe ($P = .05$) POPF. Distance to the main pancreatic duct and cystic morphology was not identified as a relevant factor for predicting overall or severe POPF.

Pancreatic zones of enucleation (Table 4)

The patient and tumor characteristics were not different among the three groups defined by the three zones. Laparoscopic approach was more often used for EN in zone #1 + 2 when compared with zone #3 ($P = .03$). We did not observe any difference in postoperative courses when comparing the EN achieved in zones #1 and #2. We noted a longer operative duration ($P = .016$), higher overall ($P = .017$) and severe ($P = .01$) POPF rates, and longer hospital stay ($P = .04$) when comparing the EN achieved in zone #3 versus that in zone #1 + 2. Patients who underwent EN in zone #3 had a relative risk [95% confidence interval] of developing a severe POPF of 3.22 [1.31–7.91] compared with patients who underwent EN in the two other pancreatic zones (Fig. 3).

Discussion

Our study identified a high-risk zone (the lower head parenchyma and uncinate process) for developing a POPF after EN, with a relative risk of 3.22 compared to the rest of the cases of pancreatic parenchyma.

POPF after EN

It is now well known that EN can lead to the same POPF rate as standard pancreatectomies (Table 1); however, EN can be considered safer in terms of its mortality rate, which might increase to 10% [21, 22] after pancreatectomies. This finding completely justifies EN as a procedure of choice in patients with benign tumors. Consequently, the patient must be informed that EN is a "mini invasive" pancreatic procedure with the advantage of preserving pancreatic parenchyma but without a reduced risk of POPF and its associated morbidity. The risk factors of overall and severe POPF have already been studied: on the one hand, several factors, such as

age [6], body mass index [10], distance to the main pancreatic duct [17], history of acute pancreatitis [6], and New York Heart Association class [14], were independently identified by a single publication each (Table 1); on the other hand, cystic morphology [6, 11] and tumor location [9, 10, 13] were identified in at least two independent series (Table 1). Our study confirmed that tumor location (i.e., the corresponding EN area) was relevant to predict POPF, but we improved the precision of this result by delimiting a particular zone with a higher risk than the rest of the pancreatic parenchyma. Despite the increasing trend, we did not observe any difference in terms of overall postoperative complications, postoperative hemorrhage, reintervention, perioperative transfusion, and readmission rates between patients who underwent EN in the high-risk zone and the others; however, these factors are clearly directly related to severe POPF, and the reduced sample of our series might be the cause of the non-significance of these results.

Pancreatic zones

As the head of the pancreas is a more difficult zone to expose and represents the intersection of the pancreatic, biliary, and digestive tracts, it was supposed to be at a higher risk of complication after EN. This has already been reported [9, 10, 13], but the uncinate process has never been studied separately from the rest of the head of the pancreas. Our pancreatic partition based on MRI was efficient for easily identifying patients at a high risk of developing a severe POPF after EN. We observed that patients who underwent EN of a tumor located in the upper part of the head (i.e., in zone #2) had a similar risk of experiencing severe POPF as did patients who underwent EN for a tumor located in the body or tail of the pancreas. We suppose that patients who underwent EN in zone #2 were carefully selected and that their tumors probably not deeply located in the head; in such cases, due to the high probability of bile duct injury, a pancreaticoduodenectomy may have been preferred preoperatively. This was confirmed by the lower number of patients (19% of our studied population) who underwent EN in zone #2 and by the higher rate of patients with a planned EN who ultimately had a standard pancreatectomy performed (36% in zone #2, 5% in zone #1, and 5% in zone #3). Thus, our study is limited by the absence of study of the tumor's depth as a risk factor of POPF, even if it has never been highlighted in another study [13].

Prevention of POPF in the high-risk zone

Our study should not discourage pancreatic surgeons from performing EN in patients with tumors located in the high-risk zone because we showed that (a) it was a safe procedure, despite its high morbidity rate

Table 4 Patients and tumor characteristics. Intraoperative data and postoperative courses according to the pancreatic zone classification risk of POPF

	Zone #1	Zone #2	P value zone#1 vs zone #2	Zone #3	P value zone#1 + 2 vs zone #3
Tumor located in the corresponding zone but patient underwent standard pancreatectomy according to intraoperative decision (%)*	1 (5)	5 (36)	.027	1 (5)	ns
n (%)	20 (43)	9 (19)	–	18 (38)	–
Male gender (%)	3 (15)	1 (11)	ns	2 (11)	ns
Age (years old)	53	52	ns	56	ns
BMI (kg/m^2)	22.8	21.5	ns	25.4	ns
Distance to Wirsung (mm)					
< 2 mm (%)	7 (35)	4 (44)	ns	10 (56)	ns
> 2 mm (%)	13 (65)	5 (56)	ns	8 (44)	ns
Tumor morphology					
Cystic (%)	10 (50)	5 (56)	ns	10 (56)	ns
Solid (%)	10 (50)	4 (44)	ns	8 (44)	ns
Tumor size (mm)	22	25	ns	22	ns
Laparoscopic approach	8 (40)	2 (22)	ns	1 (6)	.03
Operative duration (min)	170	180	ns	220	.016
POPF					
Grade A (%)	5 (25)	0	ns	3 (17)	ns
Grades B and C (%)	3 (15)	2 (22)	ns	10 (56)	.01
Total (%)	8 (40)	2 (22)	ns	13 (72)	.017
Hemorrhage (%)	0	1 (11)	ns	3 (17)	ns
Reintervention (%)	0	1 (11)	ns	4 (22)	ns
DINDO morbidity					
Grades 3–4 (%)	3 (15)	5 (56)	ns	8 (44)	ns
Overall (%)	8 (40)	5 (56)	ns	16 (89)	ns
Perioperative transfusion (%)	0	0	ns	4 (22.2)	ns
Length of hospital stay (days)	13	15		23	.04
Readmission (%)	0	0	ns	3 (17)	ns

vs versus, BMI body mass index, POPF postoperative pancreatic fistula
*These patients are not comprised in our study population

and (b) no patients required a salvage pancreatico-duodenectomy. Indeed, our findings permitted the identification of patients who should benefit from strict follow-up and possibly from POPF-preventive procedures. Some authors have described the usefulness of preoperative stenting in patients undergoing EN to reduce main pancreatic duct leakage [23]; a nasopancreatic drain can also be inserted preoperatively to intraoperatively contrast the back-fill of the main pancreatic duct [24] and thereby identify an unknown injury. If the main pancreatic duct stenting is reported as an interesting procedure for treating a prolonged POPF [25], it is correlated with a non-negligible risk of acute pancreatitis [26, 27] and cannot be proposed as a preoperative routine procedure. Indeed, when the EN of a deep tumor is planned

in the high-risk zone, a sphincterotomy followed by the insertion of a stent in the main pancreatic duct could be discussed prior to surgery. However, three arguments must be considered before routinely adopting such a policy. First, a recent randomized study did not confirm the benefit of preoperative stenting to reduce POPF [28]. However, this series was only conducted in patients who underwent distal pancreatectomy, and no data are available concerning proximal or distal EN. Second, EN in the high-risk zone also exposes the patient to other pancreatic duct injuries such as *pancreas divisum* (Type IV of the Cambridge classification; 5% of the population; risk of injury of the accessory duct) [29]; *ansa pancreatica* (Type V; 1% of the population) [29] is another duct variation in which a loop communication is made

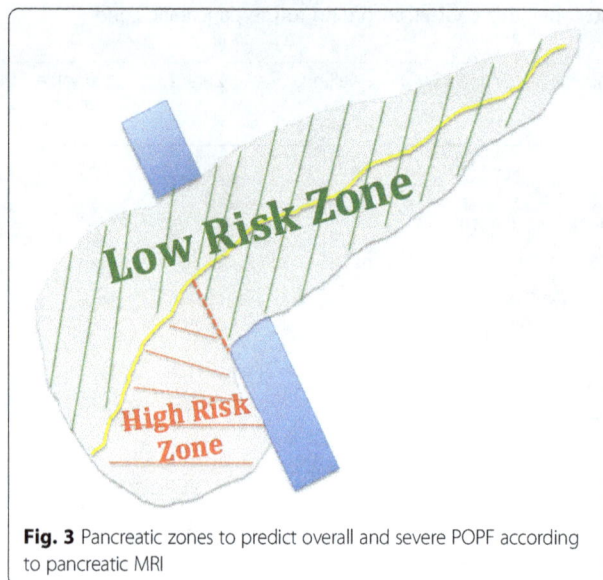

Fig. 3 Pancreatic zones to predict overall and severe POPF according to pancreatic MRI

between the main and accessory duct: stenting of the sole main duct will thus not be sufficient to prevent POPF. Third, pancreatic stenting (even after stent withdrawal) in patients diagnosed with IPMN can lead to main duct modification at imaging and impair the follow-up (modifications due to main duct IPMN or stenting). We support the idea that a careful examination of both MRI and endoscopic ultrasound could help select patients who might benefit from preoperative pancreatic stenting (the patient in the second images should have been a good candidate for preoperative stenting to avoid a lateral main duct injury despite careful ligature of the communication duct). Intraoperatively, in the case of deep EN in the high-risk zone, the pancreatic surgeon could achieve en-Roux pancreaticojejunostomy [30] or teres hepatis ligament flap plasty [31], even if such procedures have not been validated in large series to reduce POPF risk. Finally, drainage of the EN zone must be optimal to avoid pancreatic juice stagnation and favor grade A instead of severe POPF. However, drainage of the "anterior" high-risk zone is difficult ("egg cup" effect, as in the patient in the second images) and often insufficient.

Highlighted by our findings, our actual policy is to achieve a sphincterotomy with main pancreatic duct stent insertion prior to EN in the high-risk zone in patients (a) whose main pancreatic duct is found to be closer than 2 mm at MRI and/or intraoperative ultrasound and/or (b) with branch-duct IPMN consequently linked with the main pancreatic duct. Evaluation of such attitude is ongoing, and we will compare the results with those of the 18 EN achieved in the high-risk zone without preoperative stenting that we have reported in the present series.

Conclusion

Our study identifies a pancreatic zone that is at a high risk of developing a severe POPF after EN but with zero mortality. Thus, EN should be preferred to a pancreaticoduodenectomy to preserve long-term exocrine and endocrine pancreatic functions. However, we support the idea that patients who are planned for a deep EN in this zone should be selected and could benefit from some preoperative (main duct stenting) and/or intraoperative techniques (pancreaticojejunostomy and teres hepatis ligament flap plasty) to prevent severe POPF; these patients should be carefully followed up during the postoperative course, even if they have experimented with a "mini-invasive" surgery.

Additional files

Additional file 1: Figure S1. Intraoperative picture showing the enucleation (yellow arrow) of an insulinoma in the "anterior" zone #3. Please note all ligatures (a) not to have any bleeding during the parenchyma opening that could disturb the identification of main pancreatic duct and (b) preferred to coagulation to avoid thermal damage of the main pancreatic duct.

Additional file 2: Figure S2. (a) pancreatic frontal magnetic resonance imaging showing a branch-duct intrapapillary mucinous neoplasm of zone #3 (portal vein in represented in blue, pancreatic zones are delimited by interrupted red lines); the patient underwent EN in the anterior zone #3 with elective ligature of the communicant duct; (b) drainage (yellow arrow) of a deep collection in the EN zone by two double-pigtail plastic transgastric stents; (c) 24 h after drainage, the patient presented a brutal abdominal pain with hemoglobin serum level tumbling to 6 g/dL, and the CT scan showed an hematoma (red arrow) in the enucleation area without identification of the responsible artery at arteriography; consequently the patient underwent explorative laparotomy; (d) intraoperative picture showing the hematoma in zone #3 with "egg cup" effect (main part of the hematoma descending along the right mesocolon has already been removed); (e) intraoperative picture showing the ablation of the hematoma and the two double-pigtail plastic stents. Bleeding originated from the gastric wall, which was closed by an automatic stapler application after having removed the stents.

Abbreviations
EN : Enucleation; IPMN: Intraductal papillary mucinous neoplasm; MRI: Magnetic resonance imaging; POPF: Postoperative pancreatic fistula

Authors' contributions
PD and OT contributed to the study design. OT contributed to the data collection. PD and OT contributed to the data analysis and interpretation. All authors contributed to the manuscript redaction/revising. Each author has participated sufficiently in the work and agreed to be accountable for all aspects of the work in ensuring that questions related to the accuracy or integrity of any part of the work are appropriately investigated and resolved. All authors read and approved the final manuscript.

Competing interests
The authors declare that they have no competing interests.

Author details

[1]Department of Surgery, Institut Paoli-Calmettes, Marseille, France.
[2]Department of Endoscopy, Institut Paoli-Calmettes, Marseille, France.
[3]Department of Intensive Care, Institut Paoli-Calmettes, Marseille, France.
[4]Department of Surgery, Aix-Marseille University, Institut Paoli-Calmettes, CNRS, Inserm, CRCM, Marseille, France.

References

1. Beger HG. Benign tumors of the pancreas-radical surgery versus parenchyma-sparing local resection—the challenge facing surgeons. J Gastrointest Surg. 2018;22(3):562–6.
2. Zhou Y, Zhao M, Wu L, Ye F, Si X. Short- and long-term outcomes after enucleation of pancreatic tumors: an evidence-based assessment. Pancreatology. 2016;16(6):1092–8.
3. Beger HG, Siech M, Poch B, Mayer B, Schoenberg MH. Limited surgery for benign tumours of the pancreas: a systematic review. World J Surg. 2015; 39(6):1557–66.
4. Sauvanet A, Gaujoux S, Blanc B, Couvelard A, Dokmak S, Vullierme MP, et al. Parenchyma-sparing pancreatectomy for presumed noninvasive intraductal papillary mucinous neoplasms of the pancreas. Ann Surg. 2014;260(2):364–71.
5. Delannoy E, Combemale B. Pancreatic cystadenoma. Enucleation. Reconvery. Mem Acad Chir (Paris). 1964;90:521–3.
6. Wang X, Tan CL, Zhang H, Chen YH, Yang M, Ke NW, et al. Short-term outcomes and risk factors for pancreatic fistula after pancreatic enucleation: a single-center experience of 142 patients. J Surg Oncol. 2018;117(2):182–90.
7. Lu WJ, Cai HL, Ye MD, Wu YL, Xu B. Enucleation of non-invasive tumors in the proximal pancreas: indications and outcomes compared with standard resections. J Zhejiang Univ Sci B. 2017;18(10):906–16.
8. Kaiser J, Fritz S, Klauss M, Bergmann F, Hinz U, Strobel O, et al. Enucleation: a treatment alternative for branch duct intraductal papillary mucinous neoplasms. Surgery. 2017;161(3):602–10.
9. Song KB, Kim SC, Hwang DW, Lee JH, Lee DJ, Lee JW, et al. Enucleation for benign or low-grade malignant lesions of the pancreas: single-center experience with 65 consecutive patients. Surgery. 2015;158(5):1203–10.
10. Jilesen AP, van Eijck CH, Busch OR, van Gulik TM, Gouma DJ, van Dijkum EJ. Postoperative outcomes of enucleation and standard resections in patients with a pancreatic neuroendocrine tumor. World J Surg. 2016;40(3):715–28.
11. Bel O, Cherrez A, Hinz U, Mayer P, Kaiser J, Fritz S, et al. Risk of pancreatic fistula after enucleation of pancreatic tumours. Br J Surg. 2015;102(10):1258–66. https://doi.org/10.1002/bjs.9843.
12. Hüttner FJ, Koessler-Ebs J, Hackert T, Ulrich A, Büchler MW, Diener MK. Meta-analysis of surgical outcome after enucleation versus standard resection for pancreatic neoplasms. Br J Surg. 2015;102(9):1026–36.
13. Faitot F, Gaujoux S, Barbier L, Novaes M, Dokmak S, Aussilhou B, et al. Reappraisal of pancreatic enucleations: a single-center experience of 126 procedures. Surgery. 2015;158(1):201–10.
14. Zhang T, Xu J, Wang T, Liao Q, Dai M, Zhao Y. Enucleation of pancreatic lesions: indications, outcomes, and risk factors for clinical pancreatic fistula. J Gastrointest Surg. 2013;17(12):2099–104.
15. Cauley CE, Pitt HA, Ziegler KM, Nakeeb A, Schmidt CM, Zyromski NJ, et al. Pancreatic enucleation: improved outcomes compared to resection. J Gastrointest Surg. 2012;16(7):1347–53.
16. Turrini O, Schmidt CM, Pitt HA, Guiramand J, Aguilar-Saavedra JR, Aboudi S, et al. Side-branch intraductal papillary mucinous neoplasms of the pancreatic head/uncinate: resection or enucleation? HPB (Oxford). 2011; 13(2):126–31.
17. Brient C, Regenet N, Sulpice L, Brunaud L, Mucci-Hennekine S, Carrère N, et al. Risk factors for postoperative pancreatic fistulisation subsequent to enucleation. J Gastrointest Surg. 2012;16(10):1883–7.
18. Ducon Duconseil P, Turrini O, Ewald J, Soussan J, Sarran A, Gasmi M, et al. 'Peripheric' pancreatic cysts: performance of CT scan, MRI and endoscopy according to final pathological examination. HPB (Oxford). 2015;17(6):485–9.
19. Bassi C, Dervenis C, Butturini G, Fingerhut A, Yeo C, Izbicki J, et al. Postoperative pancreatic fistula: an international study group (ISGPF) definition. Surgery. 2005;138(1):8–13.
20. Dindo D, Demartines N, Clavien PA. Classification of surgical complications: a new proposal with evaluation in a cohort of 6336 patients and results of a survey. Ann Surg. 2004;240(2):205–13.
21. Nimptsch U, Krautz C, Weber GF, Mansky T, Grützmann R. Nationwide in-hospital mortality following pancreatic surgery in Germany is higher than anticipated. Ann Surg. 2016;264(6):1082–90.
22. Farges O, Bendersky N, Truant S, Delpero JR, Pruvot FR, Sauvanet A. The theory and practice of pancreatic surgery in France. Ann Surg. 2017;266(5):797–804.
23. Ide S, Uchida K, Inoue M, Koike Y, Otake K, Matsushita K, et al. Tumor enucleation with preoperative endoscopic transpapillary stenting for pediatric insulinoma. Pediatr Surg Int. 2012;28(7):707–9.
24. Misawa T, Imazu H, Fujiwara Y, et al. Efficacy of nasopancreatic stenting prior to laparoscopic enucleation of pancreatic neuroendocrine tumor. Asian J Endosc Surg. 2013;6(2):140–2.
25. Maire F, Ponsot P, Debove C, Dokmak S, Ruszniewski P, Sauvanet A. Endoscopic management of pancreatic fistula after enucleation of pancreatic tumors. Surg Endosc. 2015;29(11):3112–6.
26. Ito K, Fujita N, Kanno A, Matsubayashi H, Okaniwa S, Nakahara K, et al. Risk factors for post-ERCP pancreatitis in high risk patients who have undergone prophylactic pancreatic duct stenting: a multicenter retrospective study. Intern Med. 2011;50(24):2927–32.
27. Matsubara H, Urano F, Kinoshita Y, Okamura S, Kawashima H, Goto H, et al. Analysis of the risk factors for severity in post endoscopic retrograde cholangiopancreatography pancreatitis: the indication of prophylactic treatments. World J Gastrointest Endosc. 2017;9(4):189–95.
28. Gupta RA, Agrawal P, Doctor N, Nagral S. The effect of prophylactic transpapillary pancreatic stent insertion on clinically significant leak rate following distal pancreatectomy: results of a prospective controlled clinical trial. Ann Surg. 2015;261(3):e81.
29. Adibelli ZH, Adatepe M, Imamoglu C, Esen OS, Erkan N, Yildirim M. Anatomic variations of the pancreatic duct and their relevance with the Cambridge classification system: MRCP findings of 1158 consecutive patients. Radiol Oncol. 2016;50(4):370–7.
30. Xiao Z, Luo G, Liu Z, Jin K, Xu J, Liu C, et al. Roux-en-Y pancreaticojejunostomy reconstruction after deep enucleation of benign or borderline pancreatic lesions: a single-institution experience. HPB (Oxford). 2016;18(2):145–52.
31. Hackert T, Lozanovski VJ, Werner J, Büchler MW, Schemmer P. Teres hepatis ligament flap plasty to prevent pancreatic fistula after tumor enucleation. J Am Coll Surg. 2013;217(4):e29–34.

9

Identifying risk factors for recurrence of papillary thyroid cancer in patients who underwent modified radical neck dissection

Young Jae Ryu, Jin Seong Cho, Jung Han Yoon and Min Ho Park[*]

Abstract

Background: Papillary thyroid cancer (PTC) patients with ipsilateral neck metastatic lymph node (LN) and those with contralateral neck metastatic LN belong to N1b. Only a few studies have reported on comparisons with regard to laterality of metastatic lateral LN. The aim of this study was to evaluate predictive factors for contralateral neck LN metastasis and to determine prognostic factors for recurrence in PTC patients with N1b.

Methods: This retrospective study reviewed the medical records of 390 PTC patients who underwent total thyroidectomy and central LN dissection plus ipsilateral or bilateral modified radical neck dissection (MRND) between January 2004 and December 2012.

Results: During a median follow-up of 81 (range, 6–156) months, 84 patients had a recurrence in any lesion. Male gender, a main tumor of more than 2 cm, number of metastatic central LN, number of harvested and metastatic lateral LN, total LN ratio, multifocality, bilaterality, and gross ETE had significance in the patients who underwent bilateral MRND. In multivariate analysis according to recurrence, patients with LN ratio > 0.44 in the central compartment (hazard ratio [HR], 1.890; 95% confidence interval [CI], 1.124–3.178; $p = 0.015$), LN ratio > 0.29 in the lateral compartment (HR, 2.351; 95% CI, 1.477–3.743; $p < 0.001$), and multifocality (HR, 1.583; 95% CI, 1.030–2.431; $p = 0.036$) were associated with worse RFS. However, the type of MRND was statistically significant only in univariate analysis.

Conclusions: Recurrence in N1b PTC patients is predicted by central neck LN ratio > 0.44, lateral neck LN ratio > 0.29, and multifocality of tumors. We suggest that patients with these factors should receive short-term follow-up using image modalities like ultrasonography and computed tomography.

Keywords: Papillary thyroid cancer, Modified radical neck dissection, Recurrence

Background

Papillary thyroid carcinoma (PTC) is the most common histologic type of thyroid cancer, and its incidence has been increasing worldwide. The prognosis for PTC is better than for other types of thyroid cancer; however, the involvement of lymph nodes (LNs) is up to 80% at diagnosis [1]. It is generally accepted that the spread pattern of LN in PTC is central compartment, ipsilateral compartment, and contralateral compartment sequentially. Although the most common location of LN involvement is the central compartment, skip metastasis (lateral LN metastasis without central LN metastasis) may be observed [2]. The definition of regional LN distinguishes between N1a (levels VI, VII) and N1b (levels I, II, III, IV, V, or retropharyngeal nodes); nevertheless, recent TNM staging did not consider the location of LN involvement [3]. The size of metastatic lateral LNs in surgical specimens is often bigger than is seen with metastatic central LN; however, it is not clear whether or not the reason behind poor outcomes for PTC patients with N1b is location, size, or number of metastatic LN. Several studies revealed that patients with pathologic N1b had a worse prognosis than those with pathologic N1a [4–6]. In addition, some authors reported that

* Correspondence: mhpark@chonnam.ac.kr
Department of Surgery, Chonnam National University Medical School, 322 Seoyang-ro Hwasun-eup, Hwasun-gun Jeonnam, Gwangju 58128, South Korea

the patients with N1b disease had poorer disease-specific survival than those with N0 or N1a and the cause of death is due to distant metastasis rather than locoregional metastasis [7].

There is still debate around performing prophylactic central LN dissection for clinically LN negative PTC patients; however, it is not acceptable performing prophylactic lateral LN dissection for PTC patients without clinical N1b disease. According to recent American Thyroid Association (ATA) guidelines, comprehensive modified radical neck dissection (MRND) encompassing levels II–V was recommended for patients who were clinically N1b [8]. Few studies have compared clinocopathologic characteristics between ipsilateral MRND and bilateral MRND. Ohshima et al. reported that patients who underwent thyroidectomy and bilateral MRND had better 10-year survival rate (97.1% vs. 83.7%) and lower cancer death (5.8% vs. 28.1%) than those who underwent thyroidectomy and ipsilateral MRND [9]. On the other hand, Ito et al. revealed that N1b PTC patients, regardless of type of MRND, with metastatic lateral LNs smaller than 3 cm, with less than five metastatic lateral LNs, or without extranodal extension had similar survival outcomes compared with those N1a PTC patients [10].

The potential for detecting suspicious lateral LN with ultrasonography (US) and computed tomography (CT) is higher than that of central LN [11]. However, if suspicious contralateral LN remains, then residual or persistent disease can have potential effects on postoperative management. Thus, the aim of this study was to evaluate predictive factors for contralateral LN metastasis in PTC patients who underwent total thyroidectomy and central LN dissection, plus ipsilateral or bilateral MRND. Also, we wished to determine prognostic factors for recurrence in PTC patients with N1b.

Methods

Patients' population

We reviewed the medical records of 9135 patients who underwent thyroid surgery at Chonnam National University Hwasun Hospital between January 2004 and December 2012. Exclusion criteria were as follows: patients who had less than a 6-month follow-up period, who underwent reoperation due to suspicious residual tumor or LN within 6 months of initial surgery, who underwent thyroid surgery for reasons other than PTC, who had discordant histology between thyroid tumor and LN on the pathologic report, who did not undergo comprehensive LN dissection in the lateral neck compartment, who had only contralateral lateral metastatic LN, who did not undergo thyroidectomy and MRND concurrently, who did not achieve R0 resection, who had secondary malignancy during follow-up, who had distant metastasis at

initial diagnosis, and who had abnormal thyroid function test before first surgery. We enrolled a total 390 patients who underwent total thyroidectomy and central LN dissection plus ipsilateral or bilateral MRND in this study. This retrospective study was approved by the institutional review board in our hospital.

Operation

All patients were examined by neck US and neck CT during preoperative evaluation to scheme surgical extent, and especially to check the lateral neck compartment. We performed prophylactic central neck dissection, while MRND was not performed in the case of absence of evidence in the lateral compartment. When suspicious lateral LN was detected, fine needle aspiration cytology (FNAC) revealed the presence of absence of LN metastasis. However, in cases of uncertainty with FNAC, we performed an excisional frozen biopsy during the operation to proceed with MRND. Therefore, all patients in this study underwent therapeutic MRND. The performed surgeries included total thyroidectomy, central neck dissection, and MRND in a sequential manner. Central neck refers to level VI (pretracheal, paratracheal, prelaryngeal) or level VII (upper mediastinal LN). MRND refers to comprehensive excision of neck levels II–V with preservation of more than one in three structures: spinal accessory nerve, internal jugular vein, and sternocleidomastoid muscle. Level I dissection was not performed because it is a rare event and preoperative image modalities did not detect suspicious level I LN in enrolled patients. The boundary of LN levels were divided by operator and sent to the department of pathology. All patients were inserted with a drain after procedure.

Histopathologic examination

Surgical specimens were examined by more than two experienced pathologists. The main tumor was defined as the largest tumor. The laterality of ipsilateral MRND was consistent with the location of the main tumor. LN ratio was defined as the number of metastatic LN divided by the number of harvested LN, and skip metastases was indicated lateral LN metastasis without central LN metastasis. TNM stage and ETE were reclassified according to recent American Joint Committee on Cancer (AJCC) recommendations [3].

Postoperative follow-up

All patients received 30–100 mCi of radioactive iodine therapy 2–3 months after surgery because most patients had the possibility of more than an intermediate risk of structural disease recurrence according to recent ATA management guidelines. The patients were followed up every 3 to 6 months for 5 years and annually thereafter, if exhibiting no evidence of disease. All patients also received regular physical examination, neck US, chest radiography, whole-body iodine scanning, measurement of serum-free thyroxine, thyrotropin, thyroglobulin (Tg), and anti-thyrogobulin antibody concentrations. We defined recurrence as structural recurrence. Locoregional recurrence was confirmed by FNAC based on the result of imaging modalities such as neck US, neck CT, 18F-fluorodeoxyglucose positron emission tomography CT, and whole-body scan. Distant metastasis was confirmed by the abovementioned imaging modalities. Most patients with structural recurrence underwent reoperation; however, if the patients had an unresectable lesion or distant metastasis, radioactive iodine therapy was considered as a first option.

Complications

Hypoparathyroidism and recurrent laryngeal nerve palsy were classified as transient or permanent based on 6 months after surgery. We defined hypoparathyroidism as postoperative serum parathyroid hormone level below normal, with a concomitant low calcium level and requiring calcium and vitamin D supplementation. Patients who underwent thyroid surgery in our institution underwent examination for the level of PTH in 6 h, 24 h, and 48 h postoperatively. Patients who had a lower level of PTH were checked every 2 days during admission. The level of PTH was examined with the level of total calcium and ionized calcium. We considered recurrent laryngeal nerve palsy through flexible laryngoscopy as well as voice change after surgery. All patients in this study were not routinely examined via preoperative laryngoscopy. However, patients who had suspicious gross ETE into posterior surface of the thyroid or trachea or who had symptoms related with voice change underwent preoperative laryngoscopy. Postoperative laryngoscopy was performed selectively for patients who had preoperative experience and with symptoms regarding voice change, or with suspicion of recurrent laryngeal nerve injury. Postoperative bleeding was defined as the case which underwent the operation, and chyle leakage was defined as the case which underwent operative or conservative management.

Statistics

Disease-specific mortality was a rare event. Therefore, the primary end point was recurrence in any lesion. We defined recurrence-free survival (RFS) as the time between the first operation and confirmation of recurrence. Continuous variables are represented as median (range) or mean (standard deviation, SD), while categorical variables are shown as a number (percent). Independent t test and chi-square analysis were used to compare between ipsilateral MRND and bilateral MRND. A univariate Cox proportional hazards model was used to analyze the relationship between clinicopathologic variables and recurrence-free survival. Multivariate Cox proportional hazards regression analyses by way of backward elimination were performed using the variables with p values < 0.05 in the univariate analyses. The receiver operating characteristic curve was used to calculate optimal value of LN ratio in the central and the lateral compartment. We used the log-rank test and the Kaplan-Meier curve to calculate differences in RFS. We performed all statistical analyses using SPSS version 23.0 (IBM Inc., Armonk, NY, USA) and defined statistical significance as p less than 0.05.

Results

Patients' demographics

Of a total 390 patients, median age (range) was 46 years (17–80) and 118 patients (30.3%) were male. Patients who underwent ipsilateral MRND and bilateral MRND were 346 (88.7%) and 44 (11.3%), respectively. Mean (SD) size of the main tumor was 1.61 cm (± 0.97) and patients in which the main tumor was more than 2 cm were 93 (23.8%). Findings for T stage were as follows: T1a, 121 patients (31.0%); T1b, 109 (27.9); T2, 40 (10.3%); T3a, 4 (1.0%), T3b, 52 (13.3%); and T4a, 64 (16.4%). One hundred forty-two (36.4%) and 125 (32.1%) patients had multifocality and bilaterality of tumors. Seventy-five (19.2%) patients had minor ETE, and 116 (29.7%) patients had gross ETE of the main tumor. Mean (SD) number of harvested central LN and metastatic central LN were 7.4 (± 6.0) and 3.8 (± 4.0). Mean (SD) number of harvested central LN and metastatic lateral LN were 18.6 (± 10.3) and 4.9 (± 3.9). Skip metastasis showed in 86 (22.1%) patients. Patients with stage I were 285 (73.1%); stage II, 79 (20.3%); and stage III, 26 (6.7%). We observed chronic lymphocytic thyroiditis (CLT) in 100 (25.6%) while 20 (5.1%) patients showed lymphovascular invasion (LVI). Median follow-up was 81 (range, 6–156) months (Table 1).

Recurrence

Eighty-four (21.5%) patients demonstrated recurrence during the follow-up period. Among the 33 patients with recurrence in the central compartment or operative bed, 12 patients had recurrence in the lateral compartment; 1 patient, in the distant lesion; and 1 patient, in the lateral compartment and distant lesion. Forty-eight patients had recurrence only in the lateral compartment. Three patients showed only distant metastasis. The most common organ of distant metastasis is the lung (4 patients) followed by the bone (1 patient) (Table 2). Of 84 patients who had a recurrence, 79 (94.0%) patients had a recurrence within 5 years after surgery.

Table 1 Patients' demographics

Variables	Number (%)
Age (years)[§]	46 (17–80)
≤ 55 years	285 (73.1)
Male	118 (30.3)
Hypertension	62 (15.9)
Diabetes	26 (6.7)
Modified radical neck dissection	
Ipsilateral	346 (88.7)
Bilateral	44 (11.3)
Main tumor size (cm)[*]	1.61 ± 0.97
> 2 cm	93 (23.8)
T stage	
T1a	121 (31.0)
T1b	109 (27.9)
T2	40 (10.3)
T3a	4 (1.0)
T3b	52 (13.3)
T4a	64 (16.4)
Multifocality	142 (36.4)
Bilaterality	125 (32.1)
Extrathyroidal extension	
No	199 (51.0)
Minor	75 (19.2)
Gross	116 (29.7)
Number of central lymph node	
Harvested[§, *]	6 (2–65), 7.4 ± 6.0
Metastatic[§, *]	3 (0–29), 3.8 ± 4.0
Number of lateral lymph node	
Harvested[§, *]	16 (8–62), 18.6 ± 10.3
Metastatic[§, *]	4 (1–23), 4.9 ± 3.9
Skip metastases	86 (22.1)
Stage	
I	285 (73.1)
II	79 (20.3)
III	26 (6.7)
Lymphovascular invasion	20 (5.1)
Chronic lymphocytic thyroiditis	100 (25.6)
Recurrence	84 (21.5)
Follow-up[§]	81 months (6–156)
Total patients	390

[§]Median and range
[*]Mean and standard deviation

Comparison according to MRND type

Between patients who underwent unilateral MRND and the patients with bilateral MRND, male gender, larger than a 2 cm main tumor, number of metastatic central LN, number of harvested and metastatic lateral LN, total LN ratio, multifocality, bilaterality, and gross ETE had significance in patients who underwent bilateral MRND.

Table 2 Distribution of recurrence site

	Number
Central LN or operative bed	33
Only central LN or op bed	19
+ Lateral LN	12
+ Distant metastasis	1
+ Lateral LN + distant metastasis	1
Only lateral LN	48
Only distant metastasis	3

LN lymph node

There was no statistical association with age, CLT, LVI, and TNM stage (Table 3).

Uni- and multivariate analyses according to recurrence

In univariate analysis of associations with recurrence, larger than 2 cm main tumor ($p = 0.025$), LN ratio > 0.44 in the central compartment ($p < 0.001$) and LN ratio > 0.29 in the lateral compartment ($p < 0.001$), bilateral MRND ($p = 0.004$), multifocality ($p = 0.012$), no CLT ($p = 0.037$), and gross ETE ($p = 0.040$) showed statistically significant differences. However, there were no differences in RFS with age, sex, skip metastasis, bilaterality, LVI, or stage (Table 4, Fig. 1a–c).

In multivariate analysis, LN ratio > 0.44 in the central compartment (vs. ≤ 0.44; hazard ratio [HR], 1.890; 95% confidence interval [CI], 1.124–3.178; $p = 0.015$), LN ratio > 0.29 in the lateral compartment (vs. ≤ 0.29; HR, 2.351; 95% CI, 1.477–3.743; $p < 0.001$), and multifocality (vs. no multifocality; HR, 1.583; 95% CI, 1.030–2.431; $p = 0.036$) were associated with worse RFS (Table 5).

Postoperative complications

Of the 390 patients, the incidence of transient and permanent hypoparathyroidism were 16 (4.1%) and 3 (0.8%) patients, respectively. We observed transient and permanent recurrent laryngeal nerve palsy in 23 (5.9%) and 14 (3.6%) patients (Table 6). Among 29 patients with invasion to recurrent laryngeal nerve, 24 patients underwent shaving operation and 5 patients underwent re-anastomosis of recurrent laryngeal nerve; no patients underwent concurrent tracheostomy. Two patients underwent reoperation due to postoperative bleeding during admission after initial surgery; two patients showed chyle leakage, one of these patients underwent operative treatment and the remaining patient recovered after conservative management.

Discussion

Among PTC patients with N1b in this study, 44 (12.7%) had contralateral neck metastatic LNs. Contralateral neck LN metastasis was associated with male gender, more than 2 cm size of main tumor, a high number of

Table 3 Comparison of MRND type and clinicopathologic characteristics

Variables	Ipsilateral MRND N = 346	Bilateral MRND N = 44	p
Age	46.2 ± 13.3	48.1 ± 15.6	0.369
≤ 55 years	255 (73.7)	30 (68.2)	0.471
> 55 years	91 (26.3)	14 (31.8)	
Sex			< 0.001
Female	252 (72.8)	20 (45.5)	
Male	94 (27.2)	24 (54.5)	
Main tumor size (cm)	1.54 ± 0.91	2.20 ± 1.21	< 0.001
≤ 2 cm	272 (78.6)	25 (56.8)	0.002
> 2 cm	74 (21.4)	19 (43.2)	
Number of central lymph node			
Harvested	7.2 ± 5.9	8.4 ± 6.2	0.210
Metastatic	3.4 ± 3.5	6.3 ± 6.0	< 0.001
Number of lateral lymph node			< 0.001
Harvested	16.6 ± 8.1	33.6 ± 13.3	< 0.001
Metastatic	4.2 ± 2.9	10.5 ± 5.5	
Skip metastases	80 (23.1)	6 (13.6)	0.179
LN ratio	0.34 ± 0.19	0.41 ± 0.21	0.012
Multifocality	114 (32.9)	28 (63.6)	< 0.001
Bilaterality	101 (29.2)	24 (54.5)	0.001
ETE			0.003
No/minor	252 (72.8)	22 (50.0)	
Gross	94 (27.2)	22 (50.0)	
CLT	92 (26.6)	8 (18.2)	0.274
LVI	16 (4.6)	4 (9.1)	0.263
Stage			0.406
I	255 (73.7)	30 (68.2)	
II	70 (20.2)	9 (20.5)	
III	21 (6.1)	5 (11.4)	
Recurrence	67 (19.4)	17 (38.6)	0.006

MRND modified lateral neck dissection, *LN* lymph node, *ETE* extrathyroidal extension, *CLT* chronic lymphocytic thyroiditis, *LVI* lymphovascular invasion

metastatic central LN, multifocality and bilaterality of the tumors, and gross ETE. However, there was no significant relationship between type of MRND (ipsilateral MRND vs. bilateral MRND) and recurrence. LN ratio in central and lateral compartment, and multifocality of tumors were independent prognostic factors in N1b PTC patients.

According to ATA guidelines, prophylactic central LN dissection should be considered in patients with clinically central node-negative who have advanced primary tumors (T3 or T4) or clinically N1b [8]. However, prophylactic MRND is not recommended if the patients had no evidence of FANC or Tg washout measurement in the lateral compartment [8]. The sensitivity of US detection of lateral neck LN is higher than that of central

LN [11]. Meticulous evaluation of lateral neck LN using US is needed for PTC patients during the preoperative evaluation period. In a study of 135 PTC patients who underwent bilateral neck dissection, the authors found that bilaterality of tumors and tumors arising in the isthmus were associated with bilateral LN metastasis [12]. They also demonstrated that contralateral neck LN metastasis was significantly correlated with clinically node-positive in the ipsilateral neck and contralateral paratracheal LN metastasis. In another study of 1776 PTC patients who underwent thyroidectomy and ipsilateral MRND during mean follow-up of 12.1 years, 32 (1.8%) patients recurred with contralateral neck LN [13]. They concluded that risk factors for contralateral neck LN were male gender, more than 2 cm size of primary

Table 4 Univariate analysis of risk factors for recurrence

	Exp (B)	95% CI for Exp (B)	p
Age			
≤ 55 years	1		
> 55 years	1.138	0.713–1.816	0.589
Sex			
Female	1		
Male	1.037	0.653–1.648	0.877
Main tumor size			
≤ 2 cm	1		
> 2 cm	1.689	1.068–2.671	0.025
Skip metastasis			
No	1		
Yes	0.696	0.392–1.235	0.215
LN ratio (central)			
≤ 0.44	1		
> 0.44	2.492	1.508–4.118	< 0.001
LN ratio (lateral)			
≤ 0.29	1		
> 0.29	2.822	1.799–4.426	< 0.001
MRND type			
Ipsilateral	1		
Bilateral	2.158	1.267–3.676	0.004
Multifocality			
No	1		
Yes	1.735	1.131–2.662	0.012
Bilaterality			
No	1		
Yes	1.514	0.981–2.337	0.061
CLT			
NO	1		
Yes	0.542	0.305–0.962	0.037
ETE			
No/minor	1		
Gross	1.583	1.022–2.453	0.040
LVI			
No	1		
Yes	1.097	0.444–2.708	0.841
Stage			
I	1		
II	0.952	0.548–1.654	0.862
III	1.740	0.863–3.509	0.122

CI confidence interval, *LN* lymph node, *MRND* modified radical neck dissection, *CLT* chronic lymphocytic thyroiditis, *ETE* extrathyroidal extension, *LVI* lymphovascular invasion

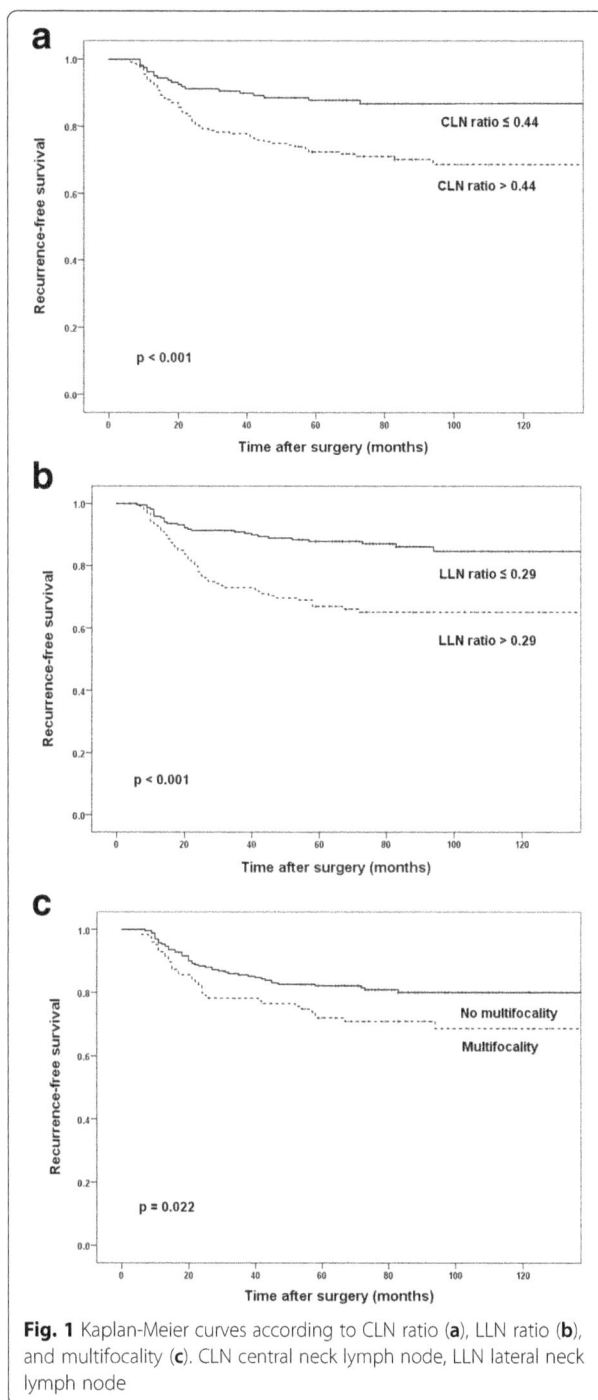

Fig. 1 Kaplan-Meier curves according to CLN ratio (**a**), LLN ratio (**b**), and multifocality (**c**). CLN central neck lymph node, LLN lateral neck lymph node

tumor, ETE, and the presence of gross nodal metastasis at the initial surgery. Therefore, they suggested that patients with the abovementioned factors may be recommended for bilateral MRND. Although N1b PTC patients with a high number of metastatic central LN, multifocality, or bilaterality, as well as those with bigger tumor or gross ETE, tended to have contralateral neck LN metastasis in this study, further study is needed to demonstrate the execution of both MRND.

Table 5 Multivariate analysis of risk factors for recurrence

	Exp (B)	95% CI for Exp (B)	p
Main tumor size			
≤ 2 cm	1		
> 2 cm	1.480	0.931–2.355	0.098
LN ratio (central)			
≤ 0.44	1		
> 0.44	1.890	1.124–3.178	0.016
LN ratio(lateral)			
≤ 0.29	1		
> 0.29	2.351	1.477–3.743	< 0.001
Multifocality			
No	1		
Yes	1.583	1.030–2.431	0.036
CLT			
No	1		
yes	0.644	0.362–1.149	0.136
MRND type			
Ipsilateral	1		
Bilateral	1.335	0.744–2.394	0.332
ETE			
No	1		
Gross	1.308	0.824–2.076	0.255

CI confidence interval, LN lymph node, CLT chronic lymphocytic thyroiditis, MRND modified radical neck dissection, ETE extrathyroidal extension

Several studies revealed that the number of metastatic LN at diagnosis were associated with recurrence in PTC [1, 14]. In addition, some studies found that LN ratio (the number of metastatic LN divided by the number of harvested LN) is related to post-treatment recurrence. A study of 198 PTC patients who underwent total thyroidectomy and neck dissection concluded that patients with LN ratio ≥ 0.3 had 3.4 times higher risk of persistent or recurrent disease than did those with ratio of 0 [15]. Schneider et al. reported that patients with LN ratio more than 0.7 showed significantly worse disease-free

Table 6 Postoperative complications

	Number (%)
Hypoparathyroidism	
Transient	16 (4.1)
Permanent	3 (0.8)
Recurrent laryngeal nerve injury	
Transient	23 (5.9)
Permanent	14 (3.6)
Postoperative bleeding	2 (0.5)
Chyle leakage	2 (0.5)

survival rates compared with those with ratio below 0.7 [16]. However, Lee et al. reported that central plus lateral LN ratio did not have an association with recurrence in patients who underwent therapeutic central and lateral neck dissection [17]. The present study separated LN status based on the location of metastatic LN: central compartment or lateral compartment. Skip metastasis, N1b without central LN metastasis, was not associated with recurrence. LN ratio > 0.44 in the central compartment and LN ratio > 0.29 in the lateral compartment were independent prognostic factors for poor RFS in patients with N1b disease. Even though the LN ratio in PTC is a useful prognostic factor for disease-free survival, multicenter studies are required to set optimal cutoffs, standardize the number and surgical extent, and supplement TNM staging.

Shattuck et al. described that individual tumor foci in multifocal PTC originate from discrete tumors independently [18]. Another study demonstrated that multifocal PTC stems from the same clone; therefore, it is important for intrathyroidal metastasis in PTC [19]. Although the reason of multifocality in PTC is not clear, multifocal PTC is not a rare event. Indeed, there is still controversy regarding multifocality in PTC and survival outcomes. Some study has reported that multifocality is not associated with recurrence [20]. Another study showed that bilaterality rather than unilateral multifocality of PTC was proven to be an independent risk factor for locoregional recurrence, distant metastasis, and cancer death [21]. On the other hand, Lin et al. revealed that multifocal PTC patients have higher recurrence rate and advanced TNM stage compared to solitary PTC patients [22]. Also, some authors described that patients with multifocal micro PTC were observed to have 5.6-fold higher LN recurrence [23]. Another study showed that the number of multifocal tumors rather than the location is significant predictive factor for disease recurrence [24]. This study showed 36.4% multifocality and 32.1% bilaterality in patients with N1b. The patients who underwent bilateral MRND tended to have multifocality and bilaterality; however, only multifocality was related to RFS.

ETE is an important prognostic factor for survival outcomes in PTC. In the sixth AJCC, ETE was classified as minor and gross [25]; however, according to recent AJCC recommendations, minor ETE was removed from the definition of T3 disease [3]. Therefore, tumors > 4 cm in greatest dimension limited to the thyroid gland is considered T3a and gross ETE with invasion only to the strap muscles is considered T3b [3]. This study did not include patients with T4b because complete resection was not achieved. The patients with gross ETE were associated with contralateral neck LN metastasis and poor RFS in univariate analysis; however, there was no statistically significance between gross ETE and RFS in multivariate analysis.

CLT is an autoimmune disease characterized by fibrosis, atrophy, and lymphocyte infiltration in thyroid tissue. CLT exhibits a thyroid-specific antigen that is represented in thyroid tumor and may be involved in the destruction of thyroid cancer. Several investigations reported that PTC patients with coexisting CLT have lower recurrence rate and better overall survival due to control of tumor growth and proliferation [26, 27]. This study showed that patients with CLT have lower recurrence rates in univariate analysis; however, there is no relation between CLT and recurrence in multivariate analysis.

In terms of the location of metastatic LN, Ito et al. revealed that the 621 N1b PTC patients with less than 3 cm metastatic lateral LN, less than five metastatic lateral LNs, or without extranodal extension had similar survival outcomes compared with those N1a PTC patients [10]. Several studies found that the location of metastatic LN rather than the number is useful for predicting risk of recurrence or distant metastasis; therefore, the distinction between N1a and N1b is extremely important for postoperative management in PTC patients [28, 29]. Even though the location of metastatic LN is not reflected in TNM stage, it is a powerful factor that affects disease-specific survival to decide the surgical extent.

According to the ATA guidelines, neck US should be performed at 6–12 months after initial surgery and then periodically depending on the risk of recurrence and Tg status [8]. A considerable number of patients had a recurrence within 5 years in this study; thus, we suggest that patients who had undergone MRND should be checked via neck US every 6 months at least for 5 years. In addition, neck CT is useful for detection of especially suspicious central LNs. Therefore, we suggest that neck CT should be performed periodically for patients with negative neck US and high level of Tg.

This study has several limitations. Study design was retrospective and conducted at a single institution. In order to determine laterality of lateral LN metastasis if the patients who underwent ipsilateral MRND had bilaterality of tumors, it was decided by the location of the bigger tumor. Therefore, selection bias is reflected in decisions regarding laterality. In addition, the decision of surgical extent might be intervened by interpretation of radiologists and surgeons of preoperative imaging modalities like neck US and neck CT. We did not consider patients with biochemical incomplete response that related to Tg and anti-Tg measurement. We are collecting more sufficient clinicopathological data for long-term follow-up of patients who underwent total thyroidectomy and MRND.

Conclusions

The patients who underwent ipsilateral MRND or bilateral MRND have the same N stage. The surgical extent of lateral neck compartment is not reflected in TNM stage. However, meticulous preoperative evaluation of contralateral LN is needed to avoid residual or persistent disease during postoperative follow-up. The factors that associated with contralateral LN metastasis were male gender, more than 2 cm size of main tumor, multifocality, bilaterality, and ETE. Recurrence in N1b PTC patients is predicted by central neck LN ratio > 0.44, lateral neck LN ratio > 0.29, and multifocality of tumors. We suggest that patients with these factors should receive short-term follow-up using image modalities like US and CT.

Abbreviations
AJCC: American Joint Committee on Cancer; ATA: American Thyroid Association; CI: Confidence interval; CLN: Central neck lymph node; CLT: Chronic lymphocytic thyroiditis; CT: Computed tomography; ETE: Extrathyroidal extension; FANC: Fine needle aspiration cytology; HR: Hazard ratio; LLN: Lateral neck lymph node; LN: Lymph node; LVI: Lymphovascular invasion; MRND: Modified radical neck dissection; PTC: Papillary thyroid cancer; RFS: Recurrence-free survival; SD: Standard deviation; US: Ultrasonography

Authors' contributions
YJR is the main author of the manuscript and has substantial contributions to the study design and data analysis. JSC and JHY contributed to the data collection and the manuscript drafting. MHP has been involved in the study design and supervision. All authors read and approved the final manuscript.

Competing interests
The authors declare that they have no competing interests.

References
1. Randolph GW, Duh QY, Heller KS, LiVolsi VA, Mandel SJ, Steward DL, et al. The prognostic significance of nodal metastases from papillary thyroid carcinoma can be stratified based on the size and number of metastatic lymph nodes, as well as the presence of extranodal extension. Thyroid. 2012;22:1144–52.
2. Machens A, Holzhausen HJ, Dralle H. Skip metastases in thyroid cancer leaping the central lymph node compartment. Arch Surg. 2004;139:43–5.
3. Amin MB, Edge S, Greene F, Byrd DR, Brookland RK, Washington MK, et al. AJCC cancer staging manual. 8th ed. New York: Springer International Publishing; 2017. p. 872–927.
4. Mazzaferri EL, Jhiang SM. Long-term impact of initial surgical and medical therapy on papillary and follicular thyroid cancer. Am J Med. 1994;97:418–28.
5. Ito Y, Miyauchi A, Jikuzono T, Higashiyama T, Takamura Y, Miya A, et al. Risk factors contributing to a poor prognosis of papillary thyroid carcinoma: validity of UICC/AJCC TNM classification and stage grouping. World J Surg. 2007;31:838–48.
6. Baek SK, Jung KY, Kang SM, Kwon SY, Woo JS, Cho SH, et al. Clinical risk factors associated with cervical lymph node recurrence in papillary thyroid carcinoma. Thyroid. 2010;20:147–52.
7. Nixon IJ, Wang LY, Palmer FL, Tuttle RM, Shaha AR, Shah JP, et al. The impact of nodal status on outcome in older patients with papillary thyroid cancer. Surgery. 2014;156:137–46.
8. Haugen BR, Alexander EK, Bible KC, Doherty GM, Mandel SJ, Nikiforov YE, et al. 2015 American Thyroid Association Management Guidelines for adult patients with thyroid nodules and differentiated thyroid cancer: the American Thyroid Association guidelines task force on thyroid nodules and differentiated thyroid cancer. Thyroid. 2016;26:1–133.

9.   Ohshima A, Yamashita H, Noguchi S, Uchino S, Watanabe S, Koike E, et al. Is a bilateral modified radical neck dissection beneficial for patients with papillary thyroid cancer? Surg Today. 2002;32:1027–30.

10. Ito Y, Fukushima M, Tomoda C, Inoue H, Kihara M, Higashiyama T, et al. Prognosis of patients with papillary thyroid carcinoma having clinically apparent metastasis to the lateral compartment. Endocr J. 2009;56:759–66.

11. Lee DW, Ji YB, Sung ES, Park JS, Lee YJ, Park DW, et al. Roles of ultrasonography and computed tomography in the surgical management of cervical lymph node metastases in papillary thyroid carcinoma. Eur J Surg Oncol. 2013;39:191–6.

12. Noguchi M, Kinami S, Kinoshita K, Kitagawa H, Thomas M, Miyazaki I, et al. Risk of bilateral cervical lymph node metastases in papillary thyroid cancer. J Surg Oncol. 1993;52:155–9.

13. Ohshima A, Yamashita H, Noguchi S, Uchino S, Watanabe S, Toda M, et al. Indications for bilateral modified radical neck dissection in patients with papillary carcinoma of the thyroid. Arch Surg. 2000;135:1194–8 discussion 9.

14. Cho SY, Lee TH, Ku YH, Kim HI, Lee GH, Kim MJ. Central lymph node metastasis in papillary thyroid microcarcinoma can be stratified according to the number, the size of metastatic foci, and the presence of desmoplasia. Surgery. 2015;157:111–8.

15. Vas Nunes JH, Clark JR, Gao K, Chua E, Campbell P, Niles N, et al. Prognostic implications of lymph node yield and lymph node ratio in papillary thyroid carcinoma. Thyroid. 2013;23:811–6.

16. Schneider DF, Mazeh H, Chen H, Sippel RS. Lymph node ratio predicts recurrence in papillary thyroid cancer. Oncologist. 2013;18:157–62.

17. Lee CW, Roh JL, Gong G, Cho KJ, Choi SH, Nam SY, et al. Risk factors for recurrence of papillary thyroid carcinoma with clinically node-positive lateral neck. Ann Surg Oncol. 2015;22:117–24.

18. Shattuck TM, Westra WH, Ladenson PW, Arnold A. Independent clonal origins of distinct tumor foci in multifocal papillary thyroid carcinoma. N Engl J Med. 2005;352:2406–12.

19. McCarthy RP, Wang M, Jones TD, Strate RW, Cheng L. Molecular evidence for the same clonal origin of multifocal papillary thyroid carcinomas. Clin Cancer Res. 2006;12:2414–8.

20. Leboulleux S, Rubino C, Baudin E, Caillou B, Hartl DM, Bidart JM, et al. Prognostic factors for persistent or recurrent disease of papillary thyroid carcinoma with neck lymph node metastases and/or tumor extension beyond the thyroid capsule at initial diagnosis. J Clin Endocrinol Metab. 2005;90:5723–9.

21. Qu N, Zhang L, Wu WL, Ji QH, Lu ZW, Zhu YX, et al. Bilaterality weighs more than unilateral multifocality in predicting prognosis in papillary thyroid cancer. Tumour Biol. 2016;37:8783–9.

22. Lin JD, Chao TC, Hsueh C, Kuo SF. High recurrent rate of multicentric papillary thyroid carcinoma. Ann Surg Oncol. 2009;16:2609–16.

23. Chow SM, Law SC, Chan JK, Au SK, Yau S, Lau WH. Papillary microcarcinoma of the thyroid - prognostic significance of lymph node metastasis and multifocality. Cancer. 2003;98:31–40.

24. Kim HJ, Sohn SY, Jang HW, Kim SW, Chung JH. Multifocality, but not bilaterality, is a predictor of disease recurrence/persistence of papillary thyroid carcinoma. World J Surg. 2013;37:376–84.

25. Greene FL, Page DL. Flemingo ID AJCC cancer staging handbook: TNM classification of malignant tumors. 6th ed. New York: Springer-Verlag; 2002.

26. Loh KC, Greenspan FS, Dong F, Miller TR, Yeo PP. Influence of lymphocytic thyroiditis on the prognostic outcome of patients with papillary thyroid carcinoma. J Clin Endocrinol Metab. 1999;84:458–63.

27. Kashima K, Yokoyama S, Noguchi S, Murakami N, Yamashita H, Watanabe S, et al. Chronic thyroiditis as a favorable prognostic factor in papillary thyroid carcinoma. Thyroid. 1998;8:197–202.

28. de Meer SG, Dauwan M, de Keizer B, Valk GD, Borel Rinkes IH, Vriens MR. Not the number but the location of lymph nodes matters for recurrence rate and disease-free survival in patients with differentiated thyroid cancer. World J Surg. 2012;36:1262–7.

29. Jeon MJ, Kim TY, Kim WG, Han JM, Jang EK, Choi YM, et al. Differentiating the location of cervical lymph node metastasis is very useful for estimating the risk of distant metastases in papillary thyroid carcinoma. Clin Endocrinol. 2014;81:593–9.

10

Clinical outcome of primary giant cell tumor of bone after curettage with or without perioperative denosumab in Japan: from a questionnaire for JCOG 1610 study

Hiroshi Urakawa[1]* , Tsukasa Yonemoto[2], Seiichi Matsumoto[3], Tatsuya Takagi[4], Kunihiro Asanuma[5], Munenori Watanuki[6], Akira Takemoto[7], Norifumi Naka[8], Yoshihiro Matsumoto[9], Akira Kawai[10], Toshiyuki Kunisada[11], Tadahiko Kubo[12], Makoto Emori[13], Hiroaki Hiraga[14], Hiroshi Hatano[15], Satoshi Tsukushi[16], Yoshihiro Nishida[1], Toshihiro Akisue[17], Takeshi Morii[18], Mitsuru Takahashi[19], Akihito Nagano[20], Hideki Yoshikawa[21], Kenji Sato[22], Masanori Kawano[23], Koji Hiraoka[24], Kazuhiro Tanaka[25], Yukihide Iwamoto[26] and Toshifumi Ozaki[27]

Abstract

Background: Giant cell tumor of bone (GCTB) is an intermediate tumor known to be locally aggressive, but rarely metastasizing. To plan a prospective study of GCTB, we performed a questionnaire survey for institutions participating in the Bone and Soft Tissue Tumor Study Group (BSTTSG) in the Japan Clinical Oncology Group (JCOG) in 2015.

Methods: We reviewed 158 consecutive patients with primary GCTB treated with curettage without perioperative denosumab from 2008 to 2010 in Japan. We investigated local and distant recurrence rates after definitive curettage. We also investigated the recurrence rate after treatment with preoperative and/or postoperative denosumab with curettage in recent years. There were 40 patients treated with perioperative denosumab, and the factors affecting recurrence in them were investigated.

Results: Answers were available from 24 of 30 institutions (80.0%) participating in JCOG BSTTSG. Thirty (19.0%) and 4 (2.5%) of 158 patients developed local and distant recurrence after curettage without perioperative denosumab from 2008 to 2010, respectively. Campanacci grade and embolization before surgery were significantly associated with increasing incidence of local recurrence after curettage ($p = 0.034$ and $p = 0.022$, respectively). In patients treated with perioperative desnosumab, 120 mg denosumab was administered subcutaneously for a median 6 (2–41) and 6 (1–14) times in preoperative and postoperative settings, respectively. The recurrence rates were 6 of 21 (28.6%), 2 of 9 (22.2%), and 0 of 10 (0.0%) in the preoperative, postoperative, and both pre- and postoperative denosumab treatment groups, respectively. With all of the preoperative treatments, administration exceeding five times was significantly associated with a decreased incidence of local recurrence after curettage ($p < 0.001$).

Conclusion: The recurrence rate of GCTB was still high after curettage, especially in Campanacci grade III, and improvements in the therapeutic strategy are needed in this cohort. There is a possibility that a sufficient dose of preoperative denosumab can reduce recurrence after curettage. Recently, we have started a clinical trial, JCOG1610, to investigate the efficacy of preoperative denosumab in patients who can be treated with curettage in GCTB.

Keywords: Giant cell tumor of bone, Outcome, Denosumab, Japan

* Correspondence: urakawa@med.nagoya-u.ac.jp
[1]Department of Orthopaedic Surgery, Nagoya University, 65 Tsurumai, Showa-ku, Nagoya, Aichi 466-8550, Japan
Full list of author information is available at the end of the article

Background

Giant cell tumor of bone (GCTB) is an intermediate tumor known to be locally aggressive, but rarely metastasizing in the WHO classification [1]. GCTB possibly originates from the metaphyseal region [2], and accounts for 4–5% of all skeletal neoplasms in Japan. Local and distant recurrence rates were reported in 24.8–30.8% [3–6] and 2% [7, 8] of the patients after curettage, respectively. To reduce local recurrence and preserve the adjacent joint, adjuvant treatments such as high-speed burr [3], phenol [5, 9], ethanol, liquid nitrogen [5], and polymethyl methacrylate (PMMA) [3, 5, 9] have been reported. Even though there were some reports of GCTB in Japan [7, 10, 11], the recent clinical results of GCTB after curettage in multiple institutions in Japan have not been well documented.

Denosumab is a fully human monoclonal antibody that inhibits the receptor activator of NF-κB (RANK) ligand (RANKL) and then interrupts RANK-RANKL interactions. In GCTB, the stromal cells and osteoclast-like giant cells express RANKL and RANK, respectively, and the RANK-RANKL interaction is considered to be necessary for the differentiation and activation of osteoclasts [12]. Therefore, the RANK-RANKL interaction has a critical role for bone destruction in GCTB, and dramatic change was observed after treatment of denosumab in GCTB. Multinucleated osteoclast-like giant cells and stromal cells were decreased after denosumab treatment for GCTB [13]. A recent phase 2 study demonstrated the effects of denosumab for patients with unresectable GCTB and salvageable GCTB whose surgery was associated with severe morbidity [14]. Denosumab was accepted for health insurance coverage in Japan in 2014. However, the role of denosumab in patients with GCTB who can be treated by curettage has not been well defined.

We performed a questionnaire survey for institutions participating in the Bone and Soft Tissue Tumor Study Group (BSTTSG) in the Japan Clinical Oncology Group (JCOG) in 2015 for planning a clinical trial of JCOG1610, a randomized phase III study of preoperative denosumab with curettage for GCTB. The first aim of the present study was to identify the historical outcome after curettage for GCTB without perioperative desnosumab in Japan. The second purpose was to identify the clinical use of perioperative denosumab and the factors influencing local recurrence after perioperative denosumab with curettage.

Methods

Patients

We reviewed 158 patients with GCTB treated by curettage without perioperative desnosumab from 2008 to 2010 in institutions participating in the JCOG BSTTSG.

We also reviewed 40 patients with GCTB treated with curettage and perioperative denosumab.

Methods

We performed a questionnaire survey for institutions participating in the BSTTSG in JCOG in April and June 2015. This questionnaire survey was performed for planning a clinical trial of JCOG 1610 (UMIN000029451), a randomized phase III study of preoperative denosumab with curettage for GCTB. We retrospectively reviewed clinical records and filled out the questionnaire. The questionnaire included standard treatments (e.g., local adjuvant, reconstruction) of curettage for GCTB in each institution, details (e.g., number of extremities, Campanacci grade, pathological fracture at presentation, and embolization before surgery) of GCTB treated with curettage from 2008 to 2010, and clinical results (e.g., number of local recurrences, distant recurrences, and death) after the curettage, and details (e.g., sites, Campanacci grade, pathological fracture at presentation, time to the recurrence, final joint preservation, and embolization before surgery) of the patients with local recurrence. We also asked about perioperative use of denosumab for GCTB. The questionnaire included the indications of denosumab for GCTB in each institution, the number of patients treated with preoperative, postoperative, and both pre- and postoperative denosumab, respectively, number of times of perioperative denosumab administration, and clinical results of local recurrence after the perioperative denosumab with curettage. This study was approved by the ethics committee of Nagoya University Graduate School and School of Medicine (Nagoya, Japan) and a waiver of informed consent was provided.

Statistics

A chi-square test was used to analyze the correlation of various clinical factors with recurrence. Clinical factors such as sites (extremity, trunk), Campanacci grade (I, II, III), pathological fracture at presentation (yes, no), timing of denosumab (preoperative only vs postoperative only, both preoperative and postoperative vs preoperative or postoperative, preoperative only vs both preoperative and postoperative, postoperative only vs both preoperative and postoperative), and number of times of denosumab administration ($5>$, $5\leq$) were analyzed as related to the frequency of recurrence. p values of < 0.05 were considered significant. Statistical analysis was done using IBM SPSS Statistics 24.0 software (IBM, Armonk, NY, USA).

Results

Responses to the questionnaire were available from 24 of 30 institutions (80.0%) participating to JCOG BSTTSG. Standard treatments of curettage for GCTB in the 24 institutions are summarized in Table 1. As a local adjuvant

Table 1 Standard treatments with curettage for GCTB[a] in 24 institutions

Treatments	No. of institutions (%)
Local adjuvants	
High-speed burr	22 (92%)
Ethanol	8 (33%)
Liquid nitrogen	6 (25%)
Phenol	3 (13%)
Reconstruction after curettage	
Autologous bone graft	18 (75%)
PMMA[b]	17 (71%)
β-TCP[c]	11 (46%)
Hydroxyapatite	10 (42%)
Allogeneic bone graft	2 (8%)

[a]*GCTB* giant cell tumor of bone
[b]*PMMA*, polymethyl methacrylate
[c]*β-TCP*, β tricalcium phosphate; some of the replies by responded institutions are overlapped

therapy, high-speed burr was used after curettage in 22 of 24 (92%) institutions followed by ethanol (8 of 24 institutions, 33%), liquid nitrogen (6 of 24 institutions, 25%), and phenol (3 of 24 institutions, 13%). Autologous bone graft and polymethyl methacrylate (PMMA) were used for reconstruction after curettage in 18 (75%) and 17 (71%) of 24 institutions, respectively. Characteristics of the patients with GCTB were summarized in Table 2. Primary tumor sites were in an extremity in 151 of 158 (96%) patients and trunk in 7 of 158 (4%). Sixteen of 158

Table 2 Characteristics of patients of GCTB[a] treated with curettage from 2008 to 2010

Characteristics	No. of patients (%)
Primary tumor site	
Extremity	151 (96%)
Trunk	7 (4%)
Campanacci grade	
Grade I	16 (10%)
Grade II	97 (61%)
Grade III	45 (29%)
Pathological fracture at presentation	
Yes	26 (16%)
No	132 (84%)
Do you use denosumab for this case now?	
Yes	83 (52%)
No	75 (48%)
Embolization before surgery	
Yes	8 (5%)
No	150 (95%)

[a]*GCTB*, giant cell tumor of bone

(10%) evaluated as Campanacci grade I, 97 of 158 (61%) as Campanacci grade II, and 45 of 158 (29%) as Campanacci grade III.

Thirty of 158 (19.0%) developed local recurrence, and 4 of 158 (2.5%) developed distant recurrence after curettage without perioperative denosumab. In extremities, 29 of 151 (19.2%) developed local recurrence, and 4 of 151 (2.6%) developed distant recurrence after curettage. There were no deaths after curettage. Campanacci grade and embolization before surgery were significantly associated with an increased incidence of local recurrence after curettage ($p = 0.034$ and $p = 0.022$, respectively) (Table 3). Demographics of local recurrent patients after curettage for GCTB were summarized in Table 4. Local recurrence occurred in 1 of 16 (6.2%) in Campanacci grade I, 15 of 97 (15.5%) in Campanacci grade II, and 14 of 45 (31.1%) in Campanacci grade III. Median time to local recurrence was 15.5 months (5–69 months) after curettage, and joint preservation was achieved in 26 of 30 patients (86.7%).

The indications of denosumab for GCTB at the 24 institutions are summarized in Table 5. As a general policy, denosumab was used perioperatively at 6 of 24 (25%) institutions. Actually, 40 patients were treated with perioperative denosumab in 16 institutions. The number of GCTB patients treated with perioperative denosumab and that of the institutions where they were treated were listed in Table 6. Denosumab was administered subcutaneously

Table 3 Univariate analysis of local recurrence in patients with GCTB[a] treated with curettage from 2008 to 2010. ($n = 158$)

Clinical factors	No. of local recurrence (%)	Univariate analysis p value[b]
Site		
Extremity	29/151 (19.2%)	$p = 0.746$
Trunk	1/7 (14.3%)	
Campanacci grade		
Grade I	1/16 (6.3%)	$p = 0.034$
Grade II	15/97 (15.5%)	
Grade III	14/45 (31.1%)	
Pathological fracture at presentation		
Yes	5/26 (16.7%)	$p = 0.972$
No	25/132 (18.9%)	
Do you use denosumab for this case now?		
Yes	15/83 (18.1%)	$p = 0.758$
No	15/75 (20.0%)	
Embolization before surgery		
Yes	4/8 (50%)	$p = 0.022$
No	26/150 (17.3%)	

[a]*GCTB*, giant cell tumor of bone
[b]Chi-square test

Table 4 Characteristics of local recurrent patients after curettage for GCTB[a] from 2008 to 2010

Sites	Campanacci grade	Pathological fracture at presentation	Time to recurrence (months)	Final joint preservation	Embolization before curettage
Tibia	II	No	25	Possible	No
Femur	II	No	60	Possible	Yes
Metatarsal bone	II	No	60	Impossible	Yes
Femur	III	No	6	Impossible	No
Tibia	III	No	36	Possible	Yes
Tibia	II	No	27	Possible	No
Fibula	II	No	6	Possible	No
Femur	III	No	11	Possible	No
Femur	II	No	28	Possible	No
Ulna	III	No	6	Possible	No
Femur	II	No	9	Possible	No
Tibia	II	No	21	Possible	No
Femur	II	No	24	Impossible	No
Femur	III	No	6	Possible	No
Radius	II	No	6	Impossible	No
Tibia	III	Yes	24	Possible	Yes
Tibia	III	Yes	14	Possible	No
Fibula	II	No	35	Possible	No
Femur	III	Yes	21	Possible	No
Lumbar spine	III	No	60	Not available	No
Femur	II	No	12	Possible	No
Femur	III	Yes	5	Possible	No
Femur	II	No	6	Possible	No
Talus	II	No	12	Possible	No
Femur	III	Yes	30	Possible	No
Femur	III	No	6	Possible	No
Femur	III	No	22	Possible	No
Femur	III	No	7	Possible	No
Femur	II	No	17	Possible	No
Femur	I	No	7	Possible	No

[a]*GCTB*, giant cell tumor of bone

Table 5 Indication of denosumab for GCTB[a] in 24 institutions

Indications of denosumab	No. of institutions (%)
Unresectable	21 (88%)
Difficult to joint preservation	17 (71%)
Expanding to soft tissue	11 (46%)
Adjusting the time of operation	7 (29%)
Perioperative use with curettage	6 (25%)
No experience of denosumab use	3 (13%)

[a]*GCTB*, giant cell tumor of bone; some of the replies by responded institutions are overlapped

at 120 mg, but the dosing interval was not included in the questionnaire. Median number of times of denosumab administration were 6 (2–41) and 6 (1–14) in the preoperative and postoperative settings, respectively. The local recurrences were observed in 6 of 21 (28.6%), 2 of 9 (22.2%), and 0 of 10 (0.0%) patients treated with the preoperative, postoperative, and both preoperative and postoperative denosumab, respectively. In 31 patients treated with any preoperative denosumab, administration exceeding 5 times was significantly associated with a decreased incidence of local recurrence after curettage ($p < 0.001$) (Table 7). Question for toxicity or side effects during perioperative denosumab were not included in the questionnaire survey.

Table 6 No. of patients and institutions treated with perioperative denosumab for GCTB[a]

Timing of perioperative denosumab	No. of patients (%)	No. of institutions (%)
Preoperative only	21 (53%)	10 (63%)
Postoperative only	9 (23%)	5 (31%)
Both pre- and postoperative	10 (25%)	5 (31%)
Total	40	16[*]

[a]GCTB, giant cell tumor of bone
*Some institutions performed denosumab at different timing

Discussion

To plan a clinical trial JCOG 1610, a randomized phase III study of preoperative denosumab with curettage for GCTB, we conducted a questionnaire survey to comprehend the historical clinical results after curettage of GCTB without perioperative denosumab. Although the clinical outcomes after curettage of GCTB have been reported sporadically in Japan [7, 10, 11], the more recent clinical results of GCTB after curettage in multiple institutions in Japan are not as clear. To determine the recent perioperative use in Japan, we also reviewed patients with GCTB

Table 7 Univariate analysis of local recurrence in patients treated with perioperative denosumab and curettage for GCTB[a] (n = 40)

Comparison of factors	No. of local recurrence (%)	Univariate analysis p value[b]
All patients (n = 40)		
Timing of denosumab		
Preoperative only	6/21 (28.6%)	p = 0.719
Postoperative only	2/9 (22.2%)	
Timing of denosumab		
Both pre- and postoperative	0/10 (0.0%)	p = 0.068
Pre- or postoperative only	8/30 (26.7%)	
Preoperative (n = 31)		
Times of denosumab administration		
5>	5/7 (71.4%)	p < 0.001
5≦	1/24 (4.2%)	
Timing of denosumab		
Preoperative only	6/21 (28.6%)	p = 0.060
Both pre- and postoperative	0/10 (18.9%)	
Postoperative (n = 19)		
Times of denosumab administration		
5>	0/7 (0.0%)	p = 0.253
5≦	2/12 (16.7%)	
Embolization before surgery		
Postoperative only	2/9 (22.2%)	p = 0.115
Both pre- and postoperative	0/10 (0.0%)	

[a]GCTB, giant cell tumor of bone
[b]Chi-square test

treated with curettage and perioperative denosumab. Even though denosumab was accepted for health insurance coverage in Japan in 2014, the risk/benefit ratio of denosumab when used for patients with GCTB who are treatable by curettage is not well defined.

There are some limitations in our study. First, because of its questionnaire format, we did not have data regarding the follow-up period after curettage. We investigated GCTB patients treated from 2008 to 2010 and performed this questionnaire survey in 2015, meaning that the follow-up period can be considered adequate given that most recurrences in GCTB occur within 5 years [3–6] and recurrent GCTB is usually treated at the same institution where the first surgery was performed. Second, there was a lack of important data such as size of tumor, detailed sites, and Campanacci grade of GCTB treated with perioperative denosumab, which could act as confounding factors. Because our study is a questionnaire survey, we could not conduct an additional survey due to unlinkable anonymizing of our data. Third, we could not perform multivariate analysis because of the small number of recurrences and lack of information regarding other important clinical factors. Finally, we could not determine whether the patients treated with preoperative denosumab were all suitable for curettage from the time of their initial consultation.

As a local adjuvant therapy, a high-speed burr was used after curettage in 92% of institutions followed by ethanol (33%), liquid nitrogen (25%), and phenol (13%) in our study. Clinical results of these local adjuvant therapies have been reported [3, 5, 9], but it is difficult to determine the advantage of each treatment. Generally, the high-speed burr is easier to use than drug therapies such as ethanol, liquid nitrogen, and phenol, accounting for its extensive use in Japan.

In our study, autologous bone graft and PMMA were used for reconstruction after curettage in 75% and 71% of institutions, respectively. Some reports demonstrated the clinical benefit of PMMA for decreasing local recurrence after curettage of GCTB [3, 4, 6, 9]. Autologous bone graft is widely used in Japan because the lack of a bone bank precludes routine use of allogenic bone.

In our study, the local recurrence rate after curettage was 19.0%. Previous reports showed local recurrence of GCTB in 24.8–30.8% after curettage [3–6], and so our local recurrence rate is slightly better than that documented in these previous reports. Past reports have shown some clinical factors affecting local recurrence such as tumor extension, surgical margin, local adjuvant therapy, Campanacci grade, use of PMMA, and soft tissue progression on multivariate analyses [4, 5, 9]. In our study, Campanacci grade was well balanced similar to previous studies [9, 15], and we ascribe the better local recurrence rate achieved in our study to the wide use of local adjuvant treatments as well as PMMA in many institutions.

In our study, Campanacci grade was significantly associated with increasing incidence of local recurrence after curettage, and this result was similar to that noted in previous studies [4]. Embolization before surgery was also significantly associated with the increasing incidence of local recurrence after curettage, but it was difficult to interpret. Since the embolization is usually used for patients with GCTB which is large and expected bleeding, there was a possibility that these factors had affected the result. However, in the present study, one of the recurrent cases after embolization had GCTB in metatarsal bone (Table 4). Our study included only a small number of cases of GCTB in the trunk and a previous report showed a high local recurrence rate of 43.3% in axial cases after curettage [4]. However, there was no difference in the local recurrence rate between location in the trunk (1 of 7 patients, 14.3%) and extremity (29 of 151 patients, 19.2%) in our study. There was no significant relation between pathological fracture at first visit and local recurrence in our study. A past report also could not demonstrate an effect of pathological fracture on local recurrence in a meta-analysis [16]. Local recurrent GCTB is known to be highly re-recurrent after curettage with rates of re-recurrence of 32 to 34% [17, 18]. Our study included no patients after recurrence, and our analysis was limited to primary tumors. Distant recurrence rate was 2.6% after curettage in our study, and this result was similar to that noted in previous studies [7, 8].

In our study, 16 of 24 (67%) institutions actually performed perioperative use of denosumab with curettage, and the recurrence rates were 6 of 21 (28.6%), 2 of 9 (22.2%), and 0 of 10 (0.0%) with preoperative, postoperative, and both pre- and postoperative treatments with curettage, respectively. One study on the perioperative use of denosumab for GCTB with curettage demonstrated local recurrence in 17 of 116 patients (15%) with a median follow-up period of 13.0 months [19]. However, the study included patients with unresectable GCTB and salvageable GCTB whose surgery was associated with severe morbidity, and the effect of denosumab for patients with GCTB who can be treated by curettage at the first visit was not clear. Our study may have also included some patients who could not be treated by curettage at first, but we could not identify those patients due to the questionnaire format used.

Median numbers of administration times of denosumab were 6 (2–41) and 6 (1–14) in the preoperative and postoperative settings, respectively in our study. Some reports demonstrated histopathological changes after 6 months treatment with denosumab [20, 21], but 6 months are thought to be too long to use it as a post-

and/or preoperative treatment in patients with GCTB which can be treated by curettage. In our study, more than five administration times was significantly associated with a decreased incidence of local recurrence after curettage in 31 patients treated with preoperative or both pre- and postoperative denosumab, meaning that a sufficiently high dose of preoperative denosumab can suppress local recurrence after curettage. When used as a running dose, five times administration of denosumab takes 3 months. This relatively short administration period is associated with major benefits, both economic and social, for patients, and this dose is specified in JCOG1610.

The clinical use of perioperative denosumab is complicated by various issues such as economic problem, side effects, and pregnancy. The cost of one-shot denosumab (120 mg) for GCTB is 46,685 yen (approximately 420 dollar) in Japan as of October 2017. In the previous phase 2 trial of GCTB, denosumab caused diverse side effects such as arthralgia (20%), headache (18%), nausea (17%), fatigue (16%), back pain (15%), extremity pain (15%), hypocalcemia (5%), and osteonecrosis of jaw (1%) of any grade [14]. The use of denosumab for pregnant women should be avoided because it was reported to increase postnatal mortality, decreased body weight gain, and decreased growth/development in a study of infants exposed in utero in cynomolgus monkeys [22]. This may affect the clinical use of denosumab for premenopausal women. In addition, there is a report that denosumab treatment in postmenopausal women with osteoporosis did not interfere with fracture healing [23], but the effects of denosumab on pathological fracture healing and final joint preservation have not been well understood in GCTB patients. Malignant transformation occurs in less than 1% of GCTB [1], and recently, malignant transformation was reported after treatment with denosumab [24] and requires particular caution. In addition, recent study showed a higher rate of recurrence in the GCTB treated with denosumab and curettage compared to historical control without denosumab in retrospective study [25]. For these reasons, perioperative treatment of denosumab should not be done unless an advantage is considered or proved in GCTB which can be treated by curettage.

At present, we have started a clinical trial, JCOG1610 (UMIN000029451), to investigate the efficacy of preoperative denosumab in patients with GCTB which can be treated with curettage. The primary aim of JCOG1610 is to confirm the effects of preoperative denosumab on recurrence after curettage. A previous report demonstrated that proliferation of stromal cells cultured from clinical specimens following denosumab treatment was approximately 50% slower than that of specimens from untreated patients [20]. Even though denosumab did not completely prevent proliferation of stromal cells which have been considered as genuine tumor cells [20], there is a possibility that preoperative denosumab may decrease local and distant recurrences after the curettage of the tumor stromal cells biologically suppressed by denosumab. Secondary endpoints of JCOG1610 include overall survival, joint-preserved survival, local relapse-free survival, metastasis-free survival, adverse events, serious adverse events, surgical and postoperative complications, and discontinuance of denosumab. Systemic denosumab treatment can affect joint-preserved survival, and both local and distant recurrence.

Conclusions

In conclusion, the recurrence rate of GCTB after curettage was 19.0% in Japan and especially high in Campanacci grade III; therefore, improvements in the therapeutic strategy are needed in this cohort. There is a possibility that a sufficient dose of preoperative denosumab can reduce recurrence after curettage. Recently, we have started JCOG1610 to investigate the efficacy of preoperative denosumab in patients with GCTB which can be treated with curettage.

Abbreviations
BSTTSG: Bone and Soft Tissue Tumor Study Group; GCTB: Giant cell tumor of bone; JCOG: Japan clinical oncology group; PMMA: Polymethyl methacrylate; RANK: Receptor activator of NF-κB; RANKL: Receptor activator of NF-κB ligand

Acknowledgements
We thank young researchers in JCOG BSTTSG, Dr. Shintaro Iwata, Dr. Makoto Endo, Dr. Tomoya Matsunobu, Dr. Tomoki Nakamura, Dr. Fumihiko Nakatani, and Dr. Kazuya Oshima for the kind advice regarding this questionnaire survey.

Funding
We do not have a funding for this questionnaire study.

Authors' contributions
HU was involved in the conception and design of the study. TY, SM, TT, KA, MW, AT, NN, YM, AK, TK, TK, ME, HH, HH, ST, YN, TA, TM, MT, AN, HY, KS, MK, and KH were responsible in the acquisition of data and HU in the analysis of data. HU drafted the article, and all authors edited and revised it for important intellectual content. HU, KT, HH, YI, and TO take responsibility for the integrity of the work as a whole, from inception to finished article. All authors approved the final version to be published.

Competing interests
None of the authors have any financial or personal relationships with any other persons or organizations that could potentially and/or inappropriately influence their work and conclusion.

Author details
[1]Department of Orthopaedic Surgery, Nagoya University, 65 Tsurumai, Showa-ku, Nagoya, Aichi 466-8550, Japan. [2]Division of Orthopaedic Surgery, Chiba Cancer Center, Chiba, Japan. [3]Department of Orthopaedic Surgery, Cancer Institute Hospital, Japanese Foundation for Cancer Research, Tokyo, Japan. [4]Department of Orthopaedic Surgery, Juntendo University, Tokyo, Japan. [5]Department of Orthopaedic Surgery, Graduate School of Medicine, Mie University, Tsu, Japan. [6]Department of Orthopaedic Surgery, Tohoku University Hospital, Sendai, Japan. [7]Department of Orthopaedic Surgery, School of Medicine, Yokohama City University, Yokohama, Japan. [8]Musculoskeletal Oncology Service, Osaka International Cancer Institute, Osaka, Japan. [9]Department of Orthopaedic Surgery, Kyushu University, Fukuoka, Japan. [10]Department of Orthopaedic Surgery, National Cancer Center, Tokyo, Japan. [11]Department of Medical Materials for Musculoskeletal Reconstruction, Graduate School of Medicine, Dentistry, and Pharmaceutical Sciences, Okayama University, Okayama, Japan. [12]Department of Orthopaedic Surgery, Hiroshima University, Hiroshima, Japan. [13]Department of Orthopaedic Surgery, Sapporo Medical University, Sapporo, Japan. [14]Department of Orthopaedic Surgery, Hokkaido Cancer Center, Sapporo, Japan. [15]Department of Orthopaedic Surgery, Niigata Cancer Center Hospital, Niigata, Japan. [16]Department of Orthopaedic Surgery, Aichi Cancer Center, Nagoya, Japan. [17]Department of Orthopaedic Surgery, Kobe University, Kobe, Japan. [18]Department of Orthopaedic Surgery, Kyorin University, Mitaka, Japan. [19]Department of Orthopaedic Surgery, Shizuoka Cancer Center, Shizuoka, Japan. [20]Department of Orthopaedic Surgery, Gifu University, Gifu, Japan. [21]Department of Orthopaedic Surgery, Osaka University, Osaka, Japan. [22]Department of Orthopaedic Surgery, Teikyo University, Tokyo, Japan. [23]Department of Orthopaedic Surgery, Oita University, Oita, Japan. [24]Department of Orthopaedic Surgery, Kurume University, Kurume, Japan. [25]Department of Endoprosthetic Surgery, Oita University, Oita, Japan. [26]Kyushu Rosai Hospital, Kitakyushu, Japan. [27]Department of Orthopaedic Surgery, Graduate School of Medicine, Dentistry, and Pharmaceutical Sciences, Okayama University, Okayama, Japan.

References
1.　Fletcher CDM. WHO classification of tumours of soft tissue and bone. 4th ed. Lyon: IARC Press; 2013.
2.　Futamura N, Urakawa H, Tsukushi S, Arai E, Kozawa E, Ishiguro N, Nishida Y. Giant cell tumor of bone arising in long bones possibly originates from the metaphyseal region. Oncol Lett. 2016;11:2629–34.
3.　Balke M, Schremper L, Gebert C, Ahrens H, Streitbuerger A, Koehler G, Hardes J, Gosheger G. Giant cell tumor of bone: treatment and outcome of 214 cases. J Cancer Res Clin Oncol. 2008;134:969–78.
4.　Gaston CL, Bhumbra R, Watanuki M, Abudu AT, Carter SR, Jeys LM, Tillman RM, Grimer RJ. Does the addition of cement improve the rate of local recurrence after curettage of giant cell tumours in bone? J Bone Joint Surg Br. 2011;93:1665–9.
5.　van der Heijden L, van der Geest IC, Schreuder HW, van de Sande MA, Dijkstra PD. Liquid nitrogen or phenolization for giant cell tumor of bone?: a comparative cohort study of various standard treatments at two tertiary referral centers. J Bone Joint Surg Am. 2014;96:e35.
6.　Gao ZH, Yin JQ, Xie XB, Zou CY, Huang G, Wang J, Shen JN. Local control of giant cell tumors of the long bone after aggressive curettage with and without bone cement. BMC Musculoskelet Disord. 2014;15:330.
7.　Masui F, Ushigome S, Fujii K. Giant cell tumor of bone: a clinicopathologic study of prognostic factors. Pathol Int. 1998;48:723–9.
8.　Siebenrock KA, Unni KK, Rock MG. Giant-cell tumour of bone metastasising to the lungs. A long-term follow-up. J Bone Joint Surg Br. 1998;80:43–7.
9.　Arbeitsgemeinschaft K, Becker WT, Dohle J, Bernd L, Braun A, Cserhati M, Enderle A, Hovy L, Matejovsky Z, Szendroi M, et al. Local recurrence of giant cell tumor of bone after intralesional treatment with and without adjuvant therapy. J Bone Joint Surg Am. 2008;90:1060–7.
10.　Muramatsu K, Ihara K, Taguchi T. Treatment of giant cell tumor of long bones: clinical outcome and reconstructive strategy for lower and upper limbs. Orthopedics. 2009;32:491.

11. Oda Y, Miura H, Tsuneyoshi M, Iwamoto Y. Giant cell tumor of bone: oncological and functional results of long-term follow-up. Jpn J Clin Oncol. 1998;28:323–8.

12. Atkins GJ, Haynes DR, Graves SE, Evdokiou A, Hay S, Bouralexis S, Findlay DM. Expression of osteoclast differentiation signals by stromal elements of giant cell tumors. J Bone Miner Res. 2000;15:640–9.

13. Branstetter DG, Nelson SD, Manivel JC, Blay JY, Chawla S, Thomas DM, Jun S, Jacobs I. Denosumab induces tumor reduction and bone formation in patients with giant-cell tumor of bone. Clin Cancer Res. 2012;18:4415–24.

14. Chawla S, Henshaw R, Seeger L, Choy E, Blay JY, Ferrari S, Kroep J, Grimer R, Reichardt P, Rutkowski P, et al. Safety and efficacy of denosumab for adults and skeletally mature adolescents with giant cell tumour of bone: interim analysis of an open-label, parallel-group, phase 2 study. Lancet Oncol. 2013;14:901–8.

15. Campanacci M, Baldini N, Boriani S, Sudanese A. Giant-cell tumor of bone. J Bone Joint Surg Am. 1987;69:106–14.

16. Salunke AA, Chen Y, Chen X, Tan JH, Singh G, Tai BC, Khin LW, Puhaindran ME. Does pathological fracture affect the rate of local recurrence in patients with a giant cell tumour of bone?: a meta-analysis. Bone Joint J. 2015;97-B:1566–71.

17. Takeuchi A, Tsuchiya H, Niu X, Ueda T, Jeon DG, Wang EH, Asavamongkolkul A, Kusuzaki K, Sakayama K, Kang YK. The prognostic factors of recurrent GCT: a cooperative study by the Eastern Asian Musculoskeletal Oncology Group. J Orthop Sci. 2011;16:196–202.

18. Klenke FM, Wenger DE, Inwards CY, Rose PS, Sim FH. Recurrent giant cell tumor of long bones: analysis of surgical management. Clin Orthop Relat Res. 2011;469:1181–7.

19. Rutkowski P, Ferrari S, Grimer RJ, Stalley PD, Dijkstra SP, Pienkowski A, Vaz G, Wunder JS, Seeger LL, Feng A, et al. Surgical downstaging in an open-label phase II trial of denosumab in patients with giant cell tumor of bone. Ann Surg Oncol. 2015;22:2860–8.

20. Mak IW, Evaniew N, Popovic S, Tozer R, Ghert M. A translational study of the neoplastic cells of Giant cell tumor of bone following neoadjuvant denosumab. J Bone Joint Surg Am. 2014;96:e127.

21. Thomas D, Henshaw R, Skubitz K, Chawla S, Staddon A, Blay JY, Roudier M, Smith J, Ye Z, Sohn W, et al. Denosumab in patients with giant-cell tumour of bone: an open-label, phase 2 study. Lancet Oncol. 2010;11:275–80.

22. Bussiere JL, Pyrah I, Boyce R, Branstetter D, Loomis M, Andrews-Cleavenger D, Farman C, Elliott G, Chellman G. Reproductive toxicity of denosumab in cynomolgus monkeys. Reprod Toxicol. 2013;42:27–40.

23. Adami S, Libanati C, Boonen S, Cummings SR, Ho PR, Wang A, Siris E, Lane J, Group FF-HW, Adachi JD, et al. Denosumab treatment in postmenopausal women with osteoporosis does not interfere with fracture-healing: results from the FREEDOM trial. J Bone Joint Surg Am. 2012;94:2113–9.

24. Aponte-Tinao LA, Piuzzi NS, Roitman P, Farfalli GL. A high-grade sarcoma arising in a patient with recurrent benign giant cell tumor of the proximal tibia while receiving treatment with denosumab. Clin Orthop Relat Res. 2015;473:3050–5.

25. Errani C, Tsukamoto S, Leone G, Righi A, Akahane M, Tanaka Y, Donati DM. Denosumab may increase the risk of local recurrence in patients with giant-cell tumor of bone treated with curettage. J Bone Joint Surg Am. 2018;100:496–504.

11

Review of the possible association between thyroid and breast carcinoma

Liangbo Dong, Jun Lu, Bangbo Zhao, Weibin Wang* and Yupei Zhao*

Abstract

Background: Thyroid and breast cancer are two of the malignant diseases with highest incidence in females. Based on clinical experience, breast and thyroid cancer often occur metachronously or synchronously. Therefore, thyroid and breast cancer might share some common etiological factors. The relationship between these diseases has attracted substantial attention, and because these two glands are both regulated by the hypothalamic-pituitary axis, such a relationship is not surprising. A study of this relationship will be useful for obtaining a better understanding of the mechanism by which these two malignancies co-occur.

Main body: This study reviewed the progress in research on the roles of iodine intake, folate metabolism, obesity, gonadal hormones, and thyroid hormone in thyroid and breast cancer. These studies evaluating the etiological roles of these factors in linking breast and thyroid cancer might also improve our understanding and identify new therapeutic approaches, such as sodium/iodide symporter-mediated radioiodine therapy and thyroid-stimulating hormone receptor antagonists, for breast cancer. In addition, some specific treatments for each cancer, such as radiotherapy for breast cancer or radioactive iodine therapy for thyroid cancer, might be risk factors for secondary malignances, including breast and thyroid cancer.

Conclusions: Studies of the precise relationship between the co-occurrence of breast and thyroid cancer will certainly improve our understanding of the biological behaviors of these two malignancies and direct evidence-based clinical practice.

Keywords: Thyroid cancer, Breast cancer, Iodine, Sodium iodide symporter, Thyroid hormone, Thyroid hormone receptor, Gonadal hormone, Obesity, Radioactive iodide therapy

Background

The thyroid and mammary glands are both regulated by the hypothalamic-pituitary axis. Based on clinical experience, patients were diagnosed with breast and thyroid cancer metachronously or synchronously more frequently than expected by accident. However, their mechanisms of action remain unknown. Are these two common malignancies in women related? Several studies have detected a possible association between these malignancies. Jee Hyun An, Yul Hwangbo, et al. carried out a retrospective case-control study that suggested that the overall risk of second primary thyroid cancer (TC) or breast cancer (BC) is significantly increased in patients who previously had BC or TC, respectively [1]. Previous studies have also

confirmed this finding [2–5]. As the genesis and development of TC and BC are associated, researchers must investigate the causes of these types of multiple primary tumors (MPTs). This study reviewed the recent progress in research on the roles of iodine intake, folate metabolism, obesity, gonadal hormones, thyroid hormone, and signaling pathways in thyroid and breast cancer.

Iodide

Iodide, iodine transport, and breast cancer

There is overlap between TC and BC regarding the uptake and utilization of dietary iodine. Several studies have focused on the role of iodine in BC. Hypothyroidism and low iodine intake may be important preventable etiological factors in estrogen-dependent tumors of the breast, uterus, and ovary. Iodine supplementation may lead to a decreased incidence of these cancers in future generations. The sodium/iodine symporter (NIS), a large integral

* Correspondence: wwb_xh@163.com; zhao8028@263.net
Department of General Surgery, Peking Union Medical College Hospital, Chinese Academy of Medical Science and Peking Union Medical College, Beijing 100730, People's Republic of China

plasma membrane glycoprotein that mediates iodide up-take, is expressed at its highest levels in the thyroid and lactating breast [6–8]. Over 40 years ago, BC tissues were shown to take up radioactive iodine; in contrast, uptake does not occur in normal, non-lactating breast tissues [9]. 25 years later, NIS mRNA was first detected in breast cancer specimens [10]. In 2001, Moon DH, Lee SH, et al. studied the correlation between the expression of the human NIS mRNA and the uptake of 99mTc-pertechnetate in 25 breast tumors. However, compared with NIS mRNA expression, the level of iodide uptake was relatively low [11]. Later, in 2003, the NIS protein was shown to be predominantly expressed in the intracellular space, whereas NIS in lactating mammary glands is located on the basolateral membrane [6]. Therefore, researchers have hypothesized that the mislocalization of NIS protein may lead to the disparity between the NIS expression level and observed radioiodide uptake. Based on endocrinological studies, iodine deficiency may stimulate the gonadotrophin secretion and then result in a hyperestrogenic state, which possesses characteristics of relatively high production of estrone and estradiol and a relatively low estriol to estrone and estradiol ratio. This alteration in endocrine state may increase the risk of BC [12]. In addition, strategies that increase dietary iodine intake may reduce the risk of BC [13] (Fig. 1). Conversely, excess iodide intake also plays an unfavorable role in BC by

stimulating ER-α transcriptional activity [14]. Malya FU et al. reported a high urine-iodine concentration (UIC) in a significantly larger portion of BC patients than controls [15]. Others have also indicated that NIS can be used as an objective criterion for predicting the sensitivity of luminal B and basal BC subtypes to neoadjuvant chemotherapy, which will improve treatment outcomes in this group of patients [16].

Iodine, iodide transport, and thyroid cancer

Iodine deficiency is a well-established risk factor for the development of TC, [17] and iodine supplementation has been carried out in most areas with endemic goiter. Chronic iodine deficiency may have some protective effects on females, but no equivalent studies have detected its effect on males [18]. As shown in the study by Anne-Catherine Gerard et al., iodine deficiency induces the expression of the vascular endothelial growth factor (VEGF) mRNA in both normal thyroid cells and TC cells. This effect lasts longer in thyroid carcinoma cell lines, suggesting impairment of downregulation mechanism. Moreover, the iodine deficiency-induced VEGF expression partially depends on hypoxia-inducible factor-1 (HIF-1) instead of on reactive oxygen species. Thus, iodine deficiency may provide an angiogenic environment for abnormal proliferation of TC cells [19]. By contrast,

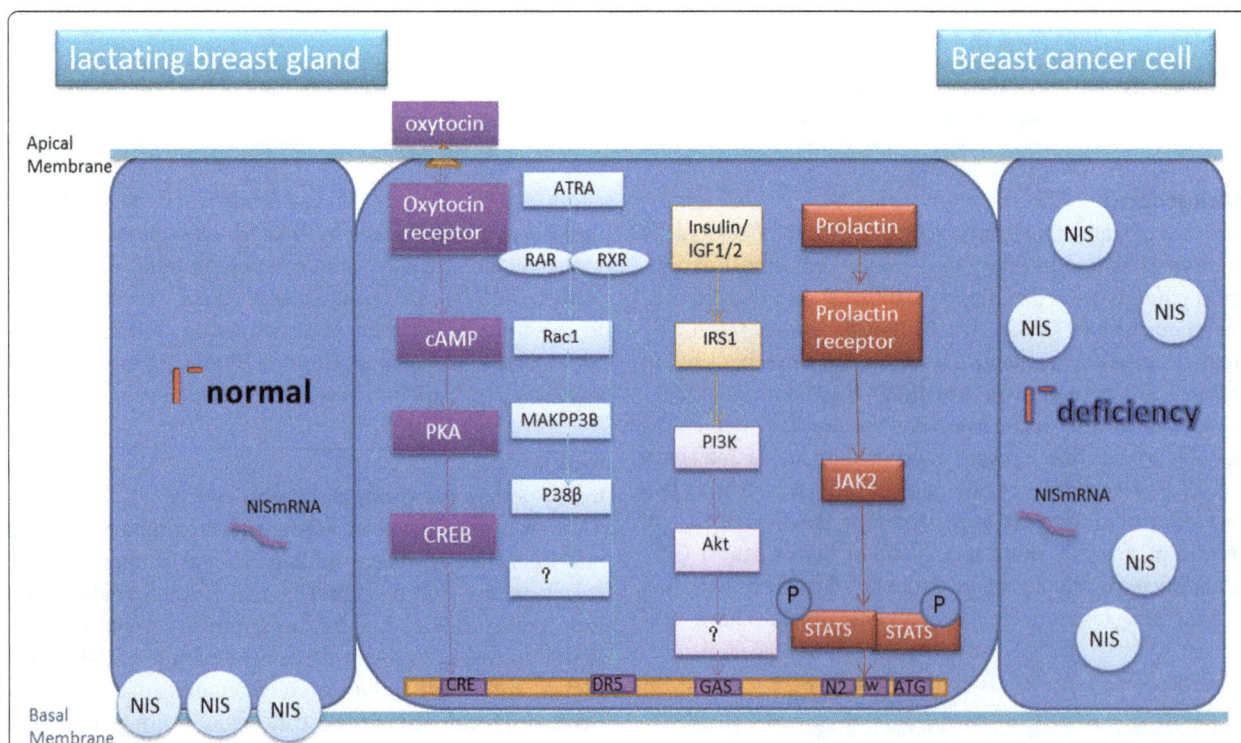

Fig. 1 Regulation and expression of the NIS gene in breast cancer. In breast cancer cells, the NIS protein is predominantly expressed in the intracellular space, whereas the protein is located on the basolateral membrane in lactating mammary glands. Mislocalization of the NIS protein may lead to a disparity between the NIS expression level and observed radioiodide uptake

excess iodine has also been connected with an increased incidence of papillary thyroid cancer (PTC). After the implementation of universal salt iodization in China in 1996, the incidence of goiter was reduced by almost 50%; however, the incidence of TC is steadily increasing [20]. Haixia Guan from Johns Hopkins Hospital and others have focused on this issue and initiated a study measuring and comparing the mutation of the T1799A BRAF in 1032 patients from five regions in China with different levels of iodine intake. As high iodine intake contributes to the occurrence of the T1799A BRAF gene mutation, it may be a risk factor for the development of PTC [21]. According to a cross-sectional study from South China, the mean UIC, an index for evaluating the nutritional status of a population, is significantly higher in patients with thyroid nodules than in healthy individuals; of these thyroid nodules, approximately 5–15% were malignant, i.e., TC [22]. However, the conclusive link between excess iodide and TC remains unclear. Others also believe that this increase in the incidence is mainly due to advances in diagnostic technology.

In conclusion, dietary iodide deficiency and intracellular iodide deficiency caused by mislocalization of NIS may play a role in the carcinogenesis of TC and BC. Iodine deficiency may cause DNA damage in the thyroid gland and promote cancer [23]. Moreover, studies on the role of iodide in BC provide promising therapeutic approaches. For instance, NIS-mediated radioiodine therapy for estrogen receptor-negative BC has been studied in more detail [24], and Kelkar MG recently reported that histone deacetylase inhibitors (HDACis) as modulators of NIS expression can significantly increase NIS expression but do not alter its intracellular localization. Thus, there is a promising future for NIS-mediated radioiodine therapy [25]. Kelkar MG, first highlighted the role of p53 as a negative transcriptional regulator of human functional NIS gene expression in BC, providing important perspectives into the promising clinical use of NIS-mediated radioiodine therapy, which may significantly impact a patient with a mutant versus wild-type p53 profile [26].

Sex hormones, reproductive factors, and thyroid cancer

Hormones induce oncogenesis by promoting cell proliferation, an essential component of carcinogenesis. In addition, their important roles have been well studied in BC and prostate cancers [27]. TC exhibits a great gender disparity; it is 2.9-fold more common in women than in men. A significant difference between men and women is their sex hormones and the influences of these hormones on multiple organs and systems. The fluctuating levels of sex hormones during a woman's menstrual cycle and pregnancy have been hypothesized to be the root cause of the gender disparity in PTC [28]. Because

TC is highly prevalent in fertile women, hormonal and reproductive factors may also be involved in its incidence [29]. As shown in the 1993 study by Inoue et al., estradiol increases proliferation of estrogen receptor (ER)-positive PTC, supporting the hypothesis that estrogen promotes the proliferation of this type of disease [30]. Estradiol also alters the expression of estrogen receptor subtypes in TC cell lines [31–33]. Guia et al. investigated the expression of estrogen receptor α (ERα) and progesterone receptor (PR) in female and male patients with PTC and connected their levels with the clinical manifestation and molecular features. ERα and PR were detected in 66.5 and 75.8% of cases, respectively. Their expression significantly relates to a larger tumor size and higher prevalence of local metastases. Furthermore, the "receptor conversion" (variation in receptor status in primary and metastatic BC) phenomenon was first observed in thyroid cancer and has subsequently been reported in BC [29]. Estrogen promotes growth through classical genomic and non-genomic pathways, which are mediated via the membrane-bound ER. This receptor is correlated to the Aurora-like serine/threonine kinase (APK) and phosphoinositol 3-kinase (PI3K) tyrosine kinase signaling pathways. However, in contrast to other carcinomas, detailed information about this regulatory mechanism has not been reported for TC [34]. As shown in the study by Rajoria et al., estrogen is associated with increased adherence, invasion, and migration of TC cell lines. Thus, the higher occurrence rate of TC in women could possibly due to the expression of a functional ER, which participates in cellular processes that contribute to the enhanced mitogenic, migratory, and invasive potential of thyroid cells. These findings will promote the future development of anti-estrogenic therapies targeting neoplasm invasion and migration, thus reducing the tendency to metastasize [35]. Membrane-bound ER is linked to the mitogen-activated protein kinase (MAPK) and PI3K tyrosine kinase signaling pathways, and in PTC, these pathways may be activated by either chromosomal rearrangement of the tyrosine receptor kinase (TRKA), RET/PTC genes, or a BRAF mutation. Additionally, these pathways may be stimulated by high estrogen levels in females. Furthermore, estrogen regulates angiogenesis and metastasis, which are crucial to the outcomes of TC [34].

Thyroid hormones (THs), TH receptor β1 (TRβ1), antibodies, and breast cancer
THs

Thyroid hormones exert diverse critical biological effects on the growth, differentiation, metabolism, and physiological function of almost all human tissues, including the mammary gland [36, 37]. However, the correlation between thyroid function and BC is uncertain. Søgaard M, Farkas

DK, et al. conducted a nationwide cohort study, which included 61,873 women with hypothyroidism and 80,343 women with hyperthyroidism, in which the women with hyperthyroidism had greater risk of developing BC, and the women with hypothyroidism had a slightly decreased incidence of BC [38]. By evaluating a large cohort of women, Journy NMY et al. also reported that the risk of BC mortality elevated in women with hyperthyroidism with hyperthyroidism after 60 years of age [39]. Others have already focused on the mechanism underlying this phenomenon. As reported in the study by Moretto FC, De Sibio MT, et al., triiodothyronine (T3) may induce the expression of HIF-1 and transform growth factor alpha (TGF) in the MCF7 breast cancer cell line. These factors are related to the genesis and development of BC. Moreover, thiiodothyronine (T3) exerts this effect by activating PI3K [40]. As shown in the 2002 study by Sumi Dinda et al., T3 may regulate the cell cycle progression and proliferation of T47D cells (an estrogen-responsive human ductal carcinoma cell line that expresses detectable levels of ER) by increasing the p53 levels and inducing pRb hyperphosphorylation via a common mechanism involving the ER and T3 receptor-mediated pathways [41]. Additionally, Hall LC et al. supported this hypothesis and reported that T3 induced activation of ER-mediated gene expression and promoted the proliferation of MCF7 cells. Although the effects were weaker than those induced by E2, T3 may play roles in BC development and progression [42]. In the 2010 study by Tosovic A et al., the T3 levels were shown to be positively and dose-dependently related to the BC risk in postmenopausal women [43]. The 2005 study by P.P. Saraiva also supported the above conclusion that high T3 levels in postmenopausal women are positively and dose-dependently correlated with the risk of BC. However, this situation was observed in postmenopausal women who had a significant increase in their thyroid/estradiol ratio. These phenomena may suggest that the imbalance between E2 and T3 promotes the genesis and development of BC [44]. In contrast, hypothyroidism has been associated with a decreased risk of BC [45]. However, the association between TH and BC is currently controversial, and conclusive evidence is lacking. In a study by Johannes LP et al., hypothyroidism and low-normal free T4 (FT4) levels were reported to be correlated to an increased risk of BC in postmenopausal women [46]. Overall, further studies are needed to investigate the precise association between thyroid function and BC.

TR

TR belongs to the nuclear hormone receptor superfamily, similar to classical biomarkers of BC, such as ER and PR. Its exact role in the genesis and progression of BC has been known for years. Several scientists investigated this question in 2014. As demonstrated in the study by Sobine Heublein, Doris Mayr, et al., TRs may be an interesting biomarker and prognostic factor for patients with BRCA1-associated BC. TRβ positivity may be positively related to the five-year or overall survival of BC patients, whereas TRα has opposing actions [47]. Jeon won Park et al. studied the mutation of TRβ, which is considered to have oncogenic activity. According to previous studies, TRβ1 may function as a tumor suppressor. However, TRβ1 expression is silenced by several mechanisms, such as hypermethylation of the promoter region and a microRNA-mediated regulatory mechanism. Additionally, TRβ1 mutations also cause it to lose its tumor suppressor function. In addition to the C-terminal frameshift mutation PV, some additional sequences in the C-terminal regions of TRβ1, such as Mkar, Mdbs, and AM, also exhibit oncogenic activity, promoting cell proliferation and suppressing differentiation and apoptosis [48]. Some researchers in China have reported that aberrant TRβ1 expression and mutations are associated with the genesis and development of BC in the Chinese population [49]. Nonetheless, the exact role of TR in the genesis of BC remains unclear. Further studies are needed to identify a new biomarker of BC and new strategies for developing targeted therapy.

As discussed above, altered TH function and dysfunction of TR contribute to the increased incidence of BC. Other factors, such as autoimmune antibodies, may also play a role in its genesis [50]. Autoimmune thyroid diseases, such as Graves' disease, are characterized by increased levels of thyroid peroxidase antibodies (TPOAbs) and thyroglobulin antibodies (TgAbs). These two autoimmune antibodies have a well-established association with BC. In addition, Pawel S. et al. in 2013 showed the TSH receptor (TSHR) antibody to be a positive determinant of BC and the only positive determinant in the analysis of age-matched patients. Thus, TSHR antagonists may potentially play a prophylactic role in BC, and additional clinical research is advisable [51].

Others

The genesis and development of both TC and BC are quite complicated. Some other factors may play a role in the co-existence of TC and BC. Radioactive iodine therapy is a routine therapy for differentiated TC in Western countries, and it is increasingly being used in China. As mentioned above, mammary gland cells also express NIS, thus, the breast tissue may also absorb radioactive iodine, and the absorption of a high dose of radioactive substances may induce carcinogenesis [52]. The results of a retrospective single-center study in Portugal suggest that the risk of developing second primary cancer is increased after radioactive iodine therapy, particularly for activities > 200 mCi [53]. However, because of the lack of statistics, this hypothesis requires further support.

Additionally, in a 2015 long-term follow-up study, radio-active iodine (RAI) therapy did not significantly increase the occurrence and recurrence of subsequent BC [54]. In 2015, Zhang YJ et al. from Peking Union Medical College conducted a meta-analysis that included 6 co-hort studies, involving 17,914 patients. The results sug-gested that the risk of secondary primary BC in TC survivors treated with RAI did not increase compared with TC survivors not treated with RAI [55]. Folate me-tabolism, which plays an essential role in DNA synthesis, is another important aspect of carcinogenesis, and it was recently shown to be involved in the increased incidence of TC and BC. As shown in a study by Zara-Lopes T, an alteration in the methylenetetrahydrofolate reductase (MTHFR) gene that participates in folate metabolism, C677T, is significantly associated with the increased inci-dence of thyroid and breast cancer. These factors may be used as potential predictive and prognostic markers for both types of cancer [56]. Obesity and a higher can-cer risk have a well-established, strong association; weight, weight gain, and obesity are responsible for ap-proximately 20% of all malignant neoplasms. TC and BC are no exception [57]. A 2016 study in Korea reported a positive association between a high body mass index (BMI) and TC incidence, and prevention efforts, such as weight gain control, may reduce the burden of TC [58]. Yunji Hwang et al. conducted a large-scale case-control study and suggested that middle-aged adults who gain weight have a higher risk of developing PTC. Although this study has some limitations, such as recall and detec-tion bias, the results still suggest that weight gain con-trol can decrease the incidence of TC [59]. A study in France also supported this hypothesis. Clavel-Chapelon F et al. identified a significant dose-dependent associ-ation between the risk of developing TC and BMI, par-ticularly in women who gained weight from menarche to adulthood [60]. Meanwhile, the role of obesity or a high BMI in the development of breast cancer has been well-known for years [61, 62]. Moreover, weight loss in-terventions are recommended for patients with BC [63].

Conclusions

In summary, the etiologies of thyroid and mammary gland cancers share common features, such as iodine intake and transport and the levels of thyroid function, TH receptors, obesity, and sex hormones. Factors that contribute to the initiation of TC, such as low dietary iodine, hypothyroidism, and other thyroid disorders, may also contribute to the in-creased risk of BC. Some factors, such as estrogen and re-productive factors that play well-established roles in BC initiation, may be associated with TC. These studies may help to explain why these two cancers occur metachro-nously or synchronously more frequently than would be ex-pected by chance. Moreover, studies on the commonalities

between these two cancers may provide new prophylactic therapeutic strategies and early diagnostic methods, such as anti-estrogen therapy for thyroid carcinoma and anti-TSHR therapy for breast carcinoma. Although further theoretical and clinical studies are still needed before these treatments are applied in the clinic, future clinical applications are promising. The precise relationship between the co-occurrence of breast and thyroid cancer remains contro-versial and inconclusive, yet studies of their co-occurrence will certainly improve our understanding of the biological behaviors of these two malignancies and direct evidence-based clinical practice.

Abbreviations
BC: Breast cancer; MPTs: Multiple primary tumors; NIS: Sodium/iodide symporter; PTC: Papillary thyroid cancer; TC: Thyroid cancer; TH: Thyroid hormone; TRβ1: TH receptor β1; TSH: Thyroid stimulating hormone; TSHR: Thyroid-stimulating hormone receptor

Funding
The Research Special Fund for the Public Welfare Industry of Health (The Translational Research of Early Diagnosis and Comprehensive Treatment in Pancreatic Cancer, 201202007).

Authors' contributions
LD, JL, and BZ wrote the paper. YZ and WW were involved in reviewing and editing the manuscript. All authors read and approved the final manuscript.

Authors' information
Zhao Yupei, male, is an academician of the Chinese Academy of Sciences, chief surgeon, 18 and 19 central alternate member, vice chairman of the China Association for Science and Technology, deputy director of the Central Health Committee, Peking Union Medical College Hospital, and vice president of the Chinese Medical Association. He has been working in the front-line of clinical work, scientific research and teaching in general surgery. He has won the second prize of national science and technology progress.

Competing interests
The authors declare that they have no competing interests.

References
1. An JH, Hwangbo Y, Ahn HY, Keam B, Lee KE, Han W, Park do J, Park IA, Noh DY, Youn YK, et al. A possible association between thyroid cancer and breast cancer. Thyroid. 2015;25:1330–8.
2. Brown AP, Chen J, Hitchcock YJ, Szabo A, Shrieve DC, Tward JD. The risk of second primary malignancies up to three decades after the treatment of differentiated thyroid cancer. J Clin Endocrinol Metab. 2008;93:504–15.
3. Subramanian S, Goldstein DP, Parlea L, Thabane L, Ezzat S, Ibrahim-Zada I, Straus S, Brierley JD, Tsang RW, Gafni A, et al. Second primary malignancy risk in thyroid cancer survivors: a systematic review and meta-analysis. Thyroid. 2007;17:1277–88.
4. Tanaka H, Tsukuma H, Koyama H, Kinoshita Y, Kinoshita N, Oshima A. Second primary cancers following breast cancer in the Japanese female population. Jpn J Cancer Res. 2001;92:1–8.

5.   Evans HS, Lewis CM, Robinson D, Bell CM, Moller H, Hodgson SV. Incidence of multiple primary cancers in a cohort of women diagnosed with breast cancer in Southeast England. Br J Cancer. 2001;84:435–40.

6.   Wapnir IL, van de Rijn M, Nowels K, Amenta PS, Walton K, Montgomery K, Greco RS, Dohan O, Carrasco N. Immunohistochemical profile of the sodium/iodide symporter in thyroid, breast, and other carcinomas using high density tissue microarrays and conventional sections. J Clin Endocrinol Metab. 2003;88:1880–8.

7.   Tazebay UH, Wapnir IL, Levy O, Dohan O, Zuckier LS, Zhao QH, Deng HF, Amenta PS, Fineberg S, Pestell RG, Carrasco N. The mammary gland iodide transporter is expressed during lactation and in breast cancer. Nat Med. 2000;6:871–8.

8.   Cho JY, Leveille R, Kao R, Rousset B, Parlow AF, Burak WE Jr, Mazzaferri EL, Jhiang SM. Hormonal regulation of radioiodide uptake activity and Na+/I-symporter expression in mammary glands. J Clin Endocrinol Metab. 2000;85:2936–43.

9.   Eskin BA, Parker JA, Bassett JG, George DL. Human breast uptake of radioactive iodine. Obstet Gynecol. 1974;44:398–402.

10. Kilbane MT, Ajjan RA, Weetman AP, Dwyer R, McDermott EW, O'Higgins NJ, Smyth PP. Tissue iodine content and serum-mediated 125I uptake-blocking activity in breast cancer. J Clin Endocrinol Metab. 2000;85:1245–50.

11. Moon DH, Lee SJ, Park KY, Park KK, Ahn SH, Pai MS, Chang H, Lee HK, Ahn IM. Correlation between 99mTc-pertechnetate uptakes and expressions of human sodium iodide symporter gene in breast tumor tissues. Nucl Med Biol. 2001;28:829–34.

12. Rappaport J. Changes in dietary iodine explains increasing incidence of breast Cancer with distant involvement in young women. J Cancer. 2017;8:174–7.

13. Smyth PP. The thyroid, iodine and breast cancer. Breast Cancer Res. 2003;5:235–8.

14. He S, Wang B, Lu X, Miao S, Yang F, Zava T, Ding Q, Zhang S, Liu J, Zava D, Shi YE. Iodine stimulates estrogen receptor singling and its systemic level is increased in surgical patients due to topical absorption. Oncotarget. 2018;9:375–84.

15. Malya FU, Kadioglu H, Hasbahceci M, Dolay K, Guzel M, Ersoy YE. The correlation between breast cancer and urinary iodine excretion levels. J Int Med Res. 2018;46:687–92.

16. Chekhun VF, Andriiv AV, Lukianova NY. Significance of iodine symporter for prognosis of the disease course and efficacy of neoadjuvant chemotherapy in patients with breast cancer of luminal and basal subtypes. Exp Oncol. 2017;39:65–8.

17. Franceschi S. Iodine intake and thyroid carcinoma–a potential risk factor. Exp Clin Endocrinol Diabetes. 1998;106(Suppl 3):S38–44.

18. Zimmermann MB, Galetti V. Iodine intake as a risk factor for thyroid cancer: a comprehensive review of animal and human studies. Thyroid Res. 2015;8:8.

19. Gerard AC, Humblet K, Wilvers C, Poncin S, Derradji H, de Ville de Goyet C, Abou-el-Ardat K, Baatout S, Sonveaux P, Denef JF, Colin IM. Iodine-deficiency-induced long lasting angiogenic reaction in thyroid cancers occurs via a vascular endothelial growth factor-hypoxia inducible factor-1-dependent, but not a reactive oxygen species-dependent, pathway. Thyroid. 2012;22:699–708.

20. Zhao W, Han C, Shi X, Xiong C, Sun J, Shan Z, Teng W. Prevalence of goiter and thyroid nodules before and after implementation of the universal salt iodization program in mainland China from 1985 to 2014: a systematic review and meta-analysis. PLoS One. 2014;9:e109549.

21. Guan H, Ji M, Bao R, Yu H, Wang Y, Hou P, Zhang Y, Shan Z, Teng W, Xing M. Association of high iodine intake with the T1799A BRAF mutation in papillary thyroid cancer. J Clin Endocrinol Metab. 2009;94:1612–7.

22. Zhao H, Tian Y, Liu Z, Li X, Feng M, Huang T. Correlation between iodine intake and thyroid disorders: a cross-sectional study from the south of China. Biol Trace Elem Res. 2014;162:87–94.

23. Maier J, van Steeg H, van Oostrom C, Paschke R, Weiss RE, Krohn K. Iodine deficiency activates antioxidant genes and causes DNA damage in the thyroid gland of rats and mice. Biochim Biophys Acta. 2007;1773:990–9.

24. Yao C, Pan Y, Li Y, Xu X, Lin Y, Wang W, Wang S. Effect of sodium/iodide symporter (NIS)-mediated radioiodine therapy on estrogen receptor-negative breast cancer. Oncol Rep. 2015;34:59–66.

25. Kelkar MG, Senthilkumar K, Jadhav S, Gupta S, Ahn BC, De A. Enhancement of human sodium iodide symporter gene therapy for breast cancer by HDAC inhibitor mediated transcriptional modulation. Sci Rep. 2016;6:19341.

26. Kelkar MG, Thakur B, Derle A, Chatterjee S, Ray P, De A. Tumor suppressor protein p53 exerts negative transcriptional regulation on human sodium iodide symporter gene expression in breast cancer. Breast Cancer Res Treat. 2017;164:603–15.

27. Pathak DR, Osuch JR, He J. Breast carcinoma etiology: current knowledge and new insights into the effects of reproductive and hormonal risk factors in black and white populations. Cancer. 2000;88:1230–8.

28. Rahbari R, Zhang L, Kebebew E. Thyroid cancer gender disparity. Future Oncol. 2010;6:1771–9.

29. Vannucchi G, De Leo S, Perrino M, Rossi S, Tosi D, Cirello V, Colombo C, Bulfamante G, Vicentini L, Fugazzola L. Impact of estrogen and progesterone receptor expression on the clinical and molecular features of papillary thyroid cancer. Eur J Endocrinol. 2015;173:29–36.

30. Inoue H, Oshimo K, Miki H, Kawano M, Monden Y. Immunohistochemical study of estrogen receptors and the responsiveness to estrogen in papillary thyroid carcinoma. Cancer. 1993;72:1364–8.

31. Lee ML, Chen GG, Vlantis AC, Tse GM, Leung BC, van Hasselt CA. Induction of thyroid papillary carcinoma cell proliferation by estrogen is associated with an altered expression of Bcl-xL. Cancer J. 2005;11:113–21.

32. Zeng Q, Chen GG, Vlantis AC, van Hasselt CA. Oestrogen mediates the growth of human thyroid carcinoma cells via an oestrogen receptor-ERK pathway. Cell Prolif. 2007;40:921–35.

33. Zeng Q, Chen G, Vlantis A, Tse G, van Hasselt C. The contributions of oestrogen receptor isoforms to the development of papillary and anaplastic thyroid carcinomas. J Pathol. 2008;214:425–33.

34. Derwahl M, Nicula D. Estrogen and its role in thyroid cancer. Endocr Relat Cancer. 2014;21:T273–83.

35. Rajoria S, Suriano R, Shanmugam A, Wilson YL, Schantz SP, Geliebter J, Tiwari RK. Metastatic phenotype is regulated by estrogen in thyroid cells. Thyroid. 2010;20:33–41.

36. Cheng SY, Leonard JL, Davis PJ. Molecular aspects of thyroid hormone actions. Endocr Rev. 2010;31:139–70.

37. Yen PM. Physiological and molecular basis of thyroid hormone action. Physiol Rev. 2001;81:1097–142.

38. Sogaard M, Farkas DK, Ehrenstein V, Jorgensen JO, Dekkers OM, Sorensen HT. Hypothyroidism and hyperthyroidism and breast cancer risk: a nationwide cohort study. Eur J Endocrinol. 2016;174:409–14.

39. Journy NMY, Bernier MO, Doody MM, Alexander BH, Linet MS, Kitahara CM. Hyperthyroidism, hypothyroidism, and cause-specific mortality in a large cohort of women. Thyroid. 2017;27:1001–10.

40. Moretto FC, De Sibio MT, Luvizon AC, Olimpio RM, de Oliveira M, Alves CA, Conde SJ, Nogueira CR. Triiodothyronine (T3) induces HIF1A and TGFA expression in MCF7 cells by activating PI3K. Life Sci. 2016;154:52–7.

41. Dinda S, Sanchez A, Moudgil V. Estrogen-like effects of thyroid hormone on the regulation of tumor suppressor proteins, p53 and retinoblastoma, in breast cancer cells. Oncogene. 2002;21:761–8.

42. Hall LC, Salazar EP, Kane SR, Liu N. Effects of thyroid hormones on human breast cancer cell proliferation. J Steroid Biochem Mol Biol. 2008;109:57–66.

43. Tosovic A, Bondeson AG, Bondeson L, Ericsson UB, Malm J, Manjer J. Prospectively measured triiodothyronine levels are positively associated with breast cancer risk in postmenopausal women. Breast Cancer Res. 2010;12:R33.

44. Saraiva PP, Figueiredo NB, Padovani CR, Brentani MM, Nogueira CR. Profile of thyroid hormones in breast cancer patients. Braz J Med Biol Res. 2005;38:761–5.

45. Cristofanilli M, Yamamura Y, Kau SW, Bevers T, Strom S, Patangan M, Hsu L, Krishnamurthy S, Theriault RL, Hortobagyi GN. Thyroid hormone and breast carcinoma. Primary hypothyroidism is associated with a reduced incidence of primary breast carcinoma. Cancer. 2005;103:1122–8.

46. Kuijpens JL, Nyklictek I, Louwman MW, Weetman TA, Pop VJ, Coebergh JW. Hypothyroidism might be related to breast cancer in post-menopausal women. Thyroid. 2005;15:1253–9.

47. Heublein S, Mayr D, Meindl A, Angele M, Gallwas J, Jeschke U, Ditsch N. Thyroid hormone receptors predict prognosis in BRCA1 associated breast Cancer in opposing ways. PLoS One. 2015;10:e0127072.

48. Park JW, Zhao L, Willingham M, Cheng SY. Oncogenic mutations of thyroid hormone receptor beta. Oncotarget. 2015;6:8115–31.

49. Ling Y, Ling X, Fan L, Wang Y, Li Q. Mutation analysis underlying the downregulation of the thyroid hormone receptor beta1 gene in the Chinese breast cancer population. Onco Targets Ther. 2015;8:2967–72.

50. Jiskra J, Limanova Z, Barkmanova J, Smutek D, Friedmannova Z. Autoimmune thyroid diseases in women with breast cancer and colorectal cancer. Physiol Res. 2004;53:693–702.

51. Szychta P, Szychta W, Gesing A, Lewinski A, Karbownik-Lewinska M. TSH receptor antibodies have predictive value for breast cancer - retrospective analysis. Thyroid Res. 2013;6:8.
52. Goldman MB, Maloof F, Monson RR, Aschengrau A, Cooper DS, Ridgway EC. Radioactive iodine therapy and breast cancer. A follow-up study of hyperthyroid women. Am J Epidemiol. 1988;127:969–80.
53. Silva-Vieira M, Carrilho Vaz S, Esteves S, Ferreira TC, Limbert E, Salgado L, Leite V. Second primary Cancer in patients with differentiated thyroid cancer: does radioiodine play a role? Thyroid. 2017;27:1068–76.
54. Ahn HY, Min HS, Yeo Y, Ma SH, Hwang Y, An JH, Choi HS, Keam B, Im SA, Park do J, et al. Radioactive iodine therapy did not significantly increase the incidence and recurrence of subsequent breast Cancer. J Clin Endocrinol Metab. 2015;100:3486–93.
55. Zhang Y, Liang J, Li H, Cong H, Lin Y. Risk of second primary breast cancer after radioactive iodine treatment in thyroid cancer: a systematic review and meta-analysis. Nucl Med Commun. 2016;37:110–5.
56. Zara-Lopes T, Gimenez-Martins AP, Nascimento-Filho CH, et al. Role of MTHFR C677T and MTR A2756G polymorphisms in thyroid and breast cancer development [J]. Genet Mol Res. 2016;15(2).
57. Wolin KY, Carson K, Colditz GA. Obesity and cancer. Oncologist. 2010;15: 556–65.
58. Shin HY, Yong HJ, Cho ER. Body mass index and incidence of thyroid cancer in Korea: the Korean cancer prevention study-II. J Cancer Res Clin Oncol. 2016; 143(1):1–7.
59. Hwang Y, Lee KE, Park YJ, Kim SJ, Kwon H, Park do J, Cho B, Choi HC, Kang D, Park SK. Annual average changes in adult obesity as a risk factor for papillary thyroid cancer: a large-scale case-control study. Medicine (Baltimore). 2016;95:e2893.
60. Clavel-Chapelon F, Guillas G, Tondeur L, Kernaleguen C, Boutron-Ruault MC. Risk of differentiated thyroid cancer in relation to adult weight, height and body shape over life: the French E3N cohort. Int J Cancer. 2010;126:2984–90.
61. Ligibel J. Obesity and breast cancer. Oncology (Williston Park). 2011;25:994–1000.
62. Yung RL, Ligibel JA. Obesity and breast cancer: risk, outcomes, and future considerations. Clin Adv Hematol Oncol. 2016;14:790–7.
63. Reeves MM, Terranova CO, Eakin EG, Demark-Wahnefried W. Weight loss intervention trials in women with breast cancer: a systematic review. Obes Rev. 2014;15:749–68.

12

Anatomical basis for the choice of laparoscopic surgery for low rectal cancer through the pelvic imaging data—a cohort study

Zhou Yang, Guo Chunhua, Yuan Huayan, Yang Jianguo and Cheng Yong[*]

Abstract

Background: Low rectal cancer surgery without anus conservation needs permanent ileostomy or colostomy which seriously affects the quality of life of patients. Therefore, low rectal cancer surgery not only pays attention to the safety of surgical treatment but also to the anus conservation.

Methods: Sixty-seven patients suffering from low rectal cancer had undergone laparoscopic surgery which was analyzed through retrospective study. They were divided into the anus-conserving and non-anus-conserving groups. Thirty-five set of pelvic data was obtained from the preoperative CT and MRI images. After that, the discriminant function was obtained to predict the surgery methods for patients with low rectal carcinoma.

Results: Anal-conserving group discriminant function $(F1) = -33.698 + 6.045 \times$ anal margin distance (cm) $+ 1.105 \times T4$; non-anus-conserving group discriminant function $(F2) = -14.125 + 3.138 \times$ anal margin distance (cm) $+ 0.804 \times T4$. If F1 is greater than F2, then the case can be treated as the anus reservation while if F2 is greater than F1 the case cannot be treated anus reservation. The accuracy of the discriminant function was evaluated which was found to be 97%.

Conclusion: The discriminant function of pelvic data provides anatomical basis for the choice of surgical methods for low rectal cancer.

Keywords: Low rectal cancer, Laparoscopic surgery, Sphincter preservation, Pelvic measurement

Background

Colorectal cancers are due to old age and lifestyle factors. There are several ways to treat rectal cancer depending on its type and stage which includes surgery, radiation therapy, and ablation or embolization therapy. Surgery plays a curative role for early rectal cancer. In recent years, there are many surgical procedures for the treatment of rectal cancer which includes Hartmann (proctosigmoidectomy), Dixon, Miles, TaTME, and ISR. But the total mesorectal excision (TME) is still the gold standard for rectal cancer surgery [1]. Apart from this, laparoscopic surgery as new techniques has been evolved for the treatment of rectal cancer to reduce postoperative complication [2]. It is widely used because of its rapid recovery of intestinal

function, little surgical trauma, less pain, and hemorrhage as well as the short time of hospitalization. Moreover, prospective randomized studies showed that the laparoscopic surgery as compared with the traditional laparotomy does not affect the surgical outcomes [3, 4].

In our present study, considering no cell invasion at lower border of tumor, the length of incisional margin, 5-year survival rate and local recurrence of rectal carcinoma had not showed any significant correlation which is currently the pathological basis of anus-conserving surgery. Preoperative chemoradiotherapy helps to enhance the chance of anus-conserving surgery by 10%–20% [5, 6]. It aims to reduce the size or extent of the cancer before using radical treatment intervention thus making procedures easier and more likely to succeed. Low rectal cancer surgery without anus conservation needs permanent ileostomy or colostomy which seriously affects the quality of

* Correspondence: chengyongcmu@sina.com
Department of Gastrointestinal Surgery, First Affiliated Hospital of Chongqing
Medical University, Chongqing 400010, China

life of patients. Therefore, low rectal cancer surgery not only pays attention to the safety of surgical treatment but also to the anus conservation [7].

Although, laparoscopic surgery has drawn more attention among the patients and doctors, the indication of laparoscopic surgery with anus conservation have been the focus of controversy about which the majority of surgeons believe that they are relevant with the tumor location, size, stage, patient gender, obesity, and other [8, 9]. The handling of this new technique requires good experience. Thus, more experienced surgeons can easily do laparoscopic low rectal cancer surgery with anus conservation, [10] but it is technically difficult for young surgeons. In this study, we found that the deep and narrow pelvis is positively associated with operation time and bleeding volume [11, 12]. Moreover, the sacrum angle and pelvic measurements were associated with making preoperative decision in TME surgery [13]. Is there any relationship between the choice of laparoscopic surgery for rectal cancer and pelvic measurements? What kind of pelvis can allow laparoscopic anus-conserving surgery? The answer to this question has been explained through our study. In this study, 67 rectal cancer patients undergoing laparoscopic surgery were examined by CT three-dimensional reconstruction and MRI images, and the relationship between pelvic data and the choice of laparoscopic rectal cancer surgery was studied.

Methods

Patients

This study had been reported in line with the STROCSS criteria [14] which included 67 cases of colonoscopy-confirmed rectal cancer patients from the anal margin less than 7 cm from August 2015 to April 2017 at department of gastrointestinal surgery of our university by the same senior surgeon. The work was retrospective and single-center. Patients with stage T4, preoperative manifestation of intestinal obstruction or perforation, tumor distance from the anal greater than 7 cm, patients after neoadjuvant chemoradiotherapy, and those who underwent laparotomy were excluded. According to the operation information of the patients, the patients were divided into anus-conserving and non-anus-conserving groups. The laparoscopic resection was performed in the anus-conserving group, and the MILES was performed in the non-anus-conserving group. Table 1 showed the clinical features and tumor characteristics of these patients. This study was approved by the medical ethics committee of Chongqing Medical University (CMU-2016501a). Informed consent was obtained from the patients for publication of this paper and any accompanying images.

Table 1 Clinical and tumor characteristics of the patients

	Operation methods		P
	Anal reservation(48)	Non-anal reservation(19)	
Age	62.38	57.84	0.230
BMI	23.36	22.65	0.359
Gender			
Male (43)	33	10	0.215
Female (24)	15	9	
Anal distance(cm)	5.286	2.587	0.000
Complication			
With (24)	15	6	0.979
Without(46)	33	13	
Tumor staging			
T1 (3)	3	0	0.128
T2 (25)	15	10	
T3 (39)	30	9	
Transverse diameter of tumor (cm)	3.417	3.425	0.651
Tumor location			
Front wall (5)	2	3	0.386
Left wall (32)	26	6	
Right wall (30)	20	10	

Anal distance, the distance from the lower edge of the tumor to the anus was measured along the central axis of the pelvic MRI. *Transverse diameter of tumor*, the maximum width of coronal plane was measured by MRI

Surgical methods

Rectal cancer patients with preoperative evaluation without surgical contraindication and with the consent of the patient and family members, laparoscopic resection was carried out by using following two methods of surgery.

Specific steps of laparoscopic anterior resection of rectal cancer are as follows: inserted five Trocar with the navel for observation hole, left middle abdomen and lower abdomen for assistant holes, and right middle abdominal and lower abdomen for operation and ultrasonic knife hole. Made the lithotomy position with trendelenburg and high left low right position, and then established 10–15 mmHg CO_2 pneumoperitoneum to push the small intestine to right upper quadrant. And then the inferior mesenteric artery trunk was separated along sigmoid mesocolon root and the inferior mesenteric artery and vein were ligated. Along the Toldts gap, the bowel was separated to sigmoid colon and descending colon junction where, according to the TME principle to isolate intestine to down edge of tumor and intraluminal stapler was used for mutilation of intestinal tube. Stopped pneumoperitoneum, taken out the separated intestinal tube from abdominal cavity by making a 4 cm oblique incision at the left lower abdomen and cut the intestinal tube at the safe distance from tumor. Pouch suturing intestinal tube and embedding anastomat were made and pneumoperitoneum was re-established. Intestinal anastomosis was performed by DST technique. According to the situation of operation, ileostomy or/and transverse colostomy were made.

MILES: surgical procedures are same with above-mentioned rectal cancer resection. But after mutilation of intestinal tube and stopped pneumoperitoneum, a 2.5–3 cm circular incision was made in the left at the first/third junction of an imaginary line between left anterior superior spine and umbilicus. Taken out, sigmoid colon cut the intestinal tube at proximal 15 cm from tumor, and sigmoid colostomy was made. In the perineal operation, a shuttle incision was made at sciatic tuberosities, midline of the perineum, and the apex of the coccyx to protect the external genitalia and the subcutaneous tissue and each layer were separated, and the anus and rectum were removed, and anastomosis was made with abdominal operation.

Free dissection of pelvic visceral fascia, internal iliac vascular sheath and paravascular lymph nodes, lymphatic tissue in the bladder cavity, and routine pathological examination of excised specimens were carried out after surgery.

Pelvic measurement

CT and MRI are relatively accurate methods for pelvic measurement [15, 16]. In preoperative evaluation, the abdominal CT and pelvic MRI examination of all 67 patients included in this study were carried out (CT model: 64 slice spiral CT, Light Speed VCT; MRI machine: MAGNETOM Avanto) and ADW 4.4 workstation was used for 3D processing of CT scan image, and 3D image construction. The pelvic MRI scan images were processed with PACS software. ADW 4.4 workstation was used to measure the parameters of the pelvis, including the pelvic entrance plane, the middle pelvic plane, and the pelvic outlet plane. The sagittal plane of the pelvis was measured with PACS software in MRI images. The measurements were completed by two radiologists without knowing the patient's clinical information. Specific measurement parameters are shown in Fig. 1.

The operation methods as the dependent variable, the single factor analysis were used to find the correlation of specific measurement parameters and operation methods. The statistically significant variables were then analyzed by discriminant analysis and used to establish prediction equations.

Statistical analysis

Excel 2003 was used to sort out the data, and SPSS 21 software was used for statistical analysis. The test data for normal distribution is checked by Shapiro-Wilk test. In univariate analysis, for the normal distribution of data, the relationship between variables and operation methods was analyzed by independent samples t test; for non-normal distribution data, Mann-Whitney U (rank) was used to examine the relationship between the study variables and operation methods. After single factor analysis showed the statistical significances, Fisher (step) analysis method was used to further study of the influencing factors of surgery, establish the discriminant function, and verify the accuracy of discriminant function ($P < 0.05$ indicated significant).

Results

In this study, 19 patients underwent Miles surgery to remove the anus, and 48 patients underwent laparoscopic anterior resection to keep the anus. The average age of the anus-conserving group was 62.38, and the non-anus-conserving was 57.84. And the mean BMI of the anus-conserving group was less than that of the non-anus-conserving group, and the anus-conserving group in the T3 phase was significantly more than that in the non-anus-conserving group. The BMI, gender, tumor staging, tumor transverse diameter, and tumor location had no effects on the surgical procedure ($P > 0.05$). The average distance of the anus-conserving group from the anal margin was 5.286 cm while of the non-anus-conserving group was 2.587 cm, which had significant difference ($P = 0.000$). See Table 1.

The operation methods as the dependent variable, the single factor analysis was used to find that anal margin (cm), suprapubic inter diameter, S3 width, sacral arc length, sacral S3, sacral T, T-S3, T tail, Subpubic T, T1, T2, T3, T4 a total of 13 independent variables were statistical significance ($P < 0.05$). See Table 2. The 13 statistically significant variables were then analyzed by discriminant analysis, and the results showed that the anal margin (cm), T4 was statistically significant for surgery methods (Wilks, lambda ≥ 0.38, $P < 0.001$). Fisher discriminant function: anus-conserving group discriminant function (F1) = $- 33.698 + 6.045 \times$ anal margin distance (cm) $+ 1.105 \times$ T4; non-anus-conserving group discriminant function (F2) = $- 14.125 + 3.138 \times$ anal margin distance (cm) $+ 0.804 \times$ T4. If F1 is greater than F2, the patients in anatomy should be treated as the anus reservation, if F2 is greater than F1, the patients in anatomy should be treated as non-anus reservation.

Table 3 showed that in the anus-conserving group, 44 of the 48 cases were correctly judged, and 18 of the 19 cases in the non-anus-conserving group were correctly judged, that is, 92.5% of the patients were correctly operated on. The accuracies of discriminant function for anus-conserving and non-conserving groups were 91.67% and 94.74%, respectively.

Discussion

The third most common type of cancer is rectal cancer worldwide with increasing incidence rate. Surgical resection is the preferred curative approach. Laparoscopic surgery is

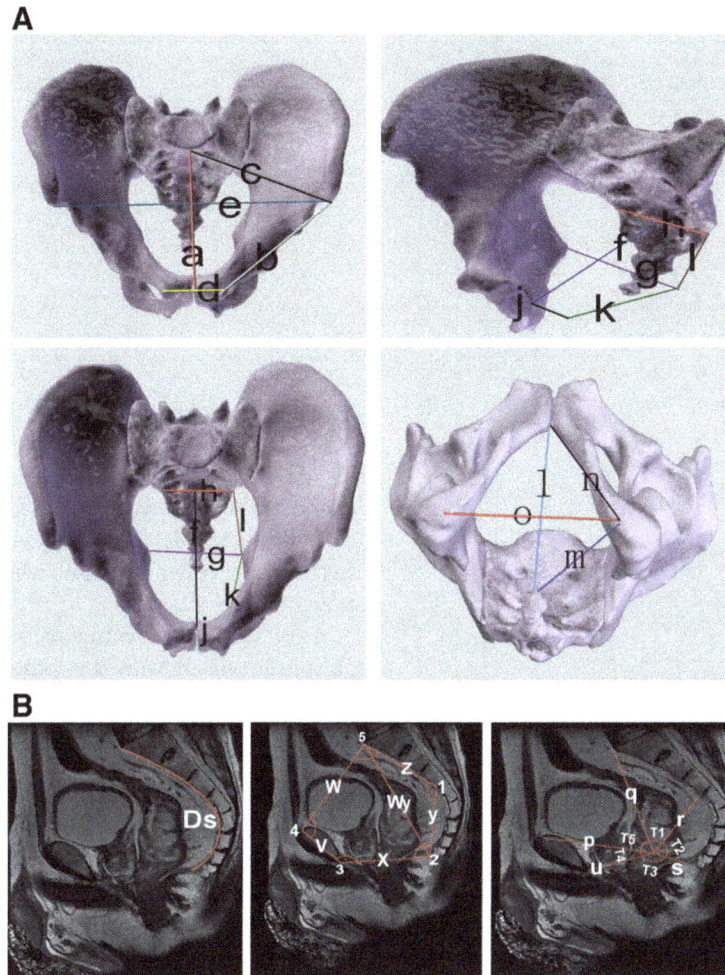

Fig. 1 a Definition of pelvic parameters assayed by CT. Pelvic inlet plane: (a) anteroposterior diameter of entrance; (b) diameter between anterior superior iliac spine and pubic bone; (c) diameter between anterior superior iliac spine and sacrum; (d) superior border diameter of pubis tubercle; (e) anterior superior iliac spine diameter. Middle pelvic plane: (f) anteroposterior diameter of middle pelvis; (g) bispinous diameter; (h) S3 width; (i) diameter of S3 and ischial spine; (j) midline diameter of pubis; (k) diameter between pubis and spinal ischiadica. Pelvic outlet plane: (l) diameter between pubic bone and coccyx; (m) diameter between ischial tuberosity and coccyx; (n) diameter between pubic and ishial tuberosity; (o) diameter of ischial tuberosity. **b** Definition of pelvic parameters assayed by MRI. (v) Suprapubic diameter; (z) sacral S3; (Wy) sacrococcygeal diameter; (Ds) caudal arc length; (y) S3 tail; (q) sacral T; (r) T-S3; (s) T tail; (p) T suprapubic; (u) T subpubic; (1) the angle between the vertex of sacral promontory and the apex of the coccyx; (2) the angle between the lower edge of the third sacral bone and the lower margin of the pubic bone; (3) the angle between the apex of the coccyx and the upper margin of pubis; (4) the angle between the vertex of sacral promontory and the lower margin of the pubic bone; (5) the angle between the vertex of sacral promontory and the lower edge of the third sacral bone; (T1) the angle between the vertex of sacral promontory and the lower edge of the third sacral bone; (T2) the angle between the lower edge of the third sacral tubercle and the apex of the coccyx; (T3) the angle between the apex of the coccyx and the lower border of the pubic bone; (T4) the angle between the lower border and upper border of the pubic bone; (T5) the angle between the upper border of the pubic bone and the vertex of sacral promontory

being used widely as compared to open surgery. With the development of surgical techniques, surgeons realized that the narrow space of the pelvis significantly restricted the operation of rectal cancer surgery, and even affected the surgical outcomes [17–19]. The nature of the tumor, the extent of the disease, and anatomical description of disease should be established prior to surgery. Pelvimeter is no longer just obstetric assessment tool, but widely used in the evaluation of rectal cancer before surgery. A lot of researches have proved that there is a link between the pelvic

measurement parameters and operation time, intraoperative bleeding volume, difficulty of operation, ring margin positive rate, surgical specimen integrity, even postoperative anastomotic fistula of rectal cancer surgery [11–13, 20]. In this study, two methods of laparoscopic surgery was used, one was laparoscopic anterior resection in which the part of the rectum containing the tumor was removed and the colon was then attached to the remaining part of the rectum so that bowels can be empty in the usual way, second was MILES which involved removal of the anus and the

Table 2 The association between measurement parameters and surgical methods

Parameters	Mean ± SD (min, max) or median (four quantile interval)	F or Z	P
Transverse diameter of tumor (cm)	3.363 (2.903, 3.825)	−0.452	0.651
Anal margin distance (cm)	4.868 (3.20, 5.69)	−6.065	0.000
a	10.97 ± 1.15 (8.20, 14.2)	−0.108	0.914
b	13.4 ± 0.83 (11.67, 15.85)	1.392	0.169
c	12.48 (12.17, 13.06)	−0.814	0.416
d	7.43 (6.48, 7.80)	−2.024	0.043
e	22.83 ± 1.63 (18.89, 26.51)	1.979	0.052
f	11.71 (11.24, 12.49)	−0.549	0.583
g	10.00 (9.12, 10.92)	−1.273	0.203
h	8.25 (7.92, 8.60)	−2.003	0.045
i	7.08 ± 0.87 (5.43, 9.29)	−0.805	0.424
j	5.32 ± 0.54 (4.39, 6.54)	1.625	0.109
k	8.92 ± 0.51 (7.82, 10.37)	0.497	0.621
l	8.53 ± 0.81 (6.73, 10.92)	−0.947	0.347
m	5.93 ± 0.97 (4.05, 8.16)	−0.595	0.554
n	9.13 ± 0.99 (6.43, 11.18)	0.366	0.716
o	11.04 ± 1.52 (7.57, 14.27)	0.389	0.698
Ds	15.04 ± 1.12 (12.98, 17.60)	3.013	0.004
v	5.00 (4.76, 5.34)	−0.529	0.597
Wy	11.83 ± 1.13 (9.16, 13.9)	1.914	0.06
z	7.76 ± 0.53 (6.36, 8.87)	2.738	0.008
y	6.27 ± 0.79 (4.21, 8.14)	1.951	0.055
1	114.14 ± 8.09 (93.37, 129.20)	−0.243	0.809
2	111.86 (32.55, 67.81)	−0.108	0.914
3	124.15 (141.48, 189.50)	−0.16	0.873
4	96.76 ± 7.25 (81.86, 113.87)	1.102	0.274
5	91.14 ± 7.99 (72.27, 113.12)	−0.92	0.361
q	11.30 ± 1.51 (7.80, 14.78)	−3.505	0.001
r	8.25 (7.31, 9.37)	−6.525	0.000
s	4.05 (3.25, 4.92)	−4.674	0.000
p	8.58 ± 1.01 (6.32, 11.18)	1.663	0.101
u	4.53 (3.94, 5.33)	−3.297	0.001

Table 2 The association between measurement parameters and surgical methods (Continued)

Parameters	Mean ± SD (min, max) or median (four quantile interval)	F or Z	P
T1	7.78 (38.1, 48.14)	−5.008	0.000
T2	43.43 (32.55, 67.81)	−5.133	0.000
T3	169.11 (141.48, 189.50)	−5.606	0.000
T4	28.70 ± 6.55 (13.31, 40.27)	4.937	0.000
T5	63.59 (59.78, 71.72)	2.676	0.009

tissues surrounding it, including the sphincter muscle and a permanent colostomy was done since the anus was removed. DST technique is considered the standard method of the rectum anastomosis [21], and we think the linear cutter into the safe distance under rectal cancer may be affected by the pelvic structure, which may affect the surgery at anatomy level.

In the 35 set of measured parameters, 10 set of them are obviously related with the location of tumor, but at the same time the structure of the whole pelvis, which can obviously reflect the relationship between the pelvic position and rectal tumor. By univariate analysis, there was statistical significance between 13 independent variables and the operation methods, and discriminant function showed that anal margin distance and T4 have significant influence on the methods of operation. Patients with larger T4 may be more likely to keep their anus, and the author thinks that this may be related to the extending angle of the linear cutter. However, in discriminant function, the distance between the tumor and the anal margin is significantly larger than the coefficient of T4, that is to say, the distance between the tumor and the anal margin is still the decisive factor for anus reservation or not.

However, this study of 67 patients in BMI ($P = 0.359$), gender ($P = 0.215$), tumor diameter ($P = 0.651$), tumor location ($P = 0.386$), and tumor stage ($P = 0.128$) had no statistical significance in the anus reservation or not, which are not consistent with other research [8, 9]. In this study, we focus on the relationship between pelvic measurement parameters and operation methods, the accuracy of function F1 and F2 for prediction of operation methods of were 91.67% and 94.74% respectively. Therefore, it was concluded that the function F1 and F2 may simply predict the surgical methods from the pelvic anatomy level. However,

Table 3 The accuracies of the discriminant function

Actual operations	Prediction		Total
	Anus reservation	Non-anus reservation	
Anus reservation	44 (91.67%)	4	48
Non-anus reservation	1	18 (94.74%)	19

the accuracies of discriminant function for anus reservation or not need to be validated on larger samples.

Conclusion

Through this study, we found that T4 plays an important role in the lower rectal cancer surgical options. The predictive accuracy of functional F1 and F2 was more than 90%. Combining with the general condition of patients and tumor, assessment of pelvic anatomy level will help to decide anus reservation or not for the low rectal cancer surgery.

Funding

This research received no specific grant from any funding agency in the public, commercial, or not-for-profit sectors.

Authors' contributions

ZY and GC carried out the studies. YH, YJ, and CY participated in the design of the study and performed the statistical analysis. All authors read and approved the final manuscript.

Competing interests

The authors declare that they have no competing interests.

References

1. Heald RJ, Husband EM, Ryall RD. The mesorectum in rectal cancer surgery—the clue to pelvic recurrence. Br J Surg. 1982;69:613–6.
2. Maglio R, Meucci M, Muzi MG, Maglio M, Masoni L. Laparoscopic total mesorectal excision for ultralow rectal cancer with transanal intersphincteric dissection as a first step: a single-surgeon experience. Am Surg. 2014;80:26–30.
3. Christoforidis D, Demartines N. Randomized clinical trial comparing laparoscopic and open surgery in patients with rectal cancer. Br J Surg. 2009;96:982–9.
4. Ng SS, Leung KL, Lee JF, Yiu RY, Li JC, Teoh AY, Leung WW. Laparoscopic-assisted versus open abdominoperineal resection for low rectal cancer:a prospective randomized trial. Ann Surg Oncol. 2008;15:2418–25.
5. M. Roh, N. Petrelli, H. Wieand, Phase III randomised trial of preoperative versus postoperative mutimodality therapy in patients with carcinoma of the rectum (NSABP R-03). J. Clin. Oncol 20 (2001) Abstract 450.
6. Sauer R, Fietkau R, Wittekind C, Rödel C, Martus P, Hohenberger W, Tschmelitsch J, Sabitzer H, Karstens JH, Becker H, Hess C, Raab R. German Rectal Cancer Group, Adjuvant vs. neoadjuvant radiochemotherapy for locally advanced rectal cancer: the German trial CAO/ARO/AIO-94. Colorectal Dis. 2003;5(2003):406–15.
7. Mulsow J, Winter DC. Sphincter preservation for distal rectal cancer - a goal worth achieving at all costs. World J Gastroenterol. 2011;17:855–61.
8. Orsenigo E, Di Palo S, Vignali A, Staudacher C. Laparoscopic intersphincteric resection for low rectal cancer,Surg. Oncologia. 2007;16:S117–20.
9. Zhou X, Su M, Hu K, Su Y, Ye Y, Huang C, Yu Z, Li X, Zhou H, Ni Y, Jiang Y. Applications of computed tomography pelvimetry and clinical-pathological parameters in sphincter preservation of mid-low rectal cancer. Int J Clin Exp Med. 2015;8:2174–81.
10. Kuo LJ, Hung CS, Wang W, Tam KW, Lee HC, Liang HH, Chang YJ, Huang MT, Wei PL. Intersphincteric resection for very low rectal cancer: clinical outcomes of open versus laparoscopic approach and multidimensional analysis of the learning curve for laparoscopic surgery. J Surg Res. 2013;524:530.
11. Boyle KM, Petty D, Chalmers AG, Quirke P, Cairns A, Finan PJ, Sagar PM, Burke D. Mri assessment of the bony pelvis may help predict resectability of rectal cancer. Color Dis. 2005;7:232–40.
12. Targarona EM, Balague C, Pernas JC, Martinez C, Berindoague R, Gich I, Trias M. Can we predict immediate outcome after laparoscopic rectal surgery? Multivariate analysis of clinical, anatomic, and pathologic features after 3-dimensional reconstruction of the pelvic anatomy. Ann Surg. 2008;247:642–9.
13. Fernández Ananín S, Targarona EM, Martinez C, Pernas JC, Hernández D, Gich I, Sancho FJ, Trias M. Predicting the pathological features of the mesorectum before the laparoscopic approach to rectal cancer. Surg. Endosc. 2014;28:3458–66.
14. Agha RA, Borrelli MR, Vella-Baldacchino M, Thavayogan R, Orgill DP. For the STROCSS Group, The STROCSS statement: strengthening the reporting of cohort studies in surgery. Int J Surg. 2017;46:198–202.
15. Keller TM, Rake A, Michel SC, Seifert B, Efe G, Treiber K, Huch R, Marincek B, Kubik-Huch RA. Obstetric pelvimetry reference values and evaluation of inter-and intraobserver error and intraindividual variability. Radiology. 2003; 227:37–43.
16. Anderson N, Humphries N, Wells JE. Measurement error in computed tomography pelvimetry, Australas. Radiol. 2005;49(2005):104–7.
17. Zhou XC, Su M, Hu KQ, Su YF, Ye YH, Huang CQ, Yu ZL, Li XY, Zhou H, Ni YZ, Jiang YI, Lou Z. CT pelvimetry and clinicopathological parameters in evaluation of the technical difficulties in performing open rectal surgery for mid-low rectal cancer. Oncol Lett. 2016;11:31–8.
18. Zur Hausen G, Gröne J, Kaufmann D, Niehues SM, Aschenbrenner K, Stroux A, Hamm B, Kreis ME, Lauscher JC. Influence of pelvic volume on surgical outcome after low anterior resection for rectal cancer. IntJ Colorectal Dis. 2017;32:1125–35.
19. Baek SJ, Kim CH, Cho MS, Bae SU, Hur H, Min BS, Baik SH, Lee KY, Kim NK. Robotic surgery for rectal cancer can overcome difficulties associated with pelvic anatomy. Surg Endosc. 2015;29:1419–24.
20. Tsuruta A, Tashiro J, Ishii T, Oka Y, Suzuki A, Kondo H, Yamaguchi S. Prediction of anastomotic leakage after laparoscopic low anterior resection in male rectal cancer by pelvic measurement in magnetic resonance imaging. Surg. Laparosc. Endosc. Percutan. Tech. 2017;27:54–9.
21. Nakayama S, Hasegawa S, Hida K, Kawada K, Sakai Y. Obtaining secure stapling of a double stapling anastomosis. J Surg Res. 2015;193:652–7.

13

Surgical management and outcome of synovial sarcoma in the spine

Minglei Yang[†], Nanzhe Zhong[†], Chenglong Zhao[†], Wei Xu, Shaohui He, Jian Zhao, Xinghai Yang[*] and Jianru Xiao[*]

Abstract

Background: Synovial sarcoma (SS) is a soft tissue sarcoma that rarely occurs in the spine, and a minimal number of cases have been reported in the literature. Spinal SS is challenging in diagnosis and treatment and has a poor prognosis. The aim of this study was to summarize and analyse the clinical features and outcomes of patients with spinal SS.

Methods: A total of 16 cases of patients with spinal SS admitted to our institution were reviewed retrospectively. General information, radiological findings and treatment strategies were collected. These patients were followed up regarding their continuing treatment, local or distant recurrence and survival.

Results: Spinal SS patients in this series ranged in age from 12 to 68 years (median, 33). Four en bloc resections and 12 piecemeal resections were performed. Improved Frankel ($P = 0.002$), visual analogue scale ($P = 0.002$) and Karnofsky Performance Status ($P = 0.002$) scores were seen postoperatively. The mean follow-up period was 35.9 ± 23.5 (median 31.5, range 4–87) months, with four local recurrences and three distant metastases detected. Eight patients (50.0%) died of disease by the last follow-up. The 1-, 3- and 5-year overall survival rates were 87.5%, 61.4% and 40.9%, respectively. Preoperative chemotherapy was used in three patients to facilitate surgical resection, and adjuvant chemotherapy and radiotherapy were used in six patients.

Conclusions: Spinal SS has a relatively high risk of local recurrence and distant metastasis. Surgical intervention can improve the neurological function and relieve pain in these patients. En bloc excision is an effective treatment strategy to improve survival and prevent local recurrence. Management of spinal SS should be under the instruction of a multidisciplinary team.

Keywords: Synovial sarcoma, Spine, Surgery, Prognosis

Background

Primary bone tumours of the spine are relatively rare, comprising only 10% or less of all bone tumours [1]. Synovial sarcoma (SS) is a malignancy that accounts for 6–9% of all soft tissue sarcomas (STSs) and is primarily seen in adolescents and young adults [2]. Two thirds of all SS cases are located in extremities, while less than 5% are found in the spine [3]. It can arise from the osseous and paravertebral soft tissues and even metastasize from other sites [4, 5]. With the enlargement of a SS, the mass can result in pain and other symptoms [6, 7]. Spinal instability, vertebral collapse and neurologic deficits may occur from the destruction of vertebrae structure and compression of nerve roots and the spinal cord [8, 9].

Surgical resection with negative margins is the initial treatment for SS [10]. However, sometimes a complete resection of lesions in the spine cannot be achieved due to the complex anatomical structure and the involved critical neurovascular tissue [11]. For unresectable SS, preoperative chemotherapy or radiotherapy could help downstage large, high-grade tumours and enable effective surgical resection. Adjuvant radiotherapy and/or chemotherapy are also recommended for patients with a microscopically positive margin or with high-grade histological types [12].

Due to its rarity, only a few SS cases involving the spine have been reported, most without follow-up or with a short follow-up period. Additionally, it is commonly accepted

* Correspondence: cnspineyang@163.com; jianruxiao83@163.com
[†]Minglei Yang, Nanzhe Zhong and Chenglong Zhao contributed equally to this work.
Department of Orthopedic Oncology, Changzheng Hospital, Second Military Medical University, 415 Fengyang Road, Shanghai 200003, China

that the diagnosis and treatment of spinal SS is challenging [13, 14]. Here, we summarize the clinical features, treatments and outcomes of 16 patients with spinal SS admitted in our institution and present our experience.

Methods
Patient samples
This study was approved by the institutional review board of the Changzheng Hospital of the Second Military Medical University. We retrospectively reviewed the clinical and follow-up data of confirmed spinal SS patients who were surgically treated in our institution from August 2008 to May 2017. General information, radiological findings, pre- and post-operative status, treatment strategies, operation details, complications and pathological findings were collected. A total of 16 patients with spinal SS were identified, including 11 men and 5 women, ranging in age from 12 to 68 years (median 33). Radiologic examinations, including a plain radiograph, computed tomography (CT) scan and magnetic resonance imaging (MRI), were used for preoperative diagnosis and disease evaluation. Histological diagnosis was confirmed by needle biopsy or open biopsy. Of the 16 cases, 5 occurred in the cervical spine, 4 in the thoracic spine, 3 in the lumbar spine and 4 in the sacrum.

Clinical features
The clinical presentations of all patients were collected. Features of radiologic examinations conducted before surgery were analysed. The Weinstein-Boriani-Biagnini (WBB) system was used for surgical staging [15]. Pre- and postoperative Frankel grading was carried out to assess the patient's neurologic status. The visual analogue scale (VAS) for assessing pain and the Karnofsky Performance Status (KPS) Scale were used before and 3 months after the operation. All patients were routinely followed up 1 and 3 months after the surgery and then at a 3-month interval for the first 1 year and then once every year thereafter. Patients' conditions were all confirmed by telephone calls at the end of the study.

Statistical analysis
Continuous variables are expressed as the mean ± standard deviation (SD). The Wilcoxon signed rank test was used to compare the Frankel grades and VAS and KPS scores pre- and post-operation. The Kaplan-Meier method was used to estimate survival. Overall survival (OS) was used as the primary end point and was defined as the interval between the first diagnosis and either death or the date of last follow-up. $P < 0.05$ was considered as statistically significant.

Results
General information
Various symptoms were recorded in these 16 spinal SS patients. Pain (15/16, 93.75%), numbness and weakness of extremities (12/16, 75.0%); limited motion of the spine (10/16, 62.5%); palpable mass (11/16, 68.75%); and disturbance of urination or defecation functions (3/16, 18.75%) were commonly observed. The mean preoperative duration of symptoms was 11.8 ± 11.8 months (median 7, range 1–42). The mean preoperative VAS and KPS scores were 5.88 ± 1.65 (median 6, range 3–9) and 45.3 ± 15.0 (median 40, range 20–70), respectively, with Frankel scores ranging from A to E (Table 1). In all 16 patients, 8 had primary lesions, while 6 had local recurrent lesions and 2 had metastatic lesions from the extremities with prior surgical treatments conducted at other institutes (Table 2).

Radiologic evaluation
Plain radiographs showed an osteolytic lesion with a well-defined soft tissue mass in 10 out of 16 patients. Based on the preoperative radiologic imaging, the average tumour size was 7.57 ± 3.33 cm. Collapse of the vertebral body was seen in one patient with a pathological fracture of T1. CT images showed osteolytic lesions in vertebral body and/or appendix (16/16), with paravertebral or epidural soft tissue masses (12/16). Most tumours were well demarcated, and tumour calcification was found in three patients. MRI revealed heterogeneous signals in T1- and T2-weighted images of the vertebral and paravertebral lesions (Figs. 1 and 2).

Table 1 Demographic data of 16 spinal SS patients

	Spinal SS, $n = 16$
Sex, M/F	11/5
Age, ≤ 30/> 30	8/8
Preoperative KPS, < 60/60–80/≥ 80	12/4/0
Preoperative Frankel scores, A–C/D–E	7/9
Preoperative VAS scores, ≤ 5/> 5	6/10
Tumour size (mean ± SD, cm)	7.57 ± 3.33
Recurrent or metastasis lesions, no/yes	8/8
Preoperative chemotherapy, no/yes	13/3
Operation time (mean ± SD, min)	292.9 ± 121.2
Intraoperative blood loss (mean ± SD, ml)	1547 ± 1152.8
Complication, no/yes	15/1
Postoperative recurrence, no/yes	12/4
Postoperative distant metastasis, no/yes	13/3
Adjuvant chemotherapy, no/yes	10/6
Adjuvant radiotherapy, no/yes	10/6

SS synovial sarcoma, VAS visual analogue scale, KPS Karnofsky Performance Status, SD standard deviation, F female, M male

Table 2 General information, treatment, and outcome of 16 patients involved

No. case	Age, years	Sex	Tumor Size, cm	Tumor sites	Recurrent case	Complications	WBB Staging	Pre-FS	Post-FS	Pre-Vas	Post-Vas	Pre-KPS
1	15	F	10*5	C3-C5	Y	N	A-B/1-3	E	E	4	1	70
2	59	M	5.7*4	right S	N	N	A-D/9-12	D	E	5	1	60
3	59	M	7*8	left S	N	wound infection	A-F/1-6	C	D	8	8	30
4	17	M	9*5	L3-S1	Y	N	A-E/7-9	C	D	5	4	40
5	53	M	14*10	L5, right S	N	N	A-E/7-12	C	D	6	6	40
6	12	M	3*3	C6-T2	Y	N	A/1-3 11-12	E	E	6	3	70
			6*5	C6-T2	Y	N	A-B/1-3 11-12	D	D	6	6	60
7	53	M	5*4	C7	N	N	A-C F/7-12	E	E	3	1	60
8	18	M	5*4	T12-L1	Y	N	A-C F/1-3 8-12	D	E	6	2	50
9	68	M	7*5	T11	N	N	A-C/1-4	D	E	6	4	30
10	20	F	4*4	C3-C5	Y	N	A-F/4-12	D	D	8	3	30
11	23	M	8*5	right S	N	N	A-E/7-12	D	E	6	1	50
12	26	M	13*10	T1	Y	T1 compression fracture[a]	A-F/7-12	B	D	8	3	30
13	13	F	5*4.5	C6-T1	N	N	A-F/1-5 11-12	C	E	4	1	40
14	58	F	4*3	C5-C7	Y	N	A-F/5-12	A	C	9	5	20
15	40	F	10*5	L3-L4	Y	N	A-F/1-3 9-12	C	D	6	6	40
16	53	M	12*7	S	N	N	A-E/1-4 10-12	D	D	4	4	50

F female, *M* male, *Y* yes, *N* no, *FS* Frankel grading score, *VAS* visual analogue scale, *KPS* =Karnofsky Performance Status, *WBB* Weinstein-Boriani-Biagnini system, *ant* anterior approach, *pst* posterior approach, *NED* no evidence of disease, *AWD* alive with disease, *DOD* died of disease, *CT* chemotherapy, *RT* radiotherapy

[a]Disease related complications: T1 pathologic fracture found pre-operatively in our institute

Table 2 General information, treatment, and outcome of 16 patients involved (Continued)

No. case	Post-KPS	Operation duration, minutes	Blood Loss, ml	Surgical approach	Surgical resection	Pre-CT	Pre-RT	Post-CT	Post-RT	Metastasis, months	Local recurrence, months	Diagnosis to event, months	Last Status
1	90	140	600	pst	En bloc	N	N	N	N	N	N	74	NED
2	80	300	1000	pst	En bloc	N	N	Y	Y	bilateral lungs, 8	N	22	AWD
3	30	330	2800	pst	Piecemeal	N	N	N	N	N	3	4	DOD
4	60	220	1200	pst	Piecemeal	N	Y	Y	Y	right lung, 24	10	47	DOD
5	40	330	4500	pst	En bloc	N	N	N	N	N	N	30	NED
6	80 / 60	180	200	pst	Piecemeal	Y	N	N	N	N	10	/	/
7	80	300	300	pst	Piecemeal	Y	N	N	N	N	8	34	DOD
8	80	360	3000	ant+pst	En bloc	N	N	Y	Y	N	N	11	NED
9	50	500	2000	pst	Piecemeal	N	Y	Y	Y	N	N	33	NED
10	80	240	400	pst	Piecemeal	N	N	N	N	N	N	6	DOD
11	80	240	1200	ant	Piecemeal	N	N	N	N	N	N	21	NED
12	50	140	300	pst	Piecemeal	N	N	Y	Y	N	N	54	NED
13	80	510	1600	ant+pst	Piecemeal	Y	Y	N	N	N	N	87	DOD
14	40	480	1200	ant+pst	Piecemeal	N	N	Y	Y	N	N	60	NED
15	40	360	2200	ant+pst	Piecemeal	N	Y	N	N	N	N	39	DOD
16	50	170	2200	pst	Piecemeal	Y	N	N	N	N	5	27	DOD
		180	1600	pst	Piecemeal	N	N	N	N	subcutaneous tissue with skin ulceration, 18	N	25	DOD

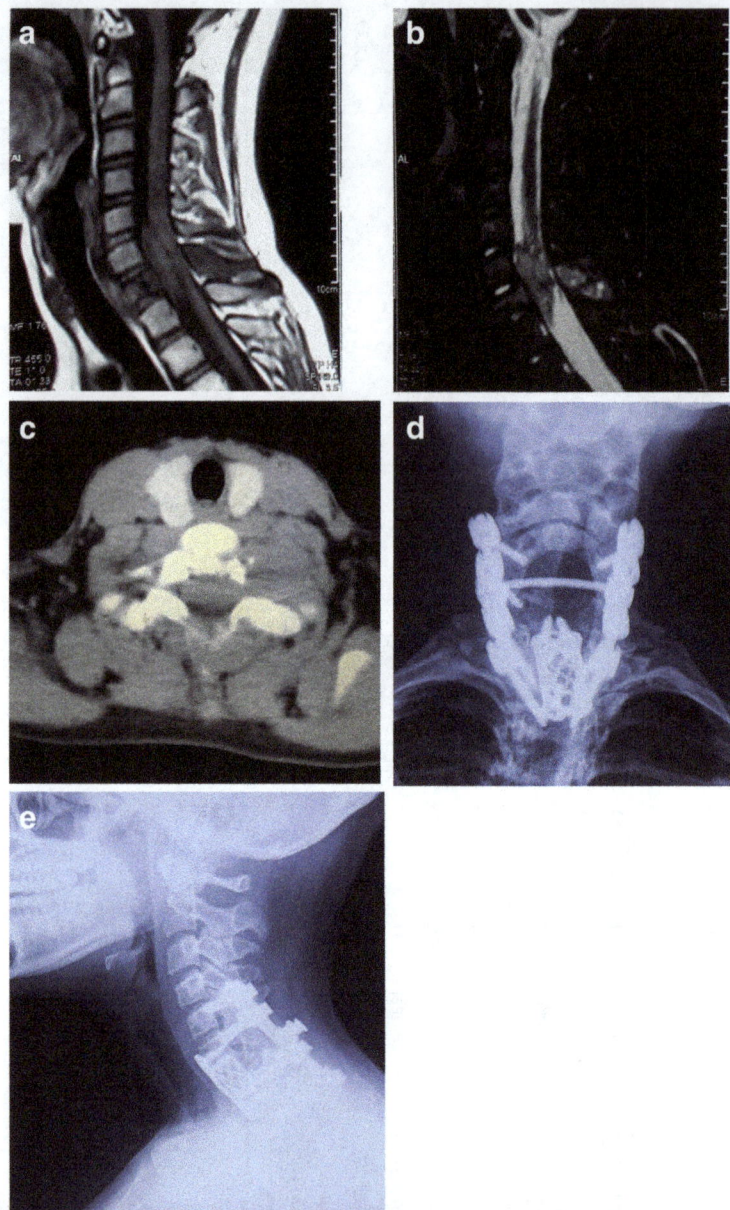

Fig. 1 Patient no. 13: MRI showing low signals in T1- (**a**) and heterogeneous signals in T2 (**b**)-weighted images of a soft tissue mass in the C7 vertebral body and appendix, with spinal cord compression from C6 to T1. CT images (**c**) showing a destructive soft tissue mass and osteolytic lesion in the C7 vertebral body and appendix. Cervical vertebra anterior and posterior (AP) (**d**) and lateral (LAT) (**e**) X-rays at the follow-up 52 months after surgery, demonstrating the maintenance of the instruments and spinal stability

Surgical intervention

All patients were surgically treated. The surgical approach and the instrumentation method were tailored for each patient. Four en bloc resections and 12 piecemeal resections were performed in the 16 spinal patients, with an average procedure time of 292.9 ± 121.2 (median 300, range 140–510) min and blood loss of 1547 ± 1152.8 (median 1200, range 200–4500) ml (Table 1). All resected specimens were proven with a negative margin by pathological examination. Intraoperatively, the surgical field was immersed with oxaliplatin. Spinal stability and balance were restored in accordance with the resection extension. Artificial vertebral bodies, titanium mesh cages and anterior titanium plates were applied to reconstruct the bony defects. Pedicle screw systems and lateral mass screw systems were used for posterior internal fixation (Figs. 1 and 2). A significant amelioration of Frankel scores was detected postoperatively ($P = 0.002$). VAS ($P = 0.002$) and KPS ($P = 0.002$) scores were also significantly improved after operation in all patients.

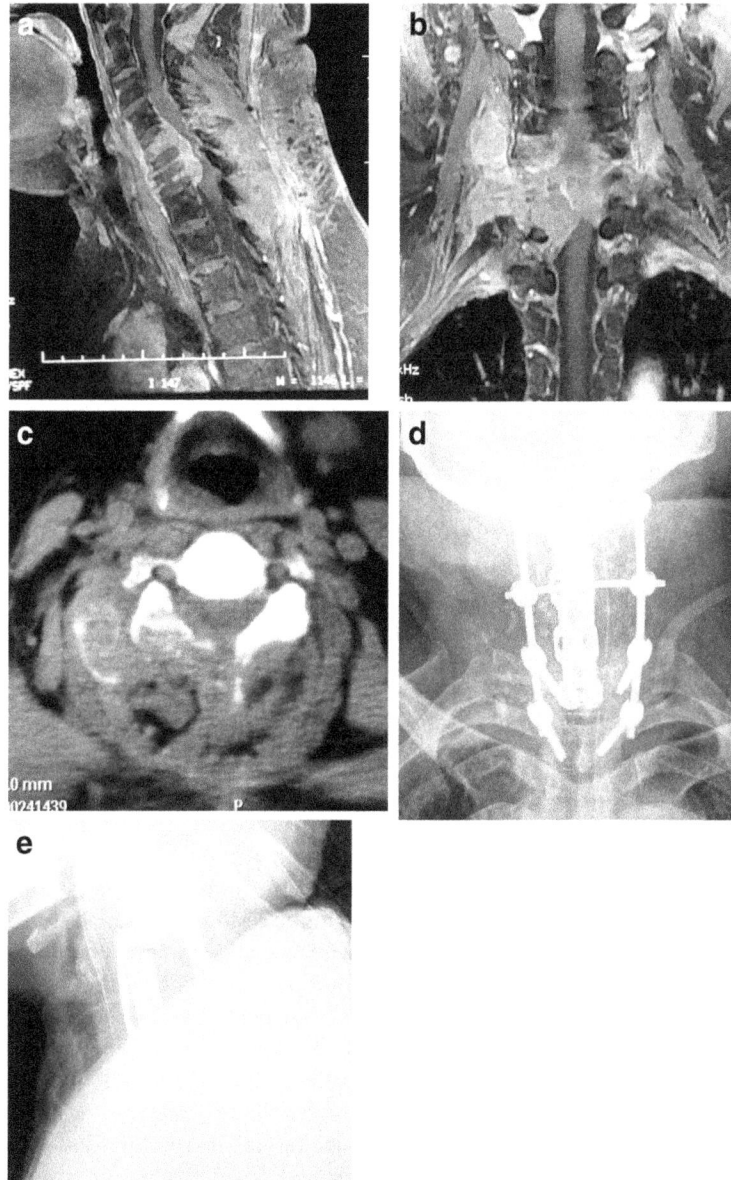

Fig. 2 Patient no. 14: MRI showing a vertebral lesion with a paraspinal mass from C5 to C7 (**a**, **b**). CT images (**c**) showing an osteolytic lesion with calcification. AP (**d**) and LAT (**e**) X-rays after surgery, showing anterior vertebral reconstruction and posterior internal fixation

Adjuvant treatment

Radiotherapy and chemotherapy were used before and/or after operation based on the tumour size, surgical findings and the general status of a patient. Because of recurrent diseases and the need to facilitate surgical resection, a total of three cases received preoperative chemotherapy. Six patients had both adjuvant chemotherapy and radiotherapy. Gamma knife was performed on the pulmonary metastasis of one patient.

Follow-up

The average time of follow-up for all 16 patients was 35.9 ± 23.5 (median 31.5, range 4–87) months. The 1-, 3-

and 5-year OS rates were 87.5%, 61.4% and 40.9%, respectively. Four of the 16 patients (25.0%) developed local recurrence 3–10 months after surgery in our institution and one of them underwent another surgical resection. All four of these patients, three of whom had a history of recurrent disease, received piecemeal resection. Three of the 16 patients (18.75%) developed distant metastasis 8–24 months after the operation, including two lung metastases and one metastasis of the subcutaneous tissue with ulceration. Eight of the 16 patients (50.00%) died during the follow-up period, with a mean survival of 33.6 ± 26.2 (median 30.5, range 4–87) months. All eight of these patients received piecemeal resection, and the causes of death included local or distant recurrence or multiple organ failure after the operation. One (6.25%) patient was alive with the disease (AWD) at last follow-up, and the other seven (43.75%) were living without evidence of disease (NED). Postoperative complications, including wound dehiscence and fat liquefaction, were observed in one patient (Table 2).

Discussion

SS is a rare and aggressive malignancy, with a predominance in adolescents and young adults [2]. Similarly, 8 of the 16 (50.0%) patients in our study were younger than 30. This type of tumour has the potential for metastasis, with the lungs being the most susceptible site [16]. In our series, there were two patients who had a lung metastasis. One patient experienced a subcutaneous tissue metastasis, which is uncommon and has only previously been reported in prior literature twice [17]. SS occurs in the extremities, most commonly near the joints, and the rarity of spinal SS limits the sample size of studies conducted on this type of cancer [18]. Most of the available knowledge on the treatment and prognosis of spinal SS comes from sporadic cases reported in previous literature (Table 3). As far as we can tell, this is the largest conducted case series that analyses the clinical features and outcomes of these patients.

Progressive chronic pain and a palpable mass are the common symptoms of SS [2, 14, 19]. In a previous report, the duration between the onset of symptoms and start of treatment could be longer than 10 years [20]. For spinal patients, numbness or weakness of the extremities and urinary or bowel dysfunction caused by nerve root irritation or spinal cord compression are commonly seen [21–23]. In our series, 81.25% patients had varying degrees of neurological deficits and almost all patients had pain in tumour sites. One patient was admitted to our institution with acute lower extremity paralysis due to a compression fracture of the T1 vertebral body. His motor and sensory functions were improved significantly after surgery. Calcification seen in plain radiographs and CT scans is thought to be one of the features of SS in approximately 30% of patients [18, 24]. In our series, the calcification feature was seen in three (18.75%) patients. On MRI, most SSs have variable and heterogeneous signals in T1- or T2-weighted images [5]. Radiologic examinations are applied to detect the tumour but are difficult to use in making a diagnosis. No definitive characteristics have been seen to distinguish SS from other diseases like nerve sheath tumours, Ewing sarcoma, chondrosarcoma and other unusual STSs.

Spinal SS has a relatively poor prognosis, with a high died of disease (DOD) risk (50.00%) and a low NED (43.75%) rate, both of which are also documented in previous studies [7, 13, 16, 25]. A total of four postoperative local recurrences and three distant metastases were detected. It has been documented that most spinal SS patients die within 3 years [18], while the 5-year OS rate of all-site SS is 25–76% [7, 26]. In the current study, the 5-year OS was 40.9%, which is consistent with the published data. Sar et al. [27] reported a patient with primary SS of the sacrum who died of this disease 94 months after surgery, which is the longest survival time in literature. In our study, the longest OS was seen in a thoracic spinal SS patient, who had an 87-month survival. There are several possible reasons of the unfavourable prognosis of spinal SS. First, nerve compression can cause neurological deficits, which impacts the quality of life of these patients. Heavy blood loss and long surgical duration also affect the general status of these patients. Second, due to the complex structures of the vertebrae and surrounding tissue, sometimes en bloc excision is hard to achieve, and potential tumour residue might occur. In our study, no local recurrences were seen in the four patients who received an en bloc excision, and they seem to have a relatively good prognosis. Therefore, any tumour residue might increase the risk of postoperative recurrence. On the other hand, the special anatomic site of spinal lesions might help refine the application and dosage of radiotherapy.

Management of spinal SS should follow the instruction of a multidisciplinary team, and surgical resection serves as the first choice, if wide excision with clear margins is possible [28–31]. Subtotal resection of the tumour might be followed shortly by a local recurrence [32]. En bloc resection is important in spinal tumours to minimize the tumour residue. Kim et al. [6] reported a C2 SS removed with negative margins, and Cao et al. [33] reported another case who underwent a T7 en bloc resection. Both patients survived without recurrence in their 2- and 1-year follow-up, respectively. In our series, a total of four patients, including two with cervical lesions, one with lumbar lesions and one with sacral lesions, received en bloc resections conducted as one-stage surgeries, and they all had favourable prognoses post-surgery. None of the four patients developed local recurrence or died of this disease during the follow-up from 11 to 74 months. A two-stage surgery with the tumour removed with negative margins may also achieve satisfying local control. Puffer et al. [18] reported a case of thoracic dumbbell SS. The tumour was grossly debulked in the first stage, and en bloc resection of the T4, 5, 6 and 7 vertebrae was performed as a second-stage operation. No evidence of tumour recurrence was observed at 67 months from the final resection. For complete tumour resection, sometimes nerve roots or vessels must be sacrificed. In a case [22] of a primitive intraneural SS of the L5 nerve root, the infiltrated root was resected for complete removal of the residual lesion. A slight sensory and motor deficit in the left leg persisted during the 5-year follow-up. The decision should be made carefully, and patients should be informed, especially

Table 3 Review of spinal SS reported in the literature by year since 2008

Literature by year	Number of cases	Age, years	Sex	Tumour sites	Treatment	Follow-up
Subramanian et al. 2018 [19]	1	47	F	T7-8	Laminectomy and total excision of the tumour followed by posterior fusion, adjuvant radiation and chemotherapy	Improvement in the neurological status and remained disease free at 6 months follow-up
Guo et al. 2016 [21]	1	10	M	T9-10	Laminotomy and total excision of the tumour, adjuvant radiation therapy and ifosfamide chemotherapy	No symptoms recurred 6 months after surgery
Yang et al. 2016 [32]	1	20	M	C2	Subtotal resection of the tumour	In situ recurrence after 6 months, patient succumbed to the disease 1 month later
Chen et al. 2016 [34]	1	20	F	T12-L2	A posterior tumour resection with decompression and postoperative radiotherapy	/
Cao et al. 2014 [33]	1	26	M	T7	T7 en bloc resection followed by radiation therapy and chemotherapy	Low back pain in 1 year after surgery
Kim et al. 2014 [6]	1	29	M	C2-3	Marginal resection followed by adjuvant radiation therapy	Disease free for 2 years
Garg et al. 2013 [24]	1	45	F	Lumbosacral paraspinal area	Wide local excision of the lump with lateral intercostal artery-based rotational flap reconstruction	/
Peia et al. 2013 [22]	1	7	F	L4-5(L5 nerve root)	Bone erosion extended and the infiltrated root resected, followed by chemotherapy	No evidence of disease after 5 years
Kim et al. 2013 [5]	1	17	M	C3	Tumour resection of C3, laminectomy of C4, partial laminectomy of C2 and posterior instrumentation of C2-C6; anterior cervical fusion of C2-C5; postoperative chemotherapy	/
Yonezawa et al. 2012 [36]	1	23	F	L3-4(cauda equina)	L2-4 left hemilaminectomy, tumour totally resected and adjuvant local radiation therapy	Free of local recurrence and metastasis 5.5 years after surgery
Naphade et al. 2011 [37]	1	14	M	C6-7	A well-defined epidural mass lesion completely excised	No signs of local recurrence or metastasis at 6 months post surgery
Zairi et al. 2011 [29]	1	36	M	C1-2	Complete resection and radiotherapeutic adjuvant treatment	Local recurrence; multiple lung metastases occurred in 6-year follow-up and died of disease
Puffer et al. 2011 [18]	3	59	F	T4-6	(1) T3-5 laminectomy with debulking of tumour, (2) en bloc resection of T4-7 with a posterior instrumented spinal fusion from T1-L1 and (3) radiation therapy and chemotherapy	No evidence of tumour recurrence or metastases at 67 months from the final resection
		54	F	Paraspinal mass centred around T10	T12-L1 laminectomy and biopsy	Died of disease 4 months later
		32	F	T5-6	Paraspinal tumour removed, dura incised and nerve root resected with negative margins; gross residual tumour in the T6 transverse process resected; followed by chemotherapy	No tumour recurrence at 6-month follow-up; suspicious lung metastases

Table 3 Review of spinal SS reported in the literature by year since 2008 (*Continued*)

Literature by year	Number of cases	Age, years	Sex	Tumour sites	Treatment	Follow-up
Foreman et al. 2011 [23]	1	29	M	C3-T1	Subtotal resection, postoperative radiation therapy and chemotherapy	6 years post resection without recurrence of the tumour
Liu et al. 2010 [35]	1	12	M	S2 and below	Tumour en bloc excision and postoperative radiation therapy	Recurrence at 6 months after surgery and died of disease 21 months after diagnosis
Arnold et al. 2010 [30]	1	26	F	C2-5	C2-3 laminectomy, posterior C2 corpectomy with occipital-C7 fixation and fusion, palliative chemoradiation	Died 6 months postoperatively of disease progression
Ravnik et al. 2009 [8]	1	32	M	T12-L2	Laminectomy with epidural mass removal; debulking surgery; following chemoradiation	Local recurrence after 12-month follow-up
Koehler et al. 2009 [4]	1	60	M	T7-10	Right-sided thoracotomy, followed by radiation therapy	No recurrence in 9-month follow-up
Barus et al.2009 [10]	1	14	F	L2-5	Marginal resection with anticipated postoperative chemotherapy and radiation	No evidence of local recurrence or distinct disease in 5 years and 9 months after surgery
Scollato et al. 2008 [31]	1	59	M	C3-5	Longitudinal myelotomy	Died of lung and hepatic metastases 3 months later

F female, *M* male

when cervical, lumbar and sacral nerve roots and vertebral arteries are entrapped and violated. In our series, in nine patients, including three with en bloc resection, the nerve roots were sacrificed.

Adjuvant therapies are beneficial for large, deep and high-grade STSs [28]. Six patients with an advanced tumour stage and relatively stable general status had chemotherapy and local radiotherapy following the operation. Of these six patients, one was DOD, one was AWD and four were alive with NED at their last follow-up. The relatively better outcomes for these patients might be affected by their better general condition. Most previously reported cases used adjuvant chemotherapy and/or radiation therapy [34–36]. Naphade et al. [37] reported a case of cervical SS where the tumour was completely excised without adjuvant treatment, and no signs of local recurrence or metastasis were detected at 6 months after surgery. There is no consensus about the role of adjuvant and preoperative chemotherapy in SS [28]. A previous study demonstrated that SS tended to have higher chemosensitivity compared to other STSs [38]. Eilber et al. [39] showed that ifosfamide-based chemotherapy offered a survival benefit to adult patients with primary extremity SS. However, Italiano et al. [12] suggested that preoperative or adjuvant chemotherapy did not improve the prognosis. Based on our study and experience, well-planned, wide surgical excision should be the cornerstone of treatment for spinal SS and the main factor indicating their prognosis. Molecular and cellular abnormalities of SS implied new therapeutic targets, and receptor tyrosine kinase inhibitors like cediranib and bevacizumab have shown promising results [40–42].

Conclusion

We presented a case series of 16 spinal SS patients, and the features of spinal SS were roughly depicted. Spinal SS has a relatively poor prognosis. Surgical management with en bloc excision is demanding yet the most effective treatment strategy to improve outcomes. Management of spinal SS should be under the instruction of a multidisciplinary team. Therefore, a multi-centred, prospective study with a large cohort is required to further investigate the therapeutic strategy for spinal SS.

Abbreviations

AWD: Alive with the disease; CT: Computed tomography; DOD: Died of disease; KPS: Karnofsky Performance Status; MRI: Magnetic resonance imaging; NED: No evidence of disease; OS: Overall survival; SS: Synovial sarcoma; STS: Soft tissue sarcomas; VAS: Visual analogue scale; WBB: Weinstein-Boriani-Biagnini

Funding

The research was generously supported by the National Natural Science Foundation of China (grant no. 81102036), the Shanghai Sailing Program (18YF1423000), and the Foundation for Young Scholars of Second Military Medical University (2017QN16, 2917QN17).

Authors' contributions

MY collected and analysed the clinical data and drafted the manuscript. NZ and CZ helped to analyse the data and draft the manuscript. WX conducted patient follow-up and reviewed the manuscript. SH and JZ conducted patient follow-up. XY and JX conducted patient follow-up, designed the study and reviewed the manuscript. All authors read and approved the final manuscript.

Competing interests

The authors declare that they have no competing interests.

References

1. Fisher CG, Keynan O, Boyd MC, Dvorak MF. The surgical management of primary tumorsof the spine: initial results of an ongoing prospective cohort study. Spine (Phila Pa 1976). 2005;30:1899–908.
2. Kerouanton A, Jimenez I, Cellier C, Laurence V, Helfre S, Pannier S, Mary P, Freneaux P, Orbach D. Synovial sarcoma in children and adolescents. J Pediatr Hematol Oncol. 2014;36:257–62.
3. Ferrari A, De Salvo GL, Oberlin O, Casanova M, De Paoli A, Rey A, Minard V, Orbach D, Carli M, Brennan B, et al. Synovial sarcoma in children and adolescents: a critical reappraisal of staging investigations in relation to the rate of metastatic involvement at diagnosis. Eur J Cancer. 2012;48:1370–5.
4. Koehler SM, Beasley MB, Chin CS, Wittig JC, Hecht AC, Qureshi SA. Synovial sarcoma of the thoracic spine. Spine J. 2009;9:e1–6.
5. Kim KW, Park SY, Won KY, Jin W, Kim SM, Park JS, Ryu KN. Synovial sarcoma of primary bone origin arising from the cervical spine. Skelet Radiol. 2013;42:303–8.
6. Kim J, Lee SH, Choi YL, Bae GE, Kim ES, Eoh W. Synovial sarcoma of the spine: a case involving paraspinal muscle with extensive calcification and the surgical consideration in treatment. Eur Spine J. 2014;23:27–31.
7. Trassard M, Le Doussal V, Hacene K, Terrier P, Ranchere D, Guillou L, Fiche M, Collin F, Vilain MO, Bertrand G, et al. Prognostic factors in localized primary synovial sarcoma: a multicenter study of 128 adult patients. J Clin Oncol. 2001;19:525–34.
8. Ravnik J, Potrc S, Kavalar R, Ravnik M, Zakotnik B, Bunc G. Dumbbell synovial sarcoma of the thoracolumbar spine: a case report. Spine (Phila Pa 1976). 2009;34:E363–6.
9. Morrison C, Wakely PJ, Ashman CJ, Lemley D, Theil K. Cystic synovial sarcoma. Ann Diagn Pathol. 2001;5:48–56.
10. Barus CE, Monsey RD, Kalof AN. Poorly differentiated synovial sarcoma of the lumbar spine in a fourteen-year-old girl. A case report. J Bone Joint Surg Am. 2009;91:1471–6.
11. Mullah-Ali A, Ramsay JA, Bourgeois JM, Hodson I, Macdonald P, Midia M, Portwine C. Paraspinal synovial sarcoma as an unusual postradiation complication in pediatric abdominal neuroblastoma. J Pediatr Hematol Oncol. 2008;30:553–7.
12. Italiano A, Penel N, Robin YM, Bui B, Le Cesne A, Piperno-Neumann S, Tubiana-Hulin M, Bompas E, Chevreau C, Isambert N, et al. Neo/adjuvant chemotherapy does not improve outcome in resected primary synovial sarcoma: a study of the French Sarcoma Group. Ann Oncol. 2009;20:425–30.
13. Singer S, Baldini EH, Demetri GD, Fletcher JA, Corson JM. Synovial sarcoma: prognostic significance of tumor size, margin of resection, and mitotic activity for survival. J Clin Oncol. 1996;14:1201–8.
14. Signorini GC, Pinna G, Freschini A, Bontempini L, Dalle OG. Synovial sarcoma of the thoracic spine. A case report. Spine (Phila Pa 1976). 1986;11:629–31.
15. Chan P, Boriani S, Fourney DR, Biagini R, Dekutoski MB, Fehlings MG, Ryken TC, Gokaslan ZL, Vrionis FD, Harrop JS, et al. An assessment of the reliability of the Enneking and Weinstein-Boriani-Biagini classifications for staging of primary spinal tumors by the Spine Oncology Study Group. Spine (Phila Pa 1976). 2009;34:384–91.
16. Ferrari A, Bisogno G, Alaggio R, Cecchetto G, Collini P, Rosolen A, Meazza C, Indolfi P, Garaventa A, De Sio L, et al. Synovial sarcoma of children and adolescents: the prognostic role of axial sites. Eur J Cancer. 2008;44:1202–9.
17. Ryan JR, Baker LH, Benjamin RS. The natural history of metastatic synovial sarcoma: experience of the Southwest Oncology group. Clin Orthop Relat Res. 1982;(164):257–60.
18. Puffer RC, Daniels DJ, Giannini C, Pichelmann MA, Rose PS, Clarke MJ. Synovial sarcoma of the spine: a report of three cases and review of the literature. Surg Neurol Int. 2011;2:18.
19. Subramanian S, Jonathan GE, Patel B, Prabhu K. Synovial sarcoma mimicking a thoracic dumbell schwannoma- a case report. Br J Neurosurg. 2018:1–4. https://doi.org/10.1080/02688697.2017.1418289.

20. Chambers LA, Lesher JM. Chronic thigh pain in a young adult diagnosed as synovial sarcoma: a case report. PM R. 2018. https://doi.org/10.1016/j.pmrj.2017.12.009. [Epub ahead of print].

21. Guo A, Guo F. Sudden onset of paraplegia secondary to an unusual presentation of pediatric synovial sarcoma. Childs Nerv Syst. 2016;32:2465–9.

22. Peia F, Gessi M, Collini P, Ferrari A, Erbetta A, Valentini LG. Pediatric primitive intraneural synovial sarcoma of L-5 nerve root. J Neurosurg Pediatr. 2013;11:473–7.

23. Foreman SM, Stahl MJ. Biphasic synovial sarcoma in the cervical spine: case report. Chiropr Man Therap. 2011;19:12.

24. Garg PK, Mohnaty D, Jain BK, Goel S, Singh B. Giant subcutaneous synovial sarcoma: an interesting case. J Clin Diagn Res. 2013;7:3014–5.

25. Ferrari A, De Salvo GL, Dall'Igna P, Meazza C, De Leonardis F, Manzitti C, De Ioris MA, Casanova M, Carli M, Bisogno G. Salvage rates and prognostic factors after relapse in children and adolescents with initially localised synovial sarcoma. Eur J Cancer. 2012;48:3448–55.

26. Spurrell EL, Fisher C, Thomas JM, Judson IR. Prognostic factors in advanced synovial sarcoma: an analysis of 104 patients treated at the Royal Marsden Hospital. Ann Oncol. 2005;16:437–44.

27. Sar C, Eralp L. Surgical treatment of primary tumors of the sacrum. Arch Orthop Trauma Surg. 2002;122:148–55.

28. Ashford RU. Expert's comment concerning Grand Rounds case entitled "synovial sarcoma of the spine: a case involving paraspinal muscle with extensive calcification and the surgical consideration in treatment" (by Junhyung Kim, Sun-Ho Lee, Yoon-La Choi, Go Eun Bae, Eun-Sang Kim, Whan Eoh). Eur Spine J. 2014;23:32–4.

29. Zairi F, Assaker R, Bouras T, Chastanet P, Reyns N. Cervical synovial sarcoma necessitating multiple neurosurgical procedures. Br J Neurosurg. 2011;25:769–71.

30. Arnold PM, Roh S, Ha TM, Anderson KK. Metastatic synovial sarcoma with cervical spinal cord compression treated with posterior ventral resection: case report. J Spinal Cord Med. 2010;33:80–4.

31. Scollato A, Buccoliero AM, Di Rita A, Gallina P, Di Lorenzo N. Intramedullary spinal cord metastasis from synovial sarcoma. Case illustration. *J Neurosurg Spine.* 2008;8:400.

32. Yang C, Fang J, Xu Y. Primary cervical intramedullary synovial sarcoma: a longitudinal observation. Spine J. 2016;16:e657–8.

33. Cao Y, Jiang C, Chen Z, Jiang X. A rare synovial sarcoma of the spine in the thoracic vertebral body. Eur Spine J. 2014;23(Suppl 2):228–35.

34. Chen Q, Shi F, Liu L, Song Y. Giant synovial sarcoma involved thoracolumbar vertebrae and paraspinal muscle. Spine J. 2016;16:e271–2.

35. Liu ZJ, Zhang LJ, Zhao Q, Li QW, Wang EB, Ji SJ, Shu H. Pediatric synovial sarcoma of the sacrum: a case report. J Pediatr Orthop B. 2010;19:207–10.

36. Yonezawa I, Saito T, Nakahara D, Won J, Wada T, Kaneko K. Synovial sarcoma of the cauda equina. J Neurosurg Spine. 2012;16:187–90.

37. Naphade PS, Desai MS, Shah RM, Raut AA. Synovial sarcoma of cervical intervertebral foramen: a rare cause of brachial weakness. Neurol India. 2011;59:783–5.

38. Karavasilis V, Seddon BM, Ashley S, Al-Muderis O, Fisher C, Judson I. Significant clinical benefit of first-line palliative chemotherapy in advanced soft-tissue sarcoma: retrospective analysis and identification of prognostic factors in 488 patients. Cancer-Am Cancer Soc. 2008;112:1585–91.

39. Eilber FC, Brennan MF, Eilber FR, Eckardt JJ, Grobmyer SR, Riedel E, Forscher C, Maki RG, Singer S. Chemotherapy is associated with improved survival in adult patients with primary extremity synovial sarcoma. Ann Surg. 2007;246:105–13.

40. Vlenterie M, Jones RL, van der Graaf WT. Synovial sarcoma diagnosis and management in the era of targeted therapies. Curr Opin Oncol. 2015;27:316–22.

41. Hong DS, Garrido-Laguna I, Ekmekcioglu S, Falchook GS, Naing A, Wheler JJ, Fu S, Moulder SL, Piha-Paul S, Tsimberidou AM, et al. Dual inhibition of the vascular endothelial growth factor pathway: a phase 1 trial evaluating bevacizumab and AZD2171 (cediranib) in patients with advanced solid tumors. Cancer-Am Cancer Soc. 2014;120:2164–73.

42. Fox E, Aplenc R, Bagatell R, Chuk MK, Dombi E, Goodspeed W, Goodwin A, Kromplewski M, Jayaprakash N, Marotti M, et al. A phase 1 trial and pharmacokinetic study of cediranib, an orally bioavailable pan-vascular endothelial growth factor receptor inhibitor, in children and adolescents with refractory solid tumors. J Clin Oncol. 2010;28:5174–81.

14

Neoadjuvant vs definitive concurrent chemoradiotherapy in locally advanced esophageal squamous cell carcinoma patients

Chih-Yi Chen[1†], Chia-Chin Li[2†] and Chun-Ru Chien[2,3,4*] (iD)

Abstract

Background: The optimal treatment for locally advanced esophageal squamous cell carcinoma remains unclear. We compared the clinical outcomes of neoadjuvant concurrent chemoradiotherapy (CCRT) followed by esophagectomy [the surgery group] and CCRT without surgery [the CCRT group] in patients with squamous cell carcinoma from an Asian population.

Methods: Eligible patients diagnosed from 2008 to 2015 were identified through the Taiwan Cancer Registry. To balance observable potential confounders, we constructed a 1:1 propensity score-matched cohort [surgery vs CCRT]. We compared the hazard ratios between the surgery and CCRT groups for death using a robust variance estimator. We also evaluated the outcomes of patients for freedom from local regional recurrence (FFLRR) and esophageal cancer-specific survival (ECSS). Extensive supplementary analyses were performed to examine the robustness of our findings.

Results: Our study population included 298 patients balanced with respect to the observed covariables. The hazard ratio of death was 0.56 [95% confidence interval 0.42~0.75] when surgery was compared to CCRT. The results remained significant in the FFLRR and ECSS outcomes. In the supplementary analyses, our results also remained significant when additional covariables were taken into consideration or when the definition of the index date was changed.

Conclusions: When compared to definitive CCRT, neoadjuvant CCRT followed by esophagectomy was associated with improved overall survival for locally advanced esophageal squamous cell carcinoma. However, given the nonrandomized nature of the study and the sensitivity to potentially unmeasured confounders, our results should be interpreted cautiously.

Keywords: Esophageal squamous cell carcinoma, Concurrent chemoradiotherapy, Esophagectomy

Background

Esophageal cancer is a common cause for cancer mortality around the world [1], and except in North America and Europe, squamous cell carcinoma (SqCC) is the major histological subtype [1].

The optimal treatment for locally advanced esophageal SqCC has remained elusive. According to the current National Comprehensive Cancer Network guidelines, esophagectomy, neoadjuvant concurrent chemoradiotherapy (CCRT) followed by esophagectomy, or definite CCRT were all possible treatment options for cT1b-4aN0-+M0 patients [2]. A seminal paper published in the New England Journal of Medicine in 2014 states that "locally advanced tumors, defined as category T3N1, are best treated with esophagectomy" [1]. However, the role of esophagectomy was questioned in a review paper published in 2017 [3]. Meta-analyses and a recent large-scale randomized

---

* Correspondence: d16181@gmail.com
†Chih-Yi Chen and Chia-Chin Li contributed equally to this work.
²Department of Radiation Oncology, China Medical University Hospital, Taichung, Taiwan
³Department of Radiation Oncology, China Medical University Hsinchu Hospital, Hsinchu, Taiwan
Full list of author information is available at the end of the article

controlled trial (RCT) reported favorable outcomes when neoadjuvant CCRT followed by esophagectomy was compared to esophagectomy alone [4, 5]. In addition, RCTs for esophageal SqCC patients from Germany and France had reported similar overall survival (OS), although better local control was obtained with neoadjuvant CCRT followed by esophagectomy compared to CCRT without surgery (also mentioned in the 2017 review paper above) [3, 6, 7]. Another RCT also reported similar OS between CCRT without surgery and upfront esophagectomy without neoadjuvant CCRT [8].

Therefore, the aim of our study was to compare neoadjuvant CCRT followed by esophagectomy to definitive CCRT for locally advanced esophageal SqCC patients in a real-world Asian population.

Methods
Data source
In our study, the primary data comes from the Taiwan Cancer Registry (TCR) and death registration. The TCR is a high-quality database [9] that provides complete information such as individual demographics, stage of disease, tumor histology, and treatment details. Some prognostic

factors, e.g., the use of positron emission tomography (PET), were also available since 2011.

Study population and study design
Our study flow chart, designed to conform to the STROBE guidelines [10], is depicted in Fig. 1. The main study population consisted of locally advanced esophageal SqCC patients diagnosed from 2008 to 2015 who received neoadjuvant CCRT [radiotherapy dose 40–50.4 Gy] before esophagectomy, or CCRT [radiotherapy dose ≥ 50.4 Gy] without surgery. The explanatory variable of interest in this study was the surgery group (neoadjuvant CCRT followed by esophagectomy) vs the CCRT group (CCRT without surgery). We collected covariables based on our experiences in clinical care and related TCR studies [11–13] for adjustment of potential nonrandomized treatment selection (as mentioned in the next section). We defined the date of diagnosis from the cancer registry as the index date and obtained the survival statuses of patients from the death registry [follow-up until Dec 31, 2016]. We then estimated propensity scores (PSs) using the covariables to construct a PS-matched sample. We used this PS-based method rather than a Cox regression model, as suggested in previous literature [14, 15].

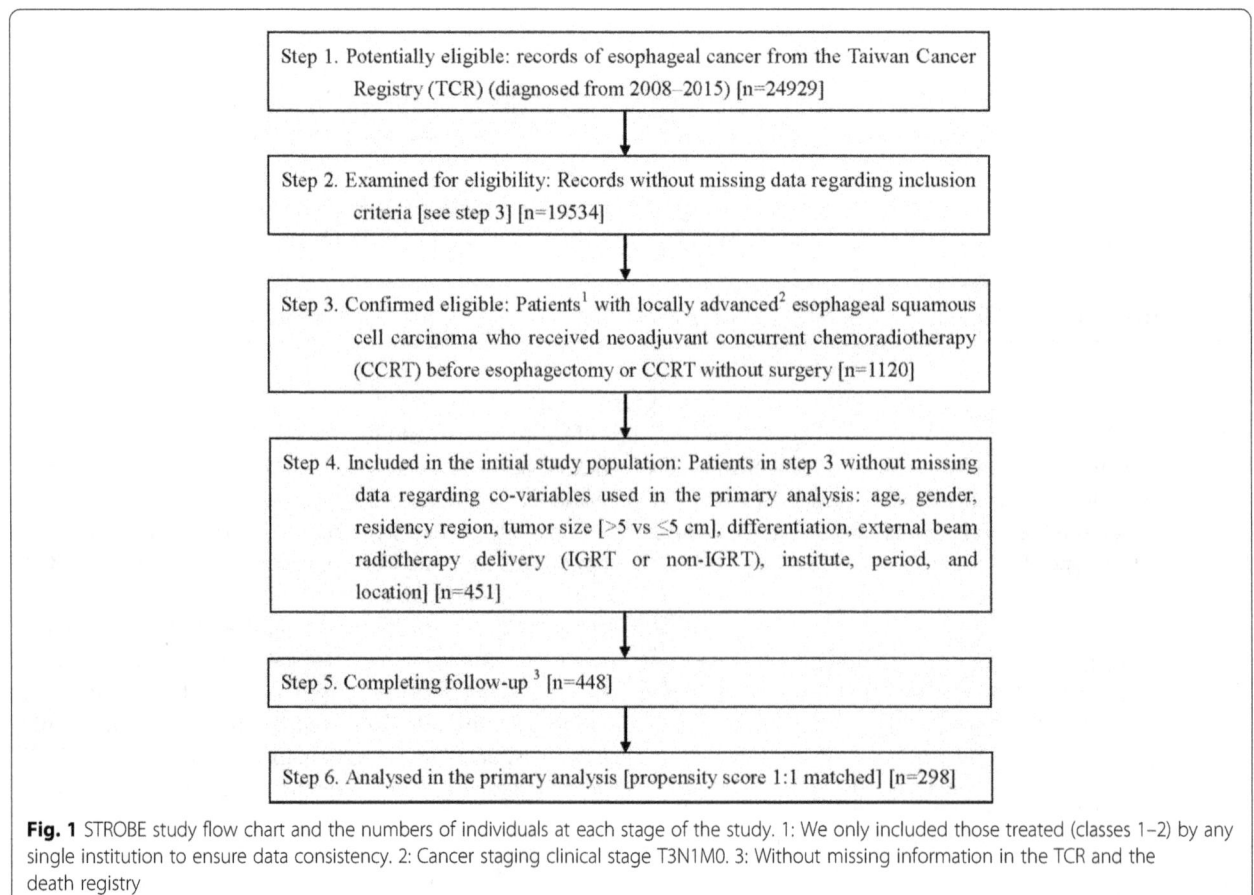

Step 1. Potentially eligible: records of esophageal cancer from the Taiwan Cancer Registry (TCR) (diagnosed from 2008–2015) [n=24929]

Step 2. Examined for eligibility: Records without missing data regarding inclusion criteria [see step 3] [n=19534]

Step 3. Confirmed eligible: Patients[1] with locally advanced[2] esophageal squamous cell carcinoma who received neoadjuvant concurrent chemoradiotherapy (CCRT) before esophagectomy or CCRT without surgery [n=1120]

Step 4. Included in the initial study population: Patients in step 3 without missing data regarding co-variables used in the primary analysis: age, gender, residency region, tumor size [>5 vs ≤5 cm], differentiation, external beam radiotherapy delivery (IGRT or non-IGRT), institute, period, and location] [n=451]

Step 5. Completing follow-up [3] [n=448]

Step 6. Analysed in the primary analysis [propensity score 1:1 matched] [n=298]

Fig. 1 STROBE study flow chart and the numbers of individuals at each stage of the study. 1: We only included those treated (classes 1–2) by any single institution to ensure data consistency. 2: Cancer staging clinical stage T3N1M0. 3: Without missing information in the TCR and the death registry

Other explanatory covariables

Patient demographics [age, gender, residency region], disease characteristics [tumor size, differentiation, tumor location], radiotherapy (RT) delivery, institution, and period were included in our primary analysis. We also considered a prognostic factor ["use of PET", available in the TCR since 2011] in the supplementary analyses. The definitions of covariables were as follows. Patient residency region was classified as northern Taiwan or elsewhere. Tumor size was classified by a diameter ≤ 5 or > 5 cm. Tumor differentiation was classified as well/moderately differentiated or poorly/undifferentiated. External beam radiotherapy delivery was classified as image-guided radiotherapy (IGRT) or non-IGRT. The hospital was classified as a high- or low-volume institute via a threshold [20 esophagectomies per year] [16]. The time period was classified as 2008–2009 or 2010–2015. Tumor location was classified as cervical or not.

Statistical analysis

We performed the statistical analysis using the software SAS 9.4 (SAS Institute, Cary, NC, USA) and STATA 12 (StataCorp LP, College Station, TX, USA). In the primary analysis, we used a logistic regression model based on covariables to evaluate the probability of receiving surgery (vs CCRT) and then used the logit of the probability as the PS in a PS-matched method. Tabulation and standardized difference [17, 18] were used to assess the balance of covariates between PS-matched groups. We used a robust variance estimator to compare the hazard ratios of events between surgery- and CCRT-matched groups during the entire follow-up period [14]. As suggested in the recent literature [19], we evaluated the robustness of our findings to potential unmeasured confounding factor(s) via the E-factor. We also evaluated the outcomes of patients for freedom from local regional recurrence (FFLRR) and esophageal cancer-specific survival (ECSS) according to the TCR and the death registry.

Supplementary analysis

In a subgroup of patients [diagnosed from 2011 to 2015] for whom additional information, i.e., use of PET, was available, we performed the first supplementary analysis (SA-1). In the second supplementary analysis (SA-2), we repeated what we did in SA-1 but limited the surgery group to those who received minimally invasive esophagectomy (MIE) because of its potential superiority [20, 21]. In the third supplementary analysis (SA-3), we reanalyzed the OS in the primary analysis when the index date was changed to the start of radiotherapy.

Results

Identification of the study population used in the primary analysis

As shown in Fig. 1, the identified initial study population consisted of 451 esophageal SqCC cancer patients divided into surgery or CCRT groups. After excluding the missing data in follow-up and applying a PS matching method, 298 patients were used as the final study population in the primary analysis. The patient characteristics are described in Table 1. All covariables after matching were well balanced with small standardized differences (< 0.25) [17].

Primary analysis

After a median follow-up of 20 months [range 3–98], death was observed for 79 patients in the surgery group and for 108 in the CCRT group. The hazard ratio (HR) of death when surgery was compared to CCRT was 0.56 [95% confidence interval (95CI) 0.42–0.75, p value < 0.001]. The observed HR 0.56 for OS could be explained by an unmeasured confounder associated with the selection of treatment (IMRT or 3DCRT) and live/death by a risk ratio of 2.35-fold each; however, weaker confounding factors could not do so. Furthermore, the confidence interval could be moved to include the null hypothesis by an unmeasured confounder by a risk ratio of 1.74, above and beyond the measured confounders; however, weaker confounding could not. The 5-year OS rate for surgery was 38% (vs 20% for CCRT). Figure 2 shows the Kaplan-Meier survival curve for OS. Surgery was also associated with better FFLRR [HR 0.17, 95CI 0.11–0.28, p value $< .001$] and ECSS [HR 0.56, 95CI 0.41–0.77, p value $< .001$].

Supplementary analyses

In the SA-1, which incorporated the use of PET into the PS model, all of the covariables were well balanced and the standardized differences were small (< 0.25) (Table 2). From this analysis, we found that surgery was still associated with improved OS compared to CCRT [HR 0.51, 95CI 0.36–0.72, p value < 0.001]. Figure 3 shows the Kaplan-Meier survival curve for OS.

In the SA-2, in which neoadjuvant CCRT followed by MIE was compared to CCRT without surgery, all of the covariables were still well balanced with small standardized differences (< 0.25) (Table 3). The HR of death when surgery [MIE] was compared to CCRT was 0.44 [95CI 0.28–0.70, p value < 0.001]. Figure 4 shows the Kaplan-Meier survival curve for OS.

In the SA-3 in which we used the RT-start date as the index date, the HR for death when surgery was compared with CCRT was similar [0.55, 95CI 0.41–0.74, p value < 0.001]. The Kaplan-Meier survival curves for OS are shown in Fig. 5.

Discussion

In this population-based study PS-matched analysis from Asia (Taiwan), we found that for locally advanced esophageal SqCC, neoadjuvant CCRT followed by esophagectomy was associated with improved OS when compared to CCRT without surgery.

Table 1 Characteristics of matched study population in the primary analysis

		Surgery Number or mean (sd)[a]	(%)[a]	CCRT Number or mean (sd)[a]	(%)[a]	Standardized difference[a]
Age		56.93 (8.65)		57.26 (10.48)		0.04
Gender	Female	8	(5)	7	(5)	0.03
	Male	141	(95)	142	(95)	
Residency	Non-north	101	(68)	100	(67)	0.01
	North	48	(32)	49	(33)	
Tumor size	≤ 5 cm	59	(40)	60	(40)	0.01
	> 5 cm	90	(60)	89	(60)	
Differentiation	Poorly/undifferentiated	46	(31)	53	(36)	0.10
	Well/moderately	103	(69)	96	(64)	
RT delivery	Non-IGRT	131	(88)	128	(86)	0.06
	IGRT	18	(12)	21	(14)	
Institution	Low volume	50	(34)	54	(36)	0.06
	High volume	99	(66)	95	(64)	
Period	2008–2009	18	(12)	19	(13)	0.02
	2010–2015	131	(88)	130	(87)	
Location	Cervical	1	(1)	1	(1)	0.00
	Noncervical	148	(99)	148	(99)	

sd standard deviation, *RT* radiotherapy, *IGRT* image-guided RT, *CCRT* concurrent chemoradiotherapy
[a]Rounded

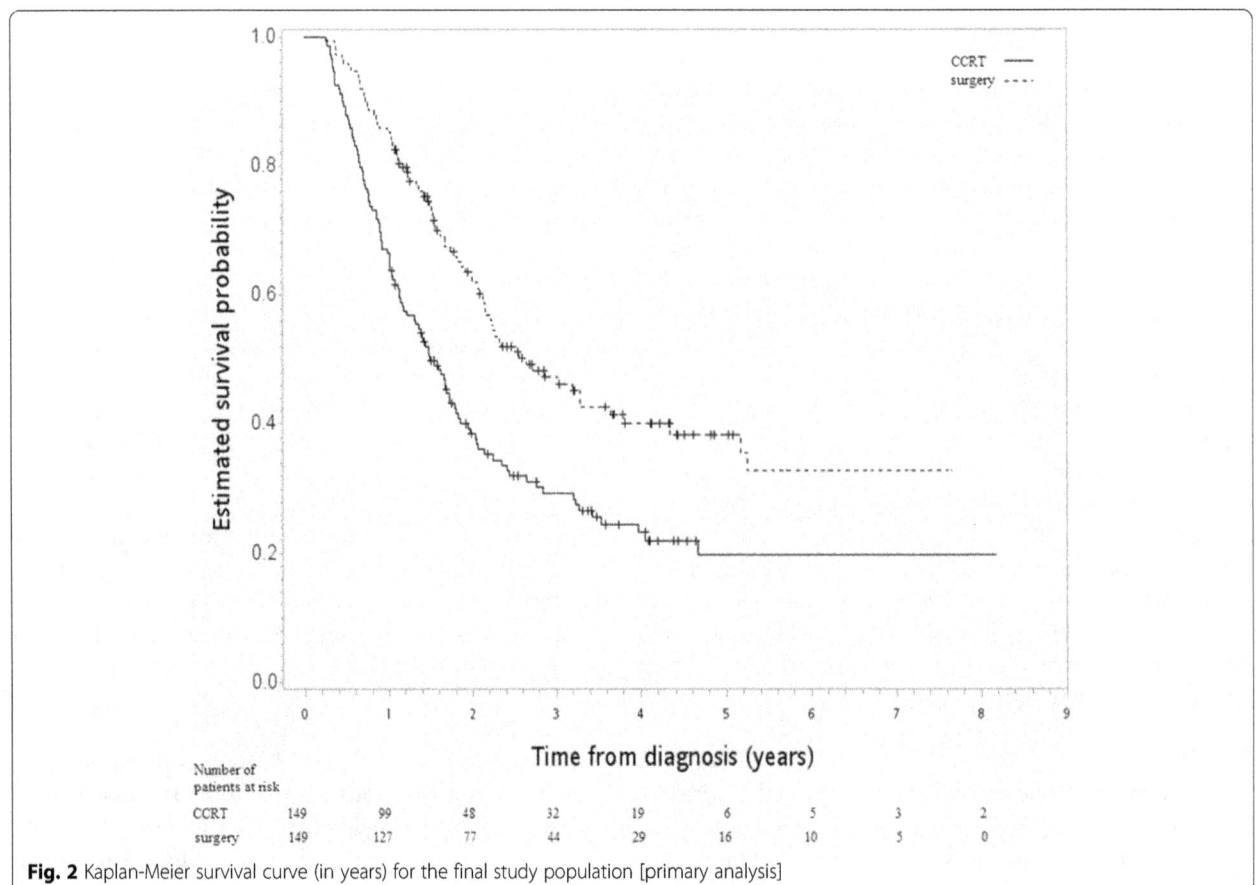

Fig. 2 Kaplan-Meier survival curve (in years) for the final study population [primary analysis]

Table 2 Characteristics of the matched study population in the SA-1

		Surgery Number or mean (sd)[a]	(%)[a]	CCRT Number or mean (sd)[a]	(%)[a]	Standardized difference[a]
Age		57.00 (7.63)		56.61 (9.62)		0.05
Gender	Female	6	(5)	3	(3)	0.14
	Male	104	(95)	107	(97)	
Residency	Non-north	76	(69)	80	(73)	0.08
	North	34	(31)	30	(27)	
Tumor size	≤ 5 cm	43	(39)	42	(38)	0.02
	> 5 cm	67	(61)	68	(62)	
Differentiation	Poorly/undifferentiated	41	(37)	42	(38)	0.02
	Well/moderately	69	(63)	68	(62)	
RT delivery	Non-IGRT	94	(85)	96	(87)	0.05
	IGRT	16	(15)	14	(13)	
Institution	Low volume	40	(36)	45	(41)	0.09
	High volume	70	(64)	65	(59)	
Use of PET	Without	12	(11)	12	(11)	0.00
	With	98	(89)	98	(89)	
Location	Cervical	1	(1)	1	(1)	0.00
	Noncervical	109	(99)	109	(99)	

sd standard deviation, *RT* radiotherapy, *IGRT* image-guided RT, *PET* positron emission tomography, *CCRT* concurrent chemoradiotherapy
[a]Rounded

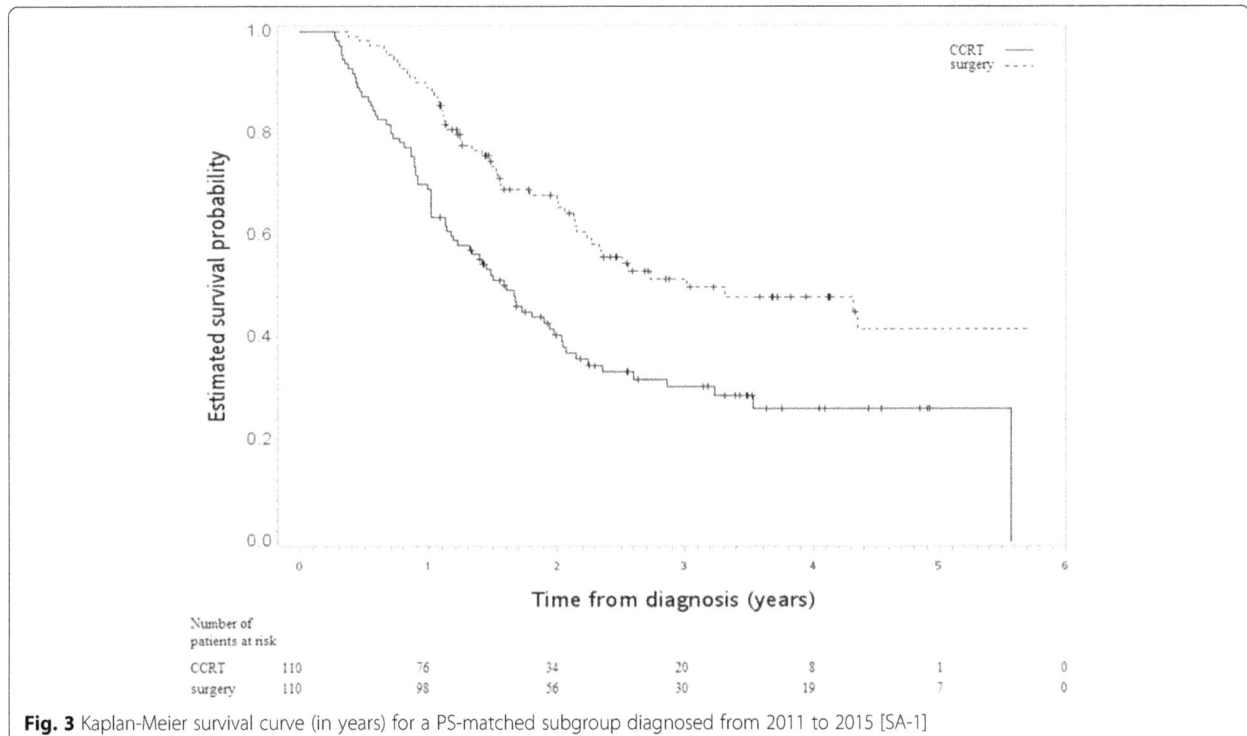

Fig. 3 Kaplan-Meier survival curve (in years) for a PS-matched subgroup diagnosed from 2011 to 2015 [SA-1]

Table 3 Characteristics of the matched study population in the SA-2

		Surgery [MIE] Number or mean (sd)[a]	(%)[a]	CCRT Number or mean (sd)[a]	(%)[a]	Standardized difference[a]
Age		56.38 (8.21)		55.35 (10.58)		0.11
Gender	Female	4	(5)	4	(5)	0.00
	Male	78	(95)	78	(95)	
Residency	Non-north	57	(70)	52	(63)	0.13
	North	25	(30)	30	(37)	
Tumor size	≤ 5 cm	31	(38)	31	(38)	0.00
	> 5 cm	51	(62)	51	(62)	
Differentiation	Poorly/undifferentiated	31	(38)	30	(37)	0.03
	Well/moderately	51	(62)	52	(63)	
RT delivery	Non-IGRT	70	(85)	68	(83)	0.07
	IGRT	12	(15)	14	(17)	
Institution	Low volume	23	(28)	25	(30)	0.05
	High volume	59	(72)	57	(70)	
Use of PET	Without	7	(9)	11	(13)	0.16
	With	75	(91)	71	(87)	

The nonoverlapped covariable (location) was not included in this matching
sd standard deviation, *RT* radiotherapy, *IGRT* image-guided RT, *PET* positron emission tomography, *MIE* minimally invasive esophagectomy, *CCRT* concurrent chemoradiotherapy
[a]Rounded

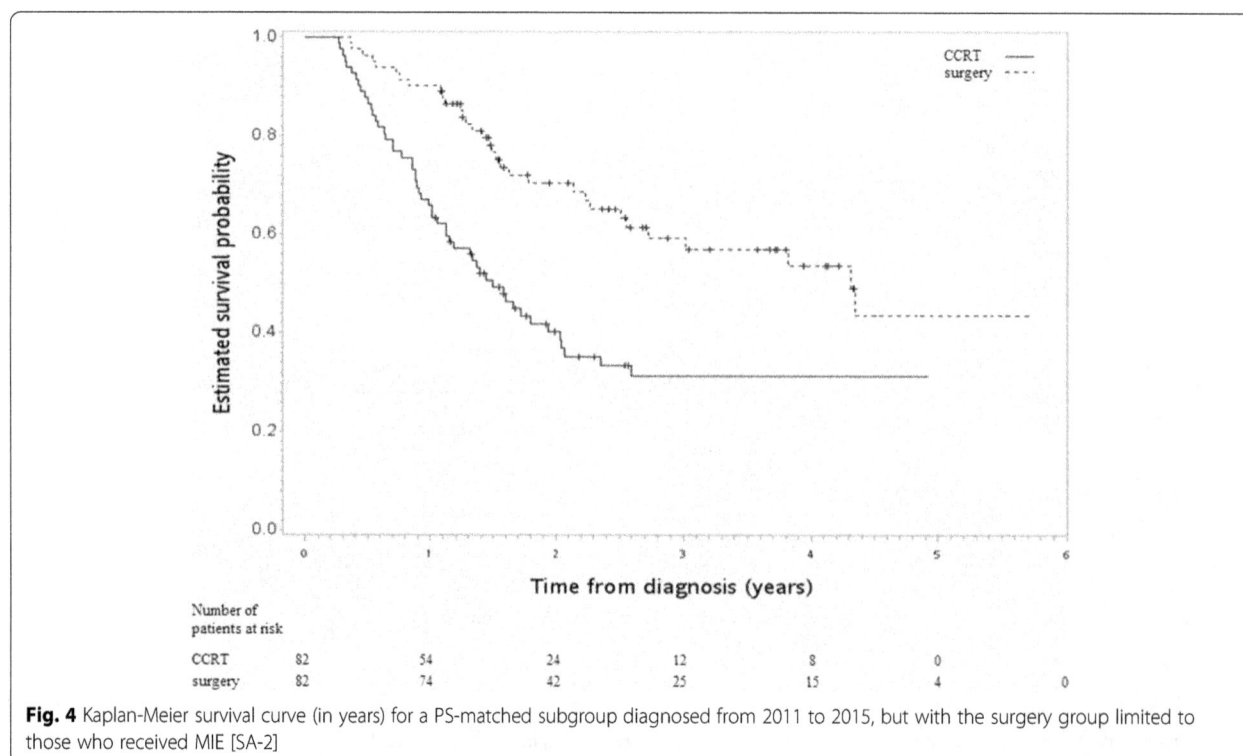

Fig. 4 Kaplan-Meier survival curve (in years) for a PS-matched subgroup diagnosed from 2011 to 2015, but with the surgery group limited to those who received MIE [SA-2]

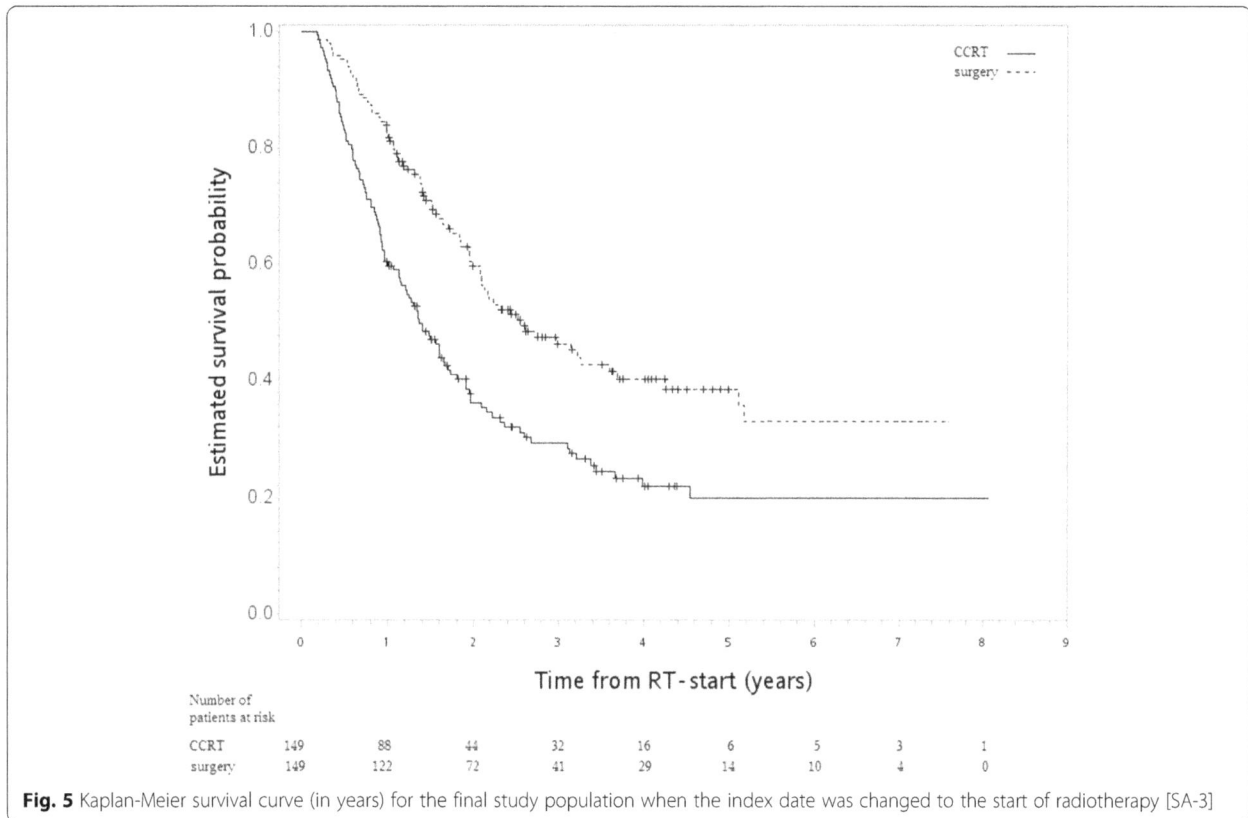

Fig. 5 Kaplan-Meier survival curve (in years) for the final study population when the index date was changed to the start of radiotherapy [SA-3]

Statistically, our results were not consistent with available RCTs [6, 7]; however, survival was actually numerically better for the surgical arm when compared to that for the nonsurgical arms in both RCTs, although not statistically significant. The 2-year OS was 39.9 vs 35.4% in the German trial [7] and 37.1 vs 36.5% [per protocol] in the French trial [6]. In our study, it was 63 vs 39%. Therefore, the outcome of CCRT in our study was similar to both RCTs, but the outcome of neoadjuvant CCRT followed by esophagectomy was higher in our study [63%] (although close to the 67% OS reported in the modern CROSS study [5]).

We feel that our findings are compatible with the prevalent concept that esophagectomy is an integral part of treatment for locally advanced esophageal cancer [1], possibly through improved disease control (demonstrated by the improved FFLRR and ECSS), as better local/regional control in the surgical arm had also been reported in the above RCTs [6, 7]. However, given the abovementioned RCTs and that our result was sensitive to potential unmeasured confounders [E-factor 1.74], we feel that our results should not be interpreted as conclusive and that further modern RCTs are needed. When we searched in "https://clinicaltrials.gov/" using ["esophagectomy" AND "concurrent chemoradiotherapy"] on May 21, 2018, we found two relevant ongoing trials [NCT02972372, NCT01740375]; however, these trials

were relevant but not identical. NCT02972372 investigated definitive CCRT vs surgery without neoadjuvant CCRT, whereas NCT01740375 investigated upfront surgery or observation for those patients who achieved complete clinical response. Therefore, the results of our study could be valuable for contemporary patient decision-making until other modern high-level evidence becomes available.

There were some limitations in our study. First, we shared the inherent limitation of observation study. Although we tried our best to follow the STROBE guidelines for observational study [10] and examined extensive supplementary analyses, potential unmeasured confounder(s), such as presenting body weight loss [6] or operability, might still threaten our results. Second, the generalizability of our finding to regions where SqCC was not the predominant histology might be questionable.

Conclusions

We found that for locally advanced esophageal SqCC, neoadjuvant CCRT followed by esophagectomy was associated with improved OS when compared to CCRT without surgery. However, given the nonrandomized nature of the study and sensitivity to potential unmeasured confounder(s), our results should be interpreted cautiously.

Abbreviations

CCRT: Concurrent chemoradiotherapy; ECSS: Esophageal cancer-specific survival; FFLRR: Freedom from local regional recurrence; IGRT: Image-guided radiotherapy; MIE: Minimally invasive esophagectomy; OS: Overall survival; PET: Positron emission tomography; PS: Propensity score; RCT: Randomized controlled trial; RT: Radiotherapy; SA: Supplementary analysis; SqCC: Squamous cell carcinoma; TCR: Taiwan Cancer Registry

Acknowledgements

The authors are thankful for the conceptual input from Dr. Tsang-Wu Liu and all of the members in the Health Promotion Administration, National Health Research Institute Esophageal Cancer Committee for their conceptual contributions. The authors thank "American Journal Experts" for editorial assistance. The corresponding author would like to thank Dr. Ya-Chen Tina Shih for her mentoring in Health Services Research.

Funding

This work was supported by the Health Promotion Administration, Ministry of Health and Welfare, Taiwan (R.O.C.) [source of this funding is the health and welfare surcharge of tobacco products] and China Medical University Hospital [CRS-106-040 to Chien C.R.].

Authors' contributions

CYC participated in the conceptualization and design of the study, interpreted data, and drafted the manuscript. CCL participated in the conceptualization and design of study, analyzed data, and drafted the manuscript. CRC participated in the conceptualization and design of study, collected the related studies, analyzed and interpreted data, and drafted the manuscript. All authors have read and approved the final manuscript.

Competing interests

The authors declare that they have no competing interests.

Author details

[1]Division of Thoracic Surgery, Department of Surgery, Chung Shan Medical University, Chung Shan Medical University Hospital, Taichung, Taiwan. [2]Department of Radiation Oncology, China Medical University Hospital, Taichung, Taiwan. [3]Department of Radiation Oncology, China Medical University Hsinchu Hospital, Hsinchu, Taiwan. [4]School of Medicine, College of Medicine, China Medical University, No.91 Hsueh-Shih Road, North District, Taichung 40402, Taiwan.

References

1. Rustgi AK, El-Serag HB. Esophageal carcinoma. N Engl J Med. 2014;371: 2499–509.
2. National Comprehensive Cancer Network. National Comprehensive Cancer Network Guidelines for esophageal and esophagogastric junction cancers, version 3.2017 [free registration required]. https://www.nccn.org/professionals/physician_gls/pdf/esophageal.pdf. Accessed 30 Sep 2017.
3. Chun SG, Skinner HD, Minsky BD. Radiation therapy for locally advanced esophageal cancer. Surg Oncol Clin N Am. 2017;26:257–76.
4. Sjoquist KM, Burmeister BH, Smithers BM, Zalcberg JR, Simes RJ, Barbour A, et al. Survival after neoadjuvant chemotherapy or chemoradiotherapy for resectable oesophageal carcinoma: an updated meta-analysis. Lancet Oncol. 2011;12:681–92.
5. Shapiro J, van Lanschot JJB, Hulshof MCCM, van Hagen P, van Berge Henegouwen MI, Wijnhoven BPL, et al. Neoadjuvant chemoradiotherapy plus surgery versus surgery alone for oesophageal or junctional cancer (CROSS): long-term results of a randomised controlled trial. Lancet Oncol. 2015;16:1090–8.
6. Bedenne L, Michel P, Bouché O, Milan C, Mariette C, Conroy T, et al. Chemoradiation followed by surgery compared with chemoradiation alone in squamous cancer of the esophagus: FFCD 9102. J Clin Oncol. 2007;25:1160–8.
7. Stahl M, Stuschke M, Lehmann N, Meyer HJ, Walz MK, Seeber S, et al. Chemoradiation with and without surgery in patients with locally advanced squamous cell carcinoma of the esophagus. J Clin Oncol. 2005;23:2310–7.
8. Chiu PW, Chan AC, Leung SF, Leong HT, Kwong KH, Li MK, et al. Multicenter prospective randomized trial comparing standard esophagectomy with chemoradiotherapy for treatment of squamous esophageal cancer: early results from the Chinese University Research Group for Esophageal Cancer (CURE). J Gastrointest Surg. 2005;9:794–802.
9. Chiang CJ, You SL, Chen CJ, Yang YW, Lo WC, Lai MS. Quality assessment and improvement of nationwide cancer registration system in Taiwan: a review. Jpn J Clin Oncol. 2015;45:291–6.
10. von Elm E, Altman DG, Egger M, Pocock SJ, Gøtzsche PC, Vandenbroucke JP, et al. The Strengthening the Reporting of Observational Studies in Epidemiology (STROBE) statement: guidelines for reporting observational studies. Int J Surg. 2014;12:1495–9.
11. Chen CY, Li CC, Chien CR. Does higher radiation dose lead to better outcome for non-operated localized esophageal squamous cell carcinoma patients who received concurrent chemoradiotherapy? A population based propensity-score matched analysis. Radiother Oncol. 2016;120:136–9.
12. Li CC, Chen CY, Chien CR. Comparative effectiveness of image-guided radiotherapy for non-operated localized esophageal squamous cell carcinoma patients receiving concurrent chemoradiotherapy: a population-based propensity score matched analysis. Oncotarget. 2016;7:71548–55.
13. Fang HY, Chen CY, Wang YC, Wang PH, Shieh SH, Chien CR. Consistently lower narcotics consumption after video-assisted thoracoscopic surgery for early stage non-small cell lung cancer when compared to open surgery: a one-year follow-up study. Eur J Cardiothorac Surg. 2013;43:783–6.
14. Austin PC. The use of propensity score methods with survival or time-to-event outcomes: reporting measures of effect similar to those used in randomized experiments. Stat Med. 2014;33:1242–58.
15. Jagsi R, Bekelman JE, Chen A, Chen RC, Hoffman K, Shih YC, et al. Considerations for observational research using large data sets in radiation oncology. Int J Radiat Oncol Biol Phys. 2014;90:11–24.
16. Gockel I, Ahlbrand CJ, Arras M, Schreiber EM, Lang H. Quality management and key performance indicators in oncologic esophageal surgery. Dig Dis Sci. 2015;60:3536–44.
17. Garrido MM, Kelley AS, Paris J, Roza K, Meier DE, Morrison RS, et al. Methods for constructing and assessing propensity scores. Health Serv Res. 2014;49:1701–20.
18. Ali MS, Groenwold RH, Belitser SV, Pestman WR, Hoes AW, Roes KC, et al. Reporting of covariate selection and balance assessment in propensity score analysis is suboptimal: a systematic review. J Clin Epidemiol. 2015;68:112–21.
19. VanderWeele TJ, Ding P. Sensitivity analysis in observational research: introducing the E-value. Ann Intern Med. 2017;167:268–74.
20. Yibulayin W, Abulizi S, Lv H, Sun W. Minimally invasive oesophagectomy versus open oesophagectomy for resectable esophageal cancer: a meta-analysis. World J Surg Oncol. 2016;14:304.
21. Straatman J, van der Wielen N, Cuesta MA, Daams F, Roig Garcia J, Bonavina L, et al. Minimally invasive versus open esophageal resection: three-year follow-up of the previously reported randomized controlled trial: the TIME trial. Ann Surg. 2017;266:232–6.

15

Uncemented, curved, short endoprosthesis stem for distal femoral reconstruction: early follow-up outcomes

Minxun Lu[1], Jie Wang[1], Cong Xiao[1,2], Fan Tang[1], Li Min[1], Yong Zhou[1], Wenli Zhang[1] and Chongqi Tu[1*]

Abstract

Background: Uncemented endoprosthetic knee replacement has become a mainstream treatment for malignant tumours of the distal femur. Most femoral stems, however, are straight and therefore poorly fit the anteriorly bowed curvature of the femur. To address this issue, we used a short, curved, uncemented press-fit femoral stem and evaluated its short-term outcomes after reconstruction of the distal femur.

Methods: Forty-two patients underwent distal femur replacement using curved press-fit stem. To assess the interface, we measured the axial length of the press-fit area and the perpendicular distance of the radiolucent area between the stem and bone on digital images obtained using tomosynthesis with Shimadzu Metal Artefact Reduction Technology (T-SMART). Postoperative complications and oncological outcomes were monitored at each follow-up visit.

Results: Of the 42 patients enrolled in the study, two had cancer-related deaths and one had local tumour recurrence. The minimum follow-up time of the surviving patients was 24 months, with no incidence of aseptic loosening or mechanical failure of the prosthesis. The average effective contact length between the press-fit stem and bone was 74.0 mm, with nearly undetectable radiolucent gaps between the implant and the bone on medial-lateral and anteroposterior views.

Conclusions: Over the short term, uncemented, curved, short stem provides a stable bone-prosthesis interface without any aseptic loosening.

Keywords: Uncemented, Curvature, Distal femur, Stem, Short

Background

Primary musculoskeletal tumours are common in the distal femur. The introduction of neo-adjuvant chemotherapy and improvement in surgical techniques and prosthesis designs have allowed an endoprosthetic replacement to become the standard method of reconstruction and limb salvage after resection of distal femoral tumours [1, 2]. However, various complications of endoprosthetic replacement are frequently encountered, including aseptic loosening, mechanical failure, infection, and periprosthetic fracture [3]. The rate of these complications is influenced by the type of fixation and the design of the prosthesis, especially for the femoral stem.

The press-fit fixation has been associated with a lower rate of aseptic loosening than cemented fixation and thus is a more reasonable method of stem fixation. However, providing adequate primary stability is a necessity for press-fit fixation. Currently, the Global Modular Replacement System [4] (GMRS, Stryker Orthopaedics, Mahwah, USA), the Kotz Modular Femur and Tibia Reconstruction System [5] (KMFTR, Howmedica GmbH, Kiel, Germany), the Modular Universal Tumour and Revision System [6] (MUTARS, Implantcast GmbH, Buxtehude, Germany), the Segmental System [7] (Zimmer Inc., Warsaw, IN, USA), and the Megasystem-C [7] (LINK GmbH, Hamburg, Germany) are acceptable choices for distal femoral reconstruction (DFR). Although these various designs do

---

* Correspondence: Tuchongqi@yeah.net
[1]Department of Orthopedics, West China Hospital, Sichuan University, No. 37 Guoxue Street, Chengdu 610041, People's Republic of China
Full list of author information is available at the end of the article

provide adequate mechanical strength and primary stability, these commercially available uncemented stems use a straight femoral stem, except the MUTARS and Segmental System. Obviously, a straight stem design is a mismatch for the anterior curvature of the medullary cavity of the femur. The MUTARS and Segmental System do provide a curved stem; its match to the anatomical femoral curvature of Chinese patients is not clear. We propose that short, curved, uncemented femoral stems with derotational fins would be a better design for femoral stems used in DFR. To our knowledge, however, the clinical outcomes of these stems for DFR implants have not previously been evaluated. Therefore, our aim in this study was to retrospectively evaluate the short-term outcomes of using short, curved, uncemented femoral stems for DFR, either after tumour resection or for DFR revision.

Methods
Ethical considerations
This study was approved by the Institutional Review Board and performed in accordance with the ethical principles of the Declaration of Helsinki. All patients provided written informed consent.

Patients
Between October 2014 and December 2017, 42 patients underwent DFR with uncemented, curved, short stems after resection of malignant tumours or for DFR revision in our Department of Orthopaedics. The study group included 25 men and 17 women, with a mean age of 29.3 years (range, 10–67 years). Among these cases, 35 were primary implantation procedures and 7 were revisions necessary due to aseptic loosening of the cemented prosthesis. Pre-operatively, the length of required resection, the percentage of resected bone required, and the radius of curvature (ROC) of the retained femur were measured on plain radiographs. Follow-up assessments were performed every 3 months, postoperatively, during the first year and at every 6 months, thereafter. Lower limb function, the condition of the bone-prosthesis interface, the presence of complications, and oncological outcomes were assessed at each follow-up visit. Lower limb function was evaluated using the Musculoskeletal Tumor Society (MSTS) scoring system [8]. The condition of the bone-prosthesis interface was assessed using digital T-SMART and plain radiography, measuring the axial length of the press-fit area and radiographic evidence of bone resorption. The axial press-fit length was defined as the distance from the distal point of the stem to the location where the perpendicular distance between the stem and the periprosthetic bone was < 1 mm, and the final axial length was calculated by averaging the axial press-fit length in the medial-lateral and anterior-posterior planes.

The periprosthetic radiolucent area, which indicates bone resorption, was evaluated at six points on the femoral stem, namely, the distal endpoint, midpoint, and proximal endpoint measured on bone anterior-posterior and medial-lateral radiographic views. We also evaluated radiographic variables of bone ingrowth into the prosthesis, including bone bridging, spot welding, and neocortex formation. Complications related to stem implantation, including infection, aseptic loosening, periprosthetic fracture, and breakage, were evaluated. All data were analysed using SPSS, version 19, software.

Stem design
All of the curved stems were fabricated by Chunlizhengda Medical Instruments (Tongzhou, Beijing, China). Of the 42 stems that were implanted, 7 were custom-made for DFR revision and 35 were standard modular stems for regular DFR. The standard stem had various diameters, ranging between 10 and 18 mm, and a length of 100 mm. The distal part of the stem was 20 mm in length and straight, with two symmetrically arranged fins (medial and lateral), with the rest of the stem having an anterior curvature (radius, 1400 mm) to match the shape of the medullary canal of the femur (Fig. 1). The stem was coated with

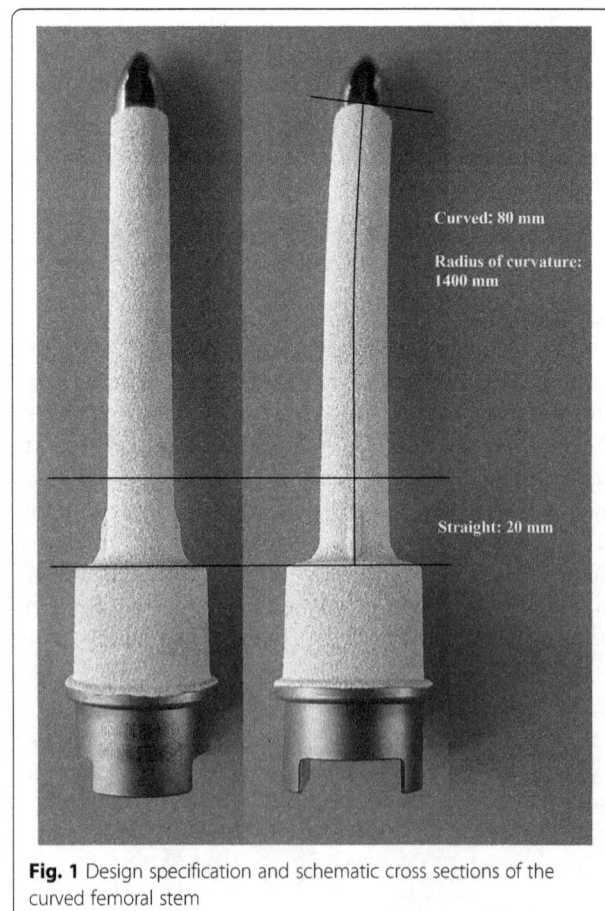

Fig. 1 Design specification and schematic cross sections of the curved femoral stem

hydroxyapatite (HA). The custom-made stems used the same standard design but were longer and/or larger.

Surgical technique

All surgeries were performed by a senior surgeon (C. Tu). The degree of tilt of the osteotomy plane was precisely controlled to minimize the potential for a misfit between the standard stem and the ROC of the femur. After segmental resection of the tumour, we used a flexible reamer, with a guide line in the centre, to enlarge the medullary cavity of the femur, maintaining its anterior curvature (Fig. 2). To minimize bone loss and maximize primary stability of the endoprosthesis, the femoral canal was under-reamed by 0.5 mm, compared to the diameter of the stem, with subsequent adjustments, in 0.5-mm increments, as needed, until a stable press-fit was achieved. After completing the reaming process, we drilled the medial and lateral tracts, using mini drill bits to minimize the risk of fracture, to allow the fins to be inserted. When implanting the stem, the rotation was easily controlled by using the position of the fins as a guide.

Postoperative management

Partial weight-bearing, using two crutches, was initiated on postoperative day 3, with active range of motion exercises of the knee also initiated on that day. Progression to full weight-bearing, using two crutches, was initiated on postoperative week 2.

Results

Of the 42 patients enrolled in the study, two died of lung metastases (average survival time, 16.5 months). The average follow-up duration for the remaining 40 patients was 30.1 months (range, 24–41 months). Three stems were inserted into the proximal femur after resection of > 60% of the length of the femur due to massive tumour resection (Fig. 3), with another 14 stems inserted into the mid-section of the femur after resection of 40–60% of the length of the femur (Fig. 4). For the remaining 23 cases, less than 40% of the length of the femur was resected (Fig. 5). The length of the resected femur ranged between 61.1 and 313.7 mm (average, 157.9 mm), with an average radius of 1347.5 mm retained (range, 820–1620 mm). Among the 40 patients who survived the period of observation, local recurrence occurred in one patient. With regard to lower limb function, the average MSTS score was $85.8 \pm 7.45\%$. Periprosthetic infection was the only complication observed, developing in three cases (7.5%; Table 1), with all three being primary implantation cases (Table 2). Of these three cases, two were treated with debridement, drainage, and antibiotics, without removal of the prosthesis. In the other case, amputation was required. There was no incidence of implant fractures, mechanical failure, or aseptic loosening.

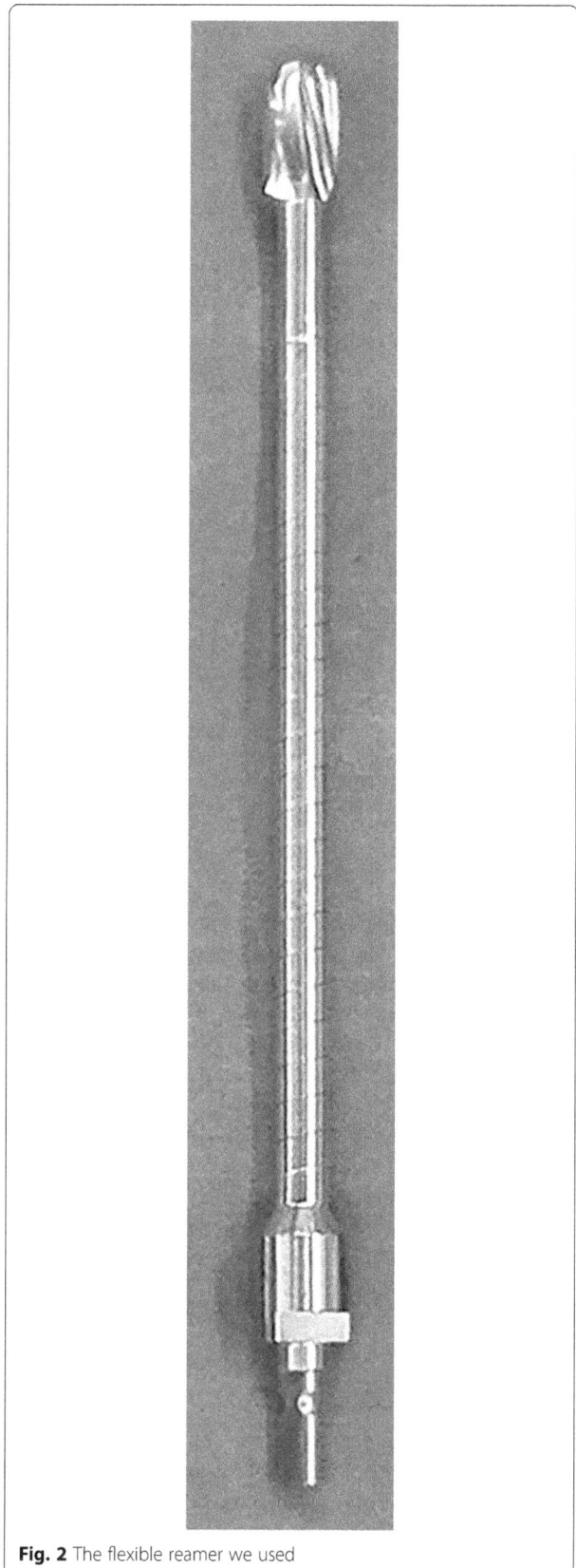

Fig. 2 The flexible reamer we used

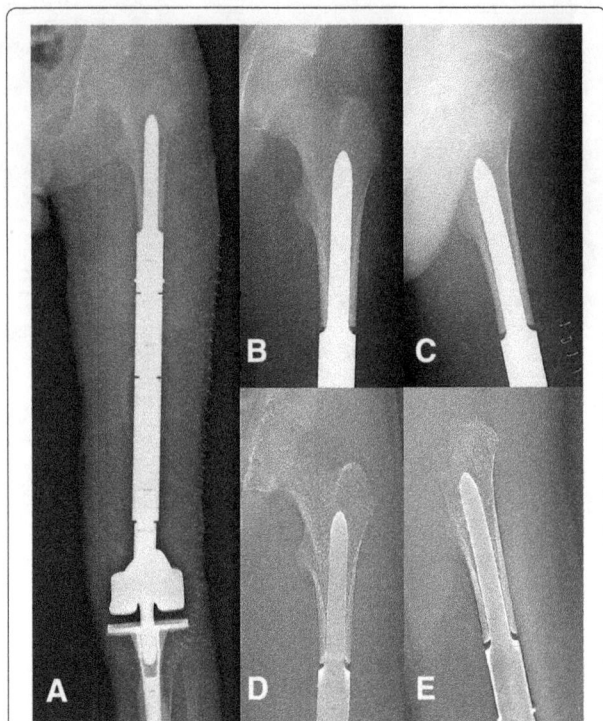

Fig. 3 A case of reconstruction of the distal femur following distal resection of 73% of the length of the femur. **a** Postero-anterior radiograph of the entire femur. **b**, **c** Postero-anterior and lateral radiographic views of the region of stem insertion of the femur. **d**, **e** Postero-anterior and lateral T-SMART views of the stem insertion region of the femur

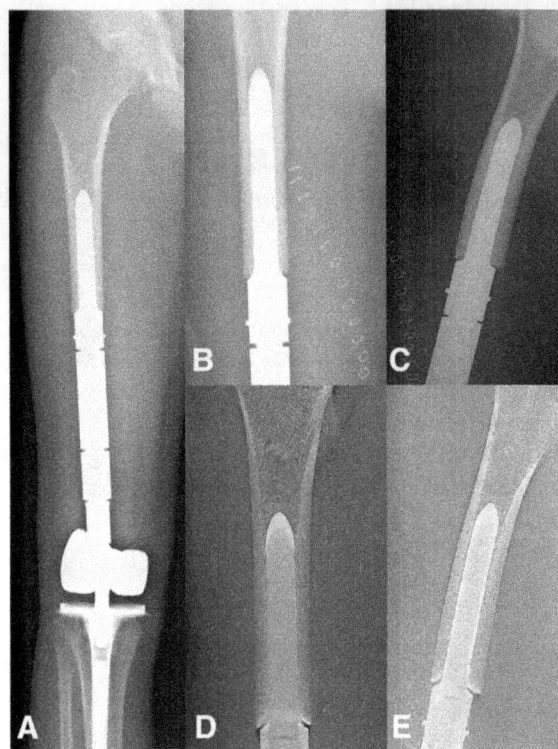

Fig. 4 A case of reconstruction of the distal femur following a distal resection of 54% of the length of the femur. **a** Postero-anterior radiograph of the entire femur. **b**, **c** Postero-anterior and lateral radiographic views of the region of stem insertion of the femur. **d**, **e** Postero-anterior and lateral T-SMART views of the stem insertion region of the femur

The average effective contact length between the press-fit stem and bone was 74.0 mm. The mean gaps between the bone and the stem in the medial and lateral planes, respectively, were as follows: distal endpoint of the stem, 0.24 and 0.16 mm; midpoint, 0.98 and 0.53 mm; and proximal endpoint, 1.09 and 0.86 mm. The mean gaps in the anterior and posterior planes, respectively, were as follows: distal endpoint of the stem, 0.61 and 0.65 mm; midpoint, 1.03 and 0.92 mm; and proximal endpoint 1.26 and 1.28 mm (Table 3). Radiographic signs of bone ingrowth were identified in all stems, with the exception of the patient who developed a periprosthetic infection requiring amputation and the patient with local tumour recurrence. A typical case of postoperative neocortex formation is shown in Fig. 6.

Discussion

Many types of cemented [3, 9–14] and uncemented [4–6, 15–19] prostheses have been used for DFR after tumour resection (Table 4). Although the optimal method of endoprosthesis fixation in the host bone is still controversial, uncemented stems are now more commonly selected than cemented stems because of the advantages they provide. Foremost, press-fit fixation of uncemented

stems can easily be achieved without the need for highly demanding bone cementation. Moreover, uncemented stems with HA coating facilitate biological bone ingrowth at the bone-prosthesis junction, as well as have a lower rate of complications [4–6, 15, 16, 18–20] than cemented stems. In the previous study, Biau et al. [9] followed up 56 patients who had undergone cemented, custom-made megaprosthesis reconstruction, between 1972 and 1994, for the treatment of distal femoral tumours. After an average follow-up of 62 months, limb function was acceptable but with femoral stem loosening reported in eight cases and stem fracture in five. In 2007, Myers et al. [12] reported on the long-term outcomes of cemented endoprosthetic replacement of the distal femur after tumours resection. Between 1973 and 2000, 335 patients underwent DFR. After a mean follow-up period of 12 years, the risk of revision for aseptic loosening of a fixed hinge was nearly 35% at 10 years, compared to 24% for a rotating hinge. Compared to cemented fixation, O'Donnell et al. [4] evaluated the early results of a custom-made, non-fluted, press-fit GMRS stem in 35 patients who had undergone DFR. Aseptic loosening and stem fracture were not observed during the minimum follow up period of

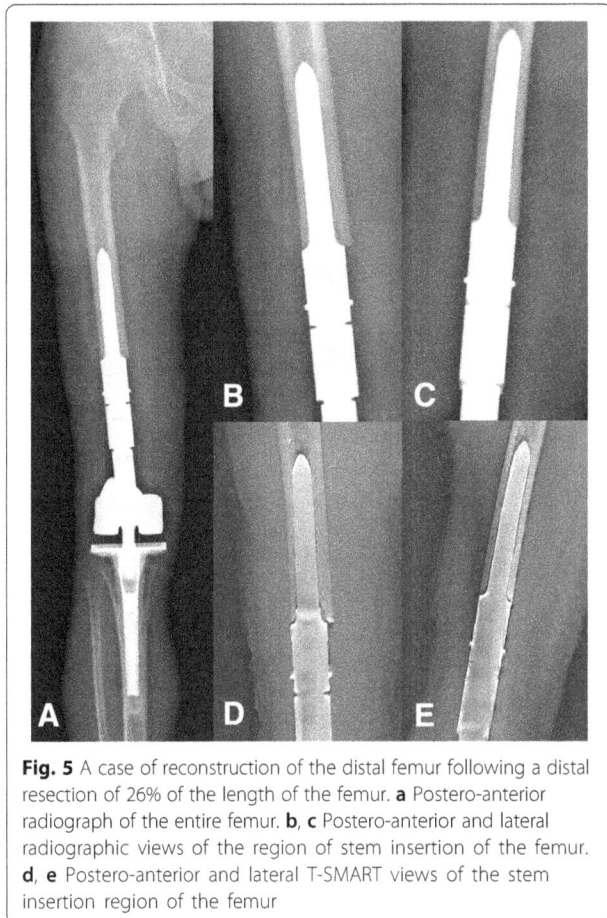

Fig. 5 A case of reconstruction of the distal femur following a distal resection of 26% of the length of the femur. **a** Postero-anterior radiograph of the entire femur. **b, c** Postero-anterior and lateral radiographic views of the region of stem insertion of the femur. **d, e** Postero-anterior and lateral T-SMART views of the stem insertion region of the femur

22 months. Additionally, a low rate of aseptic loosening or fracture in uncemented KMFTRS stems was reported by Griffin et al. [5], with femoral loosening identified in two cases (2.7%) and fracture in four (5.4%), between 1989 and 2000. Furthermore, in their 117 patients who underwent uncemented modular tumour prosthetic reconstruction (using the KMFTRS and MUTARS systems) for distal femoral tumours, Song et al. [16] reported that prosthesis removal was required in 35 cases (30%), 17 (14.5%) of these due to infection, 5 (4.2%) due to local tumour recurrence, 7 (5.9%) due to stem loosening, 4 (3.4%) due to stem fracture, and 2 (1.2%) due to periprosthetic fracture, over an average follow-up of 95 months. Our short-term outcomes on using a short, curved, femoral stem were comparable to those of previous studies using uncemented stems. The average MSTS score was good overall, with postoperative lower limb function not being a limitation to activities of daily living. Knee function was restored to a satisfactory level, even in patients who underwent massive bone resection (> 60% of the length of the femur). Over our average short-term follow-up of 30.1 months, we identified three cases of periprosthetic infection, with no radiographic evidence of aseptic loosening or breakage. As such, periprosthetic infection was the most common

complication in our study group. The previous studies reported an infection rate for primary endoprostheses of 2–20% [9, 21–23], increasing to 43% after revision surgery [24]. But, inconsistently, Pala et al. [17] reported a lower rate of infection in their case series of 98 patients who underwent revision surgery, over a mean oncologic follow-up of 4.2 years (range, 2–8 years), with infection identified in 7 cases, compared to 21 cases of infection in 197 cases of primary implantation. The findings reported by Pala et al. are comparable to ours, with no cases of infection identified in the revision group, and three in the primary implantation group. The potential risk factors of infection for oncologic patients are insufficient soft tissue coverage, immune compromising treatments, length of the procedure, and extensive surgical dissections [22, 23, 25]. Although the mean follow-up of 31 months was not sufficiently long to directly validate the rate of prosthesis-related complications, loosening is not likely to occur after bony ingrowth of a HA-coated implant has taken place for biological reconstruction [26]. However, the time to sufficient bone ingrowth, which produces a relatively high pullout force, is approximately 12 months [27]. Thus, the possibility of apparent loosening is lower in the second year after surgery than in the first year. In Pala et al.'s study [17], which focused on uncemented types of fixation for DFR, loosening contributed to endoprosthesis failure in 15 cases, requiring 2.8 years to develop, on average. Similar results were also reported by Bus et al. [6], with 15 cases of aseptic loosening identified in 89 cases of DFR performed using a MUTARS endoprosthesis, with a median time of 1.2 years. Biomechanically, it is true that the relatively high level of force would be applied on the interface between the stem and bone in the very early postoperative period for DFR because of a long lever arm of endoprostheses [4]. With insufficient bone ingrowth interface during this period, loosening or failure would be more likely to take place during this period when osteointegration is occurring rather than in the period after achieving a well-integrated interface. Thus, we believe that the majority of loosening cases would be readily apparent even at this early time point of follow-up.

Another strength of our study is our precise measurement of the radiolucent area between the periprosthetic bone and the implant, indicating potential bone resorption which may be a more prevalent complication in uncemented implants over longer follow-up periods [3, 18, 28]. We observed a slightly larger gap between the bone and the prosthesis in the anterior-posterior plane than in the medial-lateral plane, with the largest gap being 2 mm in length, which is considered a relatively slight resorption of the periprosthetic bone and unlikely to lead to loosening or breakage. Furthermore, there was minimal

Table 1 Oncology outcomes and complications related to the percentage of bone resection

Group	Number of patients	Age, years	Primary/ revision	Length of resection, mm	Percentage of bone resection, %	Radius of retained femur, mm	Oncology outcome	Amputation	Complications		
									Loosening, %	Breakage, %	Infection
< 40% resection	23	33.8 (range, 14–67)	16/7	118.7 (range, 61.1–164.2)	29.8 (range, 15–39)	1470 (range, 1230–1620)	0%	4.3% (1/23)	0	0	8.7% (2/23)
40 to 60% resection	14	22.5 (range, 10–62)	14/0	188.7 (range, 160.5–223.9)	49.2 (range, 41–58)	1210 (range, 1010–1430)	Local recurrence 7.1% (1/14)	0%	0	0	7.1% (1/14)
> 60% resection	3	26.3 (range, 14–50)	3/0	301.3 (range, 294.0–313.7)	73.4 (range, 69–78)	1050 (range, 820–1170)	0%	0%	0	0	0%
All	40	29.3 (range, 10–67)	33/7	157.9 (range, 61.1–313.7)	40.2 (range, 15–78)	1347.5 (range, 820–1620)	2.5% (1/40)	2.5% (1/40)	0	0	7.5% (3/40)

gapping at the distal endpoint and mid-section of the stem in either the medial-lateral or anterior-posterior plane, indicating that these sections of the interface were well integrated and effectively constrained the movement of the stem. It is true that having a minimal tiny gap is of beneficial to generate friction between the stem and the bone, this friction acting as a shear stress and resulting in a certain degree of stress shielding. But, considering that the interface between the stem and the bone is the first and major location bearing physical force in DFR, a minimal gap (or no gap at all) was required for press-fit fixation to produce and maintain sufficient pullout and rotation stability. Although the biomechanical outcomes related to DFR have yet to be fully characterized, we believe friction and compression to be the primary modes of load transfer between the stem and bone once bone ingrowth into the interface has developed. By contrast, during the very early postoperative period, the compressive stress placed on the collar of the stem is the main force, due to the immature formation of the bone ingrowth at the interface and a slightly larger gap caused by the drilling of a sufficient canal to insert a curved stem.

In addition to the anatomically appropriate curvature of the stem, the suitable length of the prosthesis, with sufficiently strong mechanical properties, two anti-rotational fins, and HA coating of the stem, provide a good functional outcome with a low risk of complications.

After implantation of a curved stem, strong derotational forces would be naturally generated because of space restriction. Such restraint is not available when using a straight stem as the space required for implantation is exactly the same as that allowing rotation of the stem. The curved stem, particularly with a rough surface,

provides a larger contact surface between the prosthesis and bone than a straight stem with same parameters, which generates greater friction to enhance primary pull-out and rotational stability. Lastly, the curved stem avoids unnecessary destruction of cortical bone at the proximal endpoint of the stem. Currently, the GMRS, KMFTR, MUTARS, Segmental System, and Megasystem-C are frequently used distal femoral endoprosthetic reconstruction systems with uncemented stems (Table 5). Although the MUTARS and Zimmer systems provide a curved stem, the details of the stem design are not open-source. Considering the major markets for both systems, the design of the stem is more likely to be appropriate for European and/or American populations than for Asians. A significant difference in femoral bowing between different ethnicities was reported by Maratt et al. [29]. Some studies reported that the average ROC of the femoral canal for Chinese patients ranged approximately from 1100 [30] to 1500 mm [31]. Thus, the ROC of stem we used (1400 mm) might be more suitable for the Chinese patients. According to the data related to femoral bowing we collected, there is a huge variation in the radius of the femoral curvature, ranging between 820 and 1620 mm. For all cases, we used a stem with a constant radius of 1400 mm rather than using personalized custom-made or modular stems with various radii. Although, customized and modular stems with different radius would provide a closer matching rate between the curvature of the stem and the femoral canal, designing and fabricating a customized stem requires 2 to 3 weeks, which could result in tumour progression and metastasis, while the use of modular stem with a range of radii would unnecessarily increase the cost of stems. Furthermore, we believe that any mismatch between a stem with a fixed

Table 2 Oncology outcomes and complications related to the type of implant fixation

Type of implant	Number of patients	Age/years	Oncology outcome	Amputation	Complications		
					Loosening, %	Breakage, %	Infection
Primary	33	29.0 (range, 10–67)	Local recurrence 3% (1/33)	3% (1/33)	0	0	9.1% (3/33)
Revision	7	30.7 (range, 21–45)	0%	0%	0	0	0%
All	40	29.3 (range, 10–67)	2.5% (1/40)	2.5% (1/40)	0	0	7.5% (3/40)

Uncemented, curved, short endoprosthesis stem for distal femoral reconstruction: early follow-up...

123

Table 3 Bone-implant interface evaluation related to the percentage of bone resection

Group	Number of patients	Length of retained femur, mm	Axial length of press-fit area, mm	Percentage of press-fit length in stem length, %	Vertical distance of radiolucent area					
					Anterior/posterior			Medial/lateral		
					Distal endpoint, mm	Midpoint, mm	Proximal endpoint, mm	Distal endpoint, mm	Midpoint, mm	Proximal endpoint, mm
<40% resection	23	279.8 (range, 237.7–353.6)	92.3 (range, 80.7–136.6)	91.8 (range, 80.1–97.5)	0.52/0.61	0.92/0.75	1.12/0.90	0.21/0.17	0.45/0.34	1.02/0.83
40 to 60% resection	14	195.0 (range, 150.4–246.4)	57.0 (range, 21.7–87.1)	57.0 (range, 21.7–87.1)	0.78/0.84	1.08/1.03	1.55/2.1	0.35/0.18	0.64/0.45	1.24/0.94
>60% resection	3	110.0 (range, 83.2–131.4)	20.5 (range, 15.8–24.3)	20.5 (range, 15.8–24.3)	0.63/0.3	2/2.2	N/A	0/0	2.1/2.3	N/A
All	40	236.3 (range, 83.2–353.6)	74.0 (range,15.8–136.6)	74.3 (range, 15.8–97.5)	0.61/0.65	1.03/0.92	1.26/1.28	0.24/0.16	0.98/0.53	1.09/0.86

N/A not applicable

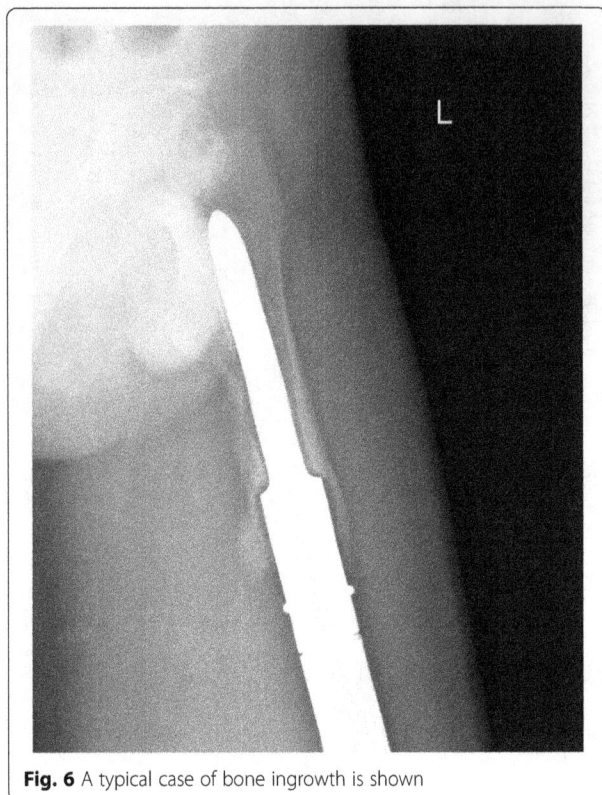

Fig. 6 A typical case of bone ingrowth is shown

for longer stem implantation. The short stem also increases the indications for limb salvage by allowing prosthesis implantation in cases with a relatively short residual proximal femur due to extensive resection. Moreover, a short stem could decrease the stress shielding effect, which is a major reason for bone resorption and even aseptic loosening. As well, Levadnyi et al. [32] reported that long stems do not effectively transmit load to bone, whereas a short stem provides a favourable environment for load transfer to the proximal region, which allows bone density to be maintained. Furthermore, the mechanical strength of a short stem is similar to that of a long stem. Zdero et al. [33] tested four different stems, including the Sigma Short Stem, Sigma Long Stem, Genesis II Short Stem, and Genesis II Long Stem, to evaluate their mechanical properties, reporting that there was no significant difference between the short and long stems in terms of axial, lateral, and torsional stiffness. Lastly, it is important to note that the insertion procedure for a short stem is much easier and quicker than for a long stem.

The short, curved stem we used has two fins, symmetrically arranged in the true medial and lateral planes of the distal end of the stem, providing guidance for implantation and an additional derotational force. Although some surgeons [4] have suggested that channels drilled into the cortical bone to allow for the insertion of fins might increase the risk of bone fracture, the fins in the stem we used are not large enough to result in such complication.

During surgical implantation, adjustment of the osteotomy plane is one of the most important components

radius of 1400 mm could be minimized through adjustment in the degree of prosthesis tilt, even in patients having the smallest femoral curvature of 820 mm.

A distinct advantage of using a short, rather than long, stem for DFR is the reduced volume of bone loss which results from the over-reaming procedure

Table 4 Previous studies for distal femur reconstruction

	Time span	Prosthesis type	Major fixation type	Number of patients*	Loosening, %	Implant fracture, %	5-year survival, %
Unwin et al. [3]	1968–1992	Custom-Stanmore	Cemented	493	9.9	3	N/A
Myers et al. [12]	1973–2000	Custom-Stanmore	Cemented	335	N/A	2	N/A
Schwartz et al. [13]	1980–2008	Custom or modular	Cemented	186	11.8	5.3	87.7
Frink et al. [10]	1983–1999	Stryker	Cemented	74	9.4	2.7	N/A
Jeys et al. [11]	1986–1996	Custom	Cemented	228	13.6	2.2	N/A
Griffin et al. [5]	1989–2000	KMFTR	Uncemented	74	2.7	5.4	N/A
Wunder et al. [15]	1986–1995	KMFTR	Uncemented	50	2	8	90
Song et al. [16]	1988–2008	KMFTR MUTARS	Uncemented	117	5.9	3.4	74
Batta et al. [19]	1994–2006	Custom	Uncemented	69	13	10	72.7
Bus et al. [6]	1995–2010	MUTARS	Uncemented	89	17	N/A	N/A
Pala et al. [17]	2003–2010	GMRS	Uncemented	187	5.3	0	N/A
O'Donnell et al. [4]	2005–2012	GMRS	Uncemented	35	0	0	N/A
Current study	2015–2017	Curved stem	Uncemented	42	0	0	N/A

GMRS Global Modular Replacement System, *KMFTR* Kotz Modular Femur and Tibia Reconstruction System, *MUTARS* Modular Universal Tumour and Revision System, *N/A* not applicable
*Number of patients who underwent distal femoral replacement

Table 5 Design features of common commercially available uncemented stems for distal femur reconstruction

Implant		GMRS Stryker	MUTARS Implantcast	Megasystem-C LINK	Segmental system Zimmer	Current study Chunli Co.
Alloy		TiAl$_6$V$_4$	TiAl$_6$V$_4$	TiAl$_6$V$_4$	CoCrMo	TiAl$_6$V$_4$
Design	Global	Straight Cylindrical	Curved Hexagonal	Straight Cylindrical	Straight/curved Conical	Partially Curved Cylindrical
	Proximal	Four fins	–	Fluted	Trabecular metal collar	Straight with two fins
	Middle	–	–	Fluted	Fluted	–
	Distal	Tapered	Cylindrical	Fluted	Fluted Double-slotted	Tapered
Radius of curvature, mm		–	–	–	–	1400
Diameter, mm		8–17	12–18	12–24	9–19	10–18
Length, mm		105–325	120/160/200	100/130/160	130/190	100/110/120
Surface	Proximal	HA-coated/porous-coated	HA-coated	Porous-coated	–	HA-coated
	Middle	Porous-coated	HA-coated	Porous-coated	–	HA-coated
	Distal	–	Polished	Porous-coated	–	Polished

GMRS Global Modular Replacement System, *MUTARS* Modular Universal Tumor and Revision System, *HA* hydroxyapatite

of the procedure to minimize the effect of mismatching between the standard stem and femoral bowing before insertion. As an example, when the radius of the retained femur is smaller than the radius of the stem, slightly more cortical bone could be removed from the anterior than posterior aspect, such that the stem would be in a slight posterior tilt and, thus, decreasing the degree of a mismatch after implantation. Similarly, the stem could be positioned in an anteverted position by resecting a greater proportion of the bone on the posterior than anterior aspect in cases in which the radius of the retained femur is larger than the radius of the stem. For press-fit implantation of the curved stem, the reaming process is another essential component of the surgical procedure. Currently, the most effective ratio between the diameter of the press-fit stem and the diameter of the reamed canal is controversial. Although some investigators have suggested that the medullary cavity should be either under-reamed by 1 to 1.5 mm or reamed to exactly match the diameter of the stem [6, 34], in our clinical experience, we have found that the canal should be reamed to be 0.5 to 1 mm larger than the diameter of the curved stem to be inserted.

This study has some limitations that should be acknowledged. The duration of follow-up was not sufficiently long to verify the long-term efficacy of this uncemented, short, curved stem we used. However, considering the relatively strong forces on the stem-bone interface because of the long lever arm of the prosthesis and lack of well-formed bone ingrowth in the very early period after the surgery, aseptic loosening or failure of the osseointegrated interface would be more likely to occur in the very early period of follow-up. Although there is a possibility that more complications might arise as we follow these patients over a longer period of time, we believe that our clinical and radiographic assessments would be helpful to estimate the long-term survival of implants. As musculoskeletal tumours are relatively rare, our study sample was small and we did not have a control group. Therefore, a larger multi-centre study is needed to compare this approach with other types of stems.

Conclusions

Reconstruction using an uncemented, curved, short stem can be an alternative treatment option DFR after resection of the primary bone or metastatic tumours of the distal femur. On the basis of our results, we suggest that selection of a short, curved stem; careful reaming and insertion without any rotation; and press-fit fixation lead to reasonable postoperative knee function and a low risk of complications.

Abbreviations
DFR: Distal femoral reconstruction; GMRS: Global Modular Replacement System; HA: Hydroxyapatite; KMFTR: Kotz Modular Femur and Tibia Reconstruction system; MSTS: Musculoskeletal Tumor Society; MUTARS: Modular Universal Tumour and Revision System; OSS: Orthopaedic Salvage System; ROC: Radius of curvature; T-SMART: Tomosynthesis with Shimadzu Metal Artefact Reduction Technology

Acknowledgements
This work was supported by the National Key Research and Development Plan (2016YFC1102003) and the National Natural Science Foundation of China (81702664).

Funding
National key research and development plan (2016YFC1102003).

Authors' contributions

MXL and CQT were involved in the concept and design of this manuscript. CX and JW were involved in the acquisition of subjects and data. MXL and CQT were involved in the design of the prosthesis. FT and CQT were involved in the postsurgical evaluation of the patients. All authors contributed toward data analysis, drafting and critically revising the paper, gave final approval of the version to be published, and agree to be accountable for all aspects of the work.

Competing interests

The authors declare that they have no competing interests.

Author details

[1]Department of Orthopedics, West China Hospital, Sichuan University, No. 37 Guoxue Street, Chengdu 610041, People's Republic of China. [2]Department of Orthopedics, The Third Hospital of Mianyang, No. 190 The East Jiannan Road, Mianyang 621000, Sichuan, People's Republic of China.

References

1. Link MP, Goorin AM, Miser AW, Green AA, Pratt CB, Belasco JB, Pritchard J, Malpas JS, Baker AR, Kirkpatrick JA, et al. The effect of adjuvant chemotherapy on relapse-free survival in patients with osteosarcoma of the extremity. N Engl J Med. 1986;314:1600–6.
2. Rougraff BT, Simon MA, Kneisl JS, Greenberg DB, Mankin HJ. Limb salvage compared with amputation for osteosarcoma of the distal end of the femur. A long-term oncological, functional, and quality-of-life study. J Bone Joint Surg Am. 1994;76:649–56.
3. Unwin PS, Cannon SR, Grimer RJ, Kemp HB, Sneath RS, Walker PS. Aseptic loosening in cemented custom-made prosthetic replacements for bone tumours of the lower limb. J Bone Joint Surg Br. 1996;78:5–13.
4. O'Donnell PW, Griffin AM, Eward WC, Sternheim A, Wunder JS, Ferguson PC. Early follow-up of a custom non-fluted diaphyseal press-fit tumour prosthesis. Int Orthop. 2014;38:123–7.
5. Griffin AM, Parsons JA, Davis AM, Bell RS, Wunder JS. Uncemented tumor endoprostheses at the knee - root causes of failure. Clin Orthop Relat Res. 2015;438:71–9.
6. Bus MP, van de Sande MA, Fiocco M, Schaap GR, Bramer JA, Dijkstra PD. What are the long-term results of MUTARS modular endoprostheses for reconstruction of tumor resection of the distal femur and proximal tibia? Clin Orthop Relat Res. 2017;475:708–18.
7. Kinkel S, Graage JD, Kretzer JP, Jakubowitz E, Nadorf J. Influence of stem design on the primary stability of megaprostheses of the proximal femur. Int Orthop. 2013;37:1877–83.
8. Enneking WF, Dunham W, Gebhardt MC, Malawar M, Pritchard DJ. A system for the functional evaluation of reconstructive procedures after surgical treatment of tumors of the musculoskeletal system. Clin Orthop Relat Res. 1993;286:241–6.
9. Biau D, Faure F, Katsahian S, Jeanrot C, Tomeno B, Anract P. Survival of total knee replacement with a megaprosthesis after bone tumor resection. J Bone Joint Surg Am. 2006;88:1285–93.
10. Frink SJ, Rutledge J, Lewis VO, Lin PP, Yasko AW. Favorable long-term results of prosthetic arthroplasty of the knee for distal femur neoplasms. Clin Orthop Relat Res. 2005;438:65–70.
11. Jeys LM, Kulkarni A, Grimer RJ, Carter SR, Tillman RM, Abudu A. Endoprosthetic reconstruction for the treatment of musculoskeletal tumors of the appendicular skeleton and pelvis. J Bone Joint Surg Am. 2008;90: 1265–71.
12. Myers GJ, Abudu AT, Carter SR, Tillman RM, Grimer RJ. Endoprosthetic replacement of the distal femur for bone tumours: long-term results. J Bone Joint Surg Br. 2007;89:521–6.
13. Schwartz AJ, Kabo JM, Eilber FC, Eilber FR, Eckardt JJ. Cemented distal femoral endoprostheses for musculoskeletal tumor: improved survival of modular versus custom implants. Clin Orthop Relat Res. 2010;468: 2198 210.
14. Sharma S, Turcotte RE, Isler MH, Wong C. Cemented rotating hinge endoprosthesis for limb salvage of distal femur tumors. Clin Orthop Relat Res. 2006;450:28–32.
15. Wunder JS, Leitch K, Griffin AM, Davis AM, Bell RS. Comparison of two methods of reconstruction for primary malignant tumors at the knee: a sequential cohort study. J Surg Oncol. 2001;77:89–99.
16. Song WS, Kong CB, Jeon DG, Cho WH, Kim JR, Cho Y, Lee SY. The impact of amount of bone resection on uncemented prosthesis failure in patients with a distal femoral tumor. J Surg Oncol. 2011;104:192–7.
17. Pala E, Henderson ER, Calabro T, Angelini A, Abati CN, Trovarelli G, Ruggieri P. Survival of current production tumor endoprostheses: complications, functional results, and a comparative statistical analysis. J Surg Oncol. 2013; 108:403–8.
18. Capanna R, Morris HG, Campanacci D, Del Ben M, Campanacci M. Modular uncemented prosthetic reconstruction after resection of tumours of the distal femur. J Bone Joint Surg Br. 1994;76:178–86.
19. Batta V, Coathup MJ, Parratt MT, Pollock RC, Aston WJ, Cannon SR, Skinner JA, Briggs TW, Blunn GW. Uncemented, custom-made, hydroxyapatite-coated collared distal femoral endoprostheses: up to 18 years' follow-up. Bone Joint J. 2014;96-B:263–9.
20. Pala E, Trovarelli G, Calabro T, Angelini A, Abati CN, Ruggieri P. Survival of modern knee tumor megaprostheses: failures, functional results, and a comparative statistical analysis. Clin Orthop Relat Res. 2015;473:891–9.
21. Bickels J, Wittig JC, Kollender Y, Henshaw RM, Kellar-Graney KL, Meller I, Malawer MM. Distal femur resection with endoprosthetic reconstruction: a long-term followup study. Clin Orthop Relat Res. 2002;400:225–35.
22. Gosheger G, Gebert C, Ahrens H, Streitbuerger A, Winkelmann W, Hardes J. Endoprosthetic reconstruction in 250 patients with sarcoma. Clin Orthop Relat Res. 2006;450:164–71.
23. Grimer RJ, Belthur M, Chandrasekar C, Carter SR, Tillman RM. Two-stage revision for infected endoprostheses used in tumor surgery. Clin Orthop Relat Res. 2002;395:193–203.
24. Hardes J, Gebert C, Schwappach A, Ahrens H, Streitburger A, Winkelmann W, Gosheger G. Characteristics and outcome of infections associated with tumor endoprostheses. Arch Orthop Trauma Surg. 2006; 126:289–96.
25. Lee SH, Oh JH, Lee KS, Yoo KH, Kim HS. Infection after prosthetic reconstruction in limb salvage surgery. Int Orthop. 2002;26:179–84.
26. Blunn GW, Briggs TW, Cannon SR, Walker PS, Unwin PS, Culligan S, Cobb JP. Cementless fixation for primary segmental bone tumor endoprostheses. Clin Orthop Relat Res. 2000;372:223–30.
27. Jeyapalina S, Beck JP, Bloebaum RD, Bachus KN. Progression of bone ingrowth and attachment strength for stability of percutaneous osseointegrated prostheses. Clin Orthop Relat Res. 2014;472:2957–65.
28. Huiskes R. The various stress patterns of press-fit, ingrown, and cemented femoral stems. Clin Orthop Relat Res. 1990;261:27–38.
29. Maratt J, Schilling PL, Holcombe S, Dougherty R, Murphy R, Wang SC, Goulet JA. Variation in the femoral bow: a novel high-throughput analysis of 3922 femurs on cross-sectional imaging. J Orthop Trauma. 2014;28:6–9.
30. Tang WM, Chiu KY, Kwan MF, Ng TP, Yau WP. Sagittal bowing of the distal femur in Chinese patients who require total knee arthroplasty. J Orthop Res. 2005;23:41–5.
31. Wang Y, Luo X, Liu C. Morphological study of marrow cavity of femur and tibia in Chinese and improvement of unreamed interlocking nail. Chinese J Orthop. 1998;18:215–8.
32. Levadnyi I, Awrejcewicz J, Gubaua JE, Pereira JT. Numerical evaluation of bone remodelling and adaptation considering different hip prosthesis designs. Clin Biomech (Bristol, Avon). 2017;50:122–9.
33. Zdero R, Saidi K, Mason SA, Schemitsch EH, Naudie DD. A biomechanical comparison of four different cementless press-fit stems used in revision surgery for total knee replacements. Proc Inst Mech Eng H. 2012;226:848–57.
34. Kinkel S, Lehner B, Kleinhans JA, Jakubowitz E, Ewerbeck V, Heisel C. Medium to long-term results after reconstruction of bone defects at the knee with tumor endoprostheses. J Surg Oncol. 2010;101:166–9.

16

Treatment options for PNET liver metastases

Giuseppe Nigri[1]*[iD], Niccolò Petrucciani[2], Tarek Debs[3], Livia Maria Mangogna[1], Anna Crovetto[1], Giovanni Moschetta[1], Raffaello Persechino[1], Paolo Aurello[1] and Giovanni Ramacciato[1]

Abstract

Background: Pancreatic neuroendocrine tumors (PNETs) are rare pancreatic neoplasms. About 40–80% of patients with PNET are metastatic at presentation, usually involving the liver (40–93%). Liver metastasis represents the most significant prognostic factor. The aim of this study is to present an up-to-date review of treatment options for patients with liver metastases from PNETs.

Methods: A systematic literature search was performed using the PubMed database to identify all pertinent studies.

Results: The literature search evaluated all the therapeutic options for patients with liver metastases of PNETs, including surgical treatment, loco-regional therapies, and pharmacological treatment. All the different treatment options showed particular indications in different presentations of liver metastases of PNET. Surgery remains the only potentially curative therapeutic option in patients with PNETs and resectable liver metastases, even if relapse rates are high. Efficacy of medical treatment has increased with advances in targeted therapies, such as everolimus and sunitinib, and the introduction of radiolabeled somatostatin analogs. Several techniques for loco-regional control of metastases are available, including chemo- or radioembolization.

Conclusions: Treatment of patients with PNET metastases should be multidisciplinary and must be personalized according to the features of individual patients and tumors.

Background

Pancreatic neuroendocrine tumors (PNETs) are rare tumors, representing 1.3 to 10.0% of all pancreatic tumors. Annual incidence of PNET is estimated to be 3.65/10,000 people per year [1–3]. Due to the recent widespread use of diagnostic techniques, there is a dramatic increase in the incidence of PNETs [4]. No differences in PNET incidence are reported between men and women. Peak of PNET's diagnosis occurs between 30 and 60 years [5]. PNETs may be classified as functioning or non-functioning tumors. Functioning PNETs are characterized by secretion of one or more biologically active peptides, inducing specific clinical syndromes. Secreting products include insulin, gastrin, glucagon, somatostatin, and vasoactive intestinal peptide (VIP). Non-functioning PNETs may secrete peptides, such as chromogranin A and neurotensin, and may be asymptomatic [6]. Diagnosis of non-functioning PNETs is usually late for the absence of specific symptoms; therefore, probability of malignancy is higher if compared with functioning PNETs and reported survival is as low as 30% [7]. PNETs are also characterized by the expression of somatostatin receptors. They may be a component of several syndromes, such as Von Hippel-Lindau syndrome, multiple endocrine neoplasia syndromes, or neurofibromatosis type I [6]. Metastases are detected at diagnosis in about 40–80% of patients with PNET [8]. The more frequent sites are the liver (40–93%), followed by the bone (12–20%) and lungs (8%–10%) [8]. The presence of liver metastases also has a negative impact on the prognosis [9, 10], and the extension of PNET liver metastases is correlated to long-term survival [11, 12]. The development of liver metastasis is related to the histological tumor type and to the site of the primary tumor [13]. Other factors with a strong prognostic impact are as

* Correspondence: giuseppe.nigri@uniroma1.it
[1]Department of Medical and Surgical Science and Translational Medicine, St. Andrea Hospital Rome, Sapienza University of Rome, Via di Grottarossa 1035, 00189 Rome, Italy
Full list of author information is available at the end of the article

follows: size of the primary tumor, mitotic index, vascular and lymphatic invasion, proliferative activity, metabolite serum concentration, and cellular atypias [14]. Treatment of metastatic PNETs is complex and requires multidisciplinary expertise including medical, interventional, and surgical specialties.

Furthermore, multidisciplinary management of metastatic PNETs is in constant evolution. Therefore, it is important to periodically review the recent acquisition, to provide up-to-date and comprehensive data to clinicians. This review, based on a systematic literature search, aims to discuss metastatic PNET's management from clinical, biochemical, and radiological diagnosis to treatment, focusing on all treatment possibilities in a multidisciplinary approach.

Methods
Search strategy and study selection
A systematic literature search was performed using the PubMed database, in order to identify all studies published up to May 2018 reporting data on patients treated for liver metastases from pancreatic neuroendocrine tumors (PNETs) undergoing surgical treatment, including liver resection or liver transplantation, interventional procedures, or medical treatment. The following MeSH search terms were used: "liver" OR "hepatic," "metastasis OR metastases," and "pancreatic neuroendocrine tumor" OR "PNET." The "related articles" function was used to broaden the search, and all the abstracts and citations of all returned studies were reviewed. The full text was examined, in case of any doubt after reading the article's abstract. Non-English language studies were excluded. Two authors (NP, LM) examined the articles to establish the inclusion in this review.

Results
Search results
Initial search retrieved 10,135 articles. Titles and abstract were analyzed to identify 476 relevant publications. Of them, 116 articles were retained to review the current literature on this topic [1–116]. PRISMA flow diagram is showed in Fig. 1. The majority of them were observational studies. Meta-analyses and review were the second most represented group.

Diagnosis and staging
The main factors determining the clinical manifestation of PNET liver metastases are the liver tumor load and the degree of endocrine activity. Usually, patients may remain asymptomatic for a long time. Development of carcinoid syndrome is possible, such as abdominal pain or discomfort. Liver malfunction or failure is a rare occurrence, even in the case of extensive liver involvement [15].

Diagnosis is done on the basis of biochemical laboratory examinations, including specific tumor markers, and on radiological imaging.

Plasmatic chromogranin A is a widely accepted tumor marker, used for diagnostic and prognostic purposes and to evaluate the response to treatment. Its specificity and sensitivity depend on tumor type and volume [16]. 5-Hydroxyindoleacetic acid is a urinary metabolite of serotonin, which may be increased in patients with metastatic PNET, and it is used for diagnosis and follow-up [17]. Other biochemical markers are less used in clinical practice, including urine serotonin, synaptophysin, neuron-specific enolase, parathyroid hormone-related protein, calcitonin, pancreatic polypeptide, and human chorionic gonadotropin [18]. On the other hand, functioning tumors secrete hormones related to a specific clinical syndrome, such as insulin (insulinoma), glucagon (glucagonoma, confirmed by serum glucagon level > 1000 pg/mL), gastrin (elevated serum gastrin and gastric acids), and vasoactive intestinal polypeptide (vipoma, VIP values > 200 pg/mL) [19–21].

Somatostatin receptor scintigraphy is frequently used for PNET imaging. Advantages include the acquisition of whole-body images with possible visualization of the primary tumor and metastases, and the possibility to identify the patients who are candidates for somatostatin receptor-based radiotherapy [22].

Positron emission tomography (PET) with DOTATOC or DOTANOC associated with the positron emitter Gallium 68 allows even better sensitivity (up to 30% higher than standard imaging) [23].

CT scan has wide diffusion and is associated with sensitivity rates up to 94–100% [24], especially if combined with PET [25]. Magnetic resonance imaging is also used in the staging and evaluation of disease progression, for its ability to detect lesions in the liver, combined with reduction of excessive radiation burden [26].

Several staging systems exist for PNET classification. The WHO, European Neuroendocrine Tumor Society (ENETS), and American Joint Committee on Cancer (AJCC) have proposed each a staging system [27–29]. The WHO classification is based on cellular proliferation (measured as mitotic count and Ki-67 expression), as shown in Table 1 [27]. The ENETS staging system (Table 2) is based on TNM classification [28], and the AJCC staging system (reported in Table 3) is developed from the TNM staging system for pancreatic adenocarcinoma [29].

Treatment options for metastatic PNETs
The therapeutic options for patients with liver metastases from pancreatic neuroendocrine tumors include surgical treatment, loco-regional therapies, and pharmacological treatment. The decision of the treatment strategy is based

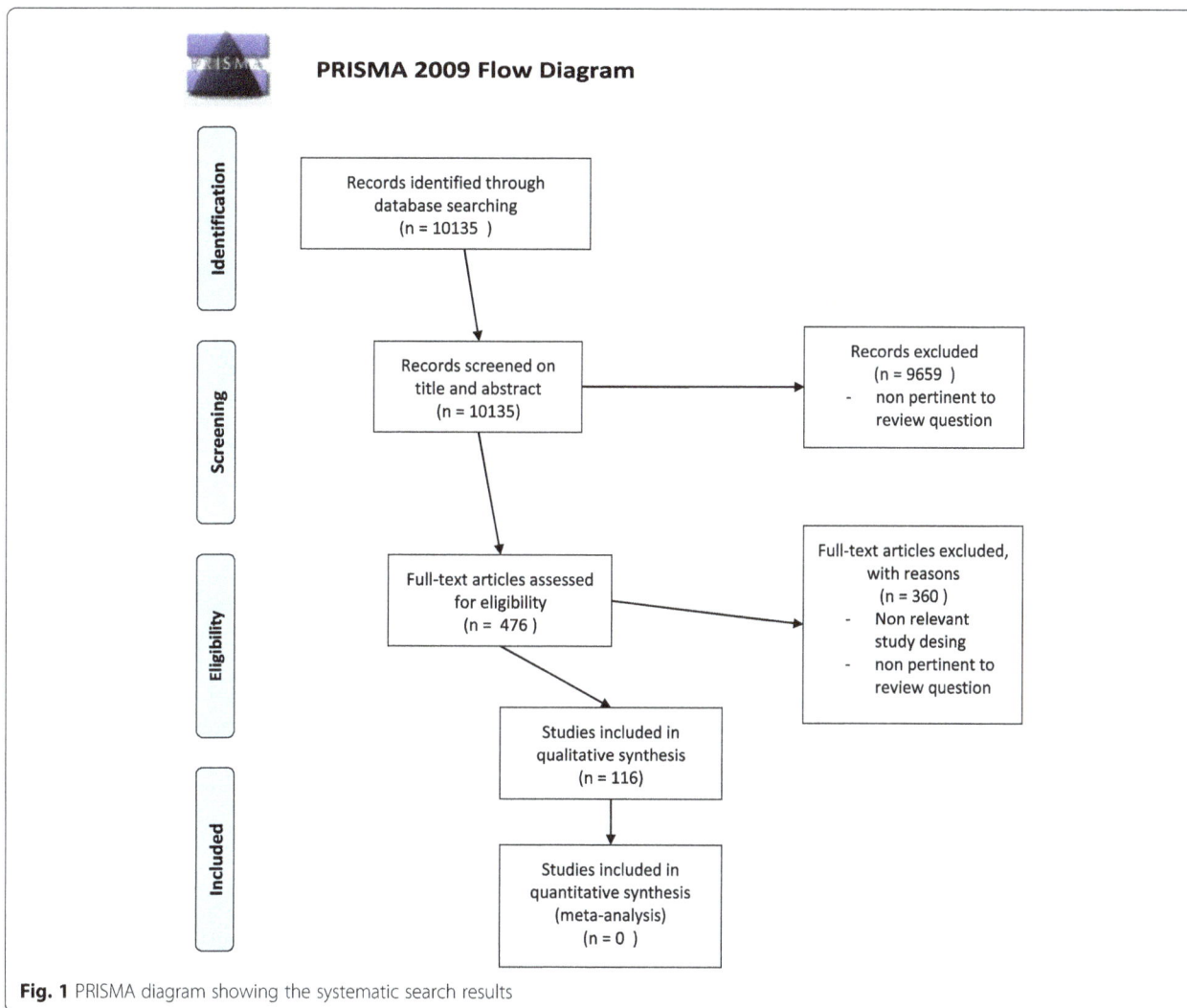

PRISMA 2009 Flow Diagram

Identification

Records identified through
database searching
(n = 10135)

Screening

Records screened on
title and abstract
(n = 10135)

Records excluded
(n = 9659)
- non pertinent to
review question

Eligibility

Full-text articles assessed
for eligibility
(n = 476)

Full-text articles excluded,
with reasons
(n = 360)
- Non relevant
study desing
- non pertinent to
review question

Included

Studies included in
qualitative synthesis
(n = 116)

Studies included in
quantitative synthesis
(meta-analysis)
(n = 0)

Fig. 1 PRISMA diagram showing the systematic search results

on the analysis of patient performance status and comorbidities, on accurate tumor staging, and on evaluation of prognostic factors. Surgery represents the only potentially curative therapy when the disease is completely resectable. In patients with advanced and unresectable disease, however, the therapeutic goal is lengthening survival with the best possible quality of life and palliation of symptoms, using a multidisciplinary approach.

Liver surgery for pancreatic neuroendocrine liver metastases

Surgery remains the treatment of choice in selected patients with PNETs and resectable liver metastases, because it may provide cure. Liver resection for neuroendocrine metastases is associated to long-term survival advantages and disease control [30, 31]. Surgery may have either curative intent, when complete resection is possible, or palliative intent, when the majority of the tumor burden is removed to control the symptoms of the disease. Due to the rarity of the disease, the majority of published articles

on surgical treatments of liver metastases from neuroendocrine tumors report data on neuroendocrine metastases from several primary sites (e.g., GEP-NET metastases).

Potentially curative surgery

Potentially curative surgery is possible in only 10–25% of patients with liver metastases [32]. Bilobar metastases may be treated with two-step resections, and preoperative portal vein embolization may be used to induce hypertrophy of the left liver lobe, as in colorectal liver metastases [33]. Concurrent or staged resection of the primary lesion and liver metastases may be considered, if surgery can remove most of the metastatic tumor volume (> 90%). Criteria helping to select patients for surgery include the presence of well-differentiated G1/ G2 tumors, absence of distant lymph node metastasis, absence of extrahepatic metastasis, absence of diffuse peritoneal metastasis, and absence of right cardiac dysfunction [34].

Table 1 WHO grading system for PNETs [27]

	Grade 1 (G1)	Grade 2 (G2)	Grade 3 (G3)
Ki-67 index	< 3%	3–20%	> 20%
Mitotic count	< 2/10 HPF	2–20/10 HPF	> 20/10 HPF
Differentiation	Well differentiated	Moderately differentiated	Poorly differentiated

WHO World Health Organization, *PNETs* pancreatic neuroendocrine tumors, *HPF* high-power field

Unfortunately, tumor relapse in the first 2 years after resection is reported in the majority of patients [35], and a relapse rate of up to 80% at 5 years has been shown [36–50]. Despite the elevated percentage of tumor recurrence, 5-year survival rates approach 85%, which is in favor of an aggressive surgical approach. Morbidity and mortality of liver resection are acceptable with the advancement in preoperative management and surgical techniques, and are comparable to liver resection for other diseases [36–51].

No randomized trials have compared the results of liver resection to other non-surgical treatments for PNET liver metastases [52]. However, retrospective comparisons of the outcomes of patients treated with medical therapies or palliative care or surgery highlight the advantages of surgical treatment. Survival outcomes of curative surgery are better than those of loco-regional therapies, such as liver chemoembolization, as reported by Elias et al., detecting a 5-year survival rate of 71% for 47 patients who underwent partial hepatectomy versus 31% for 65 patients treated with chemoembolization [41]. Furthermore, Tao et al. demonstrated that debulking surgery improves the effect of the subsequent loco-regional treatment [49].

The presence of a single liver metastasis is associated with better survival, as shown by Frilling et al. [32]. In cases of synchronous metastases, simultaneous resection of the primitive tumor and hepatectomy has been reported, with acceptable postoperative morbi-mortality. Sarmiento et al. treated 23 patients who underwent synchronous pancreatic and liver resection. Postoperative

mortality was 0%, the major complication rate 18%, and the 5-year survival was as high as 71% [42]. Bonney et al. showed comparable results, with morbidity of 25%, one death in the postoperative period, and a 5-year survival of 70% [48].

Cytoreductive surgery

Cytoreductive surgery in patients with PNET liver metastases aims to increase survival, control symptoms, and improve quality of life. Cytoreductive liver resections are indicated in patients with symptoms not controllable with medical or hormonal treatment. It consists of resection of more than 90% of the tumor mass [53, 54]. Recently, Morgan et al. proposed a threshold of > 70%, with the argument that postoperative results are comparable between debulking > 70, > 90, and 100% [55]. Reduction in tumor volume may reduce the immunosuppressive effects of the tumor and decrease the probability of development of further metastases. Surgical debulking is efficient for the symptoms in the majority of patients with functioning PNETs [44–47, 56]. Combined approaches including aggressive surgical resection, ablative therapies, and chemotherapy may be employed to obtain cytoreduction of the tumor [57].

Symptomatic benefits are achieved in 80–90% of patients submitted to curative liver resections [12, 42, 54]. The mean duration of the response to the surgical debulking is correlated with the amount of tumor removed and to the normalization of tumor markers [12]. Recurrence of symptoms occurs in the first 5 years after

Table 2 ENETS staging system for PNET [28]

Stage	T	N	M
I	T1	N0	M0
IIA	T2	N0	M0
IIB	T3	N0	M0
IIIA	T4	N0	M0
IIIB	Any T	N1	M0
IV	Any T	Any N	M1

ENETS European Neuroendocrine Tumor Society, *PNET* pancreatic neuroendocrine tumors, *T1* tumors < 2 cm limited to the pancreas, *T2* 2–4 cm limited to the pancreas, *T3* > 4 cm limited to the pancreas or invading the duodenum or common bile duct, *T4* tumor invading adjacent structures or large vessels, *N0* no regional lymph node metastases, *N1* regional lymph node metastases, *M0* no distant metastases, *M1* distant metastases

Table 3 AJCC staging system for PNETs (7th edition, 2010) [29]

Stage	T	N	M
0	Tis	N0	M0
IA	T1	N0	M0
IB	T2	N0	M0
IIA	T3	N0	M0
IIB	T1–3	N1	M0
III	T4	Any N	M0
IV	Any T	Any N	M1

AJCC American Joint Committee on Cancer, *PNET* pancreatic neuroendocrine tumors, *T1* < 2 cm limited to the pancreas, *T2* > 2 cm limited to the pancreas, *T3* tumor extends beyond the pancreas but not involving the celiac axis or SMA, *T4* tumor involves celiac axis or SMA, *N0* no regional lymph node metastases, *N1* regional lymph node metastases, *M0* no distant metastases, *M1* distant metastases

surgery in the majority of patients [42]. Reported rates of complications and mortality are considered acceptable [12, 42, 44–46, 58–60]. If > 75% of the liver parenchyma is involved, prognosis is considered unfavorable and surgical treatment should be avoided [43].

Liver transplantation

Liver transplantation represents a potentially curative treatment for liver metastases from PNETs. Early results are promising, and future development of this strategy is possible. Orthotropic liver transplantation (OLT) has been proposed for PNETs for two reasons: the less-aggressive biological behavior of neuroendocrine metastases compared to other metastases and the low percentage of patients with PNET liver metastases candidates for R0 liver resections [8, 61]. However, this indication is restricted because of the lack of donors and the perplexity in allocation of organs to oncological patients. Furthermore, the first studies on liver transplantation for metastatic neuroendocrine tumors were not concordant and reported mediocre results. This was due in part to the lack of valid and homogeneous selection criteria [61–67].

Liver transplantation is considered reasonable if expected overall survival is more than 70% at 5 years and disease-free survival is more than 50% [8]. The best candidates in this setting are young patients (< 50 years old), with no extrahepatic lesions, well-differentiated tumors, and low levels of Ki-67. Mazzaferro et al. proposed the following inclusion criteria [8]: diagnosis of low-grade NET confirmed by histological examination (with low expression of Ki-67), location of the primary tumor in an anatomic area tributary to the portal vein, primary tumor already resected with clear margins, < 50% of liver involvement, stable disease during 6 months before OLT, and age < 55 years. Recently, a comprehensive review showed encouraging 5-year survival after OLT for NET, but a high recurrence rate [68]. So at present, liver transplantation does not represent routine care in this setting and is considered investigational and allowed in the setting of clinical studies [69].

Another debated point is the indication for primary tumor resection in patients with unresectable metastatic disease. Recent retrospective studies [70] and a meta-analysis showed that the palliative resection of the primary tumor in patients with PNETs and unresectable liver metastases may increase long-term survival. The meta-analysis by Zhou and colleagues included 10 studies, with a total of 1226 patients undergoing primary tumor resection and 1623 patients who did not have surgery [71]. The results of the meta-analysis showed a significantly longer survival in patients who had surgical resection of the primary tumor (at 5 years, 35.7–83% surviving patients in the surgical group versus 5.4–50% in the non-surgical group) [71].

Liver-directed therapies

Liver-directed therapies used to treat PNET metastases include radiofrequency ablation (RFA), cryoablation, alkalization, transarterial embolization (TAE), and transarterial chemoembolization (TACE) [72].

Ablative therapies

RFA is a safe technique, generally used to treat unresectable metastases smaller than 5 cm. Associated morbidity is low and mainly consists in bleeding and abscess formation [73]. RFA is effective to treat symptoms related to liver metastases and hormone secretion, even if the tumor size represents a limiting factor. RFA is less useful for tumors > 5 cm, even if repeat ablation sessions are possible [37]. The location of the lesion should be considered, because RFA may be contraindicated for liver metastases near to vital structures or at the liver surface. Cryotherapy is another suitable option, and percutaneous ethanol injection is an alternative in cases where tumors are close to vital structures or vessels [74].

Hepatic arterial embolization

The rationale of hepatic transarterial embolization is that neuroendocrine metastases receive most of their blood supply from the hepatic artery, whereas normal liver parenchyma gets 75% of its blood supply from the portal vein flow [75]. Both TAE and TACE effectively reduce tumor size and improve patients' symptoms. No randomized studies comparing the two techniques have been published nor studies comparing embolization techniques with cytoreductive surgery in the palliative segment. Embolization is not associated with risks of tumor dissemination (this is an advantage compared to RFA). During TAE, embolization is performed using lipiodol, gem foam particles, polyvinyl alcohol foam, or bland microspheres, whereas for TACE, chemotherapeutic agents are added, leading to an intra-tumoral drug concentration over 20 times greater than those obtained with systemic administration. Furthermore, both provoke tumor ischemia. Commonly used drugs are doxorubicin, melphalan, and streptozocin. Minor side effects of the procedure are fever, leukocytosis, abdominal pain, and liver cytolysis.

Morbidity rate is low, even if serious complications, such as liver abscess, gallbladder necrosis, bowel ischemia, pleural effusion, and hepatic failure, have been reported [76]. Tumor response is objectivized in 25–86% of cases, and the duration of the response ranges from 6 to 45 months [77–79]. In a recent series, clinical improvement and tumor response were observed in 95% of patients, with median time to tumor progression of 14 ± 16 months and median overall survival of 22 ± 18 months [80].

Both TAE and TACE are considered for palliation in unresectable tumors, especially for functioning tumors with symptoms not controlled by medical therapy. Contraindications of TAE and TACE include portal vein occlusion, insufficient liver reserve, and poor performance status. In patients with previous pancreaticoduodenectomy, transarterial therapies are generally contraindicated, due to higher risks of post-procedure morbidity. Liver-directed therapies may also be proposed in patients with extrahepatic metastases to control liver disease and symptoms [80–83].

Selective internal radiotherapy (SIRT) consists of embolization with 90Yttrium microsphere, a beta-emitter that results in tissue penetration of 2.5 mm. Published data on SIRT show a response rate of 55% and stabilization of the disease in 32% of cases [84–87]. More recently, an overall disease control rate of 88.9% at 3 months after therapy has been demonstrated, confirming its effectiveness in treating unresectable PNET liver metastases [30]. SIRT is contraindicated in cases of aberrant vessels with shunt to the gastrointestinal tract, compromised portal veins, and inadequate liver functional reserve to avoid potentially serious complications.

Medical therapy

Medical therapy is indicated for advanced unresectable PNETs and includes drugs acting on hormone receptors, conventional chemotherapy, and molecular target therapy [88].

Somatostatin analogs (SSAs) act on somatostatin receptors and are effective in controlling hormonal secretion and tumor growth. Either functioning or non-functioning PNETs express at least one of the five subtypes of somatostatin receptor (SSTR). Different SSAs have specific affinity for different SSTRs [89]. Octreotide and lanreotide have high affinity for SSTR2 and bind to SSTR5, whereas the recent analog pasireotide binds with high affinity to SSTR1, SSTR2, SSTR3, and SSTR5 [89, 90]. Several studies and a randomized controlled trial advocate the use of SSAs to control tumor growth and symptoms in this setting [89, 91, 92]. The randomized controlled trial by Rinke et al. demonstrated that long-acting octreotide is efficacious on both functioning and non-functioning tumors, with a 66.7% reduction in the risk of disease progression in treated patients compared to patients taking a placebo [92]. However, these results referred to a specific setting of patients with limited liver involvement (≤ 10%) and already resected primary tumors. Further randomized trials to confirm these data in other patient categories are needed. The CLARINET (Controlled Study on Lanreotide Antiproliferative Response in NETs) study is an ongoing trial, which aims to evaluate the efficacy of lanreotide in patients with well or moderately differentiated, non-functioning NETs with Ki-67% expression < 10% [93]. A

number of other previous studies have advocated for the efficacy of SSAs on PNETs, with tumor stabilization reported in 40–80% of patients and objective tumor response (demonstrated by reduction of tumor volume) in about 10% of patients [94–96]. If treatment with SSAs at standard dose fails, management options include shortening of SSA administration intervals or augmentation of SSA dosage. For patients with progressing tumors, administration of SSAs every 21 days was compared to administration every 28 days, demonstrating a longer time to progression, better symptom control, and reduction in the serum level of tumor markers in the group with the shorter interval of administration [97]. SSAs are well tolerated and have generally mild side effects. Long-term side effects include gallbladder lithiasis (1%), glucose intolerance or diabetes, and steatorrhea [96].

Alpha-interferon may be associated with somatostatin analogs for palliation or hormonal symptoms, with tumor stabilization occurring in 30–80% of patients. Reduction of tumor volume occurs only in a small percentage of patients [98]. Side effects are frequent and include flu-like symptoms (80–90%), anorexia, weight loss, fatigue, bone marrow or liver toxicity, and autoimmune disorders.

Systemic chemotherapy is only indicated for advanced and unresectable PNETs and may consist in the administration of various cytotoxic agents, such as streptozotocin, cisplatin, dacarbazine, doxorubicin, and 5-fluorouracil [99]. The efficacy of the combination of streptozotocin with 5-fluorouracil (5-FU) and/or epirubicin in treating G1/G2 pNENs has been demonstrated, with a reported objective response rate of 20–45% [100, 101]. Alternative options include temozolomide alone or in combination with capecitabine, leading to a partial response rate of 70%, median progression-free survival (PFS) of 18 months, and 2-year survival of 92% in cases of metastatic, well-differentiated PNETs [102]. For high-grade tumors with poor differentiation, platinum-based regimes are preferred. Response rates of 42–67% have been obtained combining cisplatin and etoposide [103]. Saif et al. suggested the use of capecitabine/temozolomide (CAPTEM) regimen in patients with failure of the previous therapy [104].

Targeted therapies

Recent advancements in comprehension of the pathogenesis and molecular mechanisms of PNETs have allowed the development and introduction of novel targeted therapies in the clinical practice. The mTOR protein is a serine/threonine kinase, and a key component of a cellular pathway playing an important role in the regulation of cell growth and proliferation. mTOR is upregulated in several tumors, including PNETs [105]. Everolimus is an mTOR inhibitor that has shown efficacy in phase II and phase III studies in patients with PNETs [106]. The RADIANT3 study randomized patients with advanced PNET into two groups: patients receiving everolimus (10 mg per day) (group 1) and patients receiving a placebo (group 2). Patients treated with everolimus had significantly longer PFS (11 versus 4.6 months) than patients receiving placebo [107]. Side effects include stomatitis, rash, fatigue, diarrhea, hyperglycemia, and hematological and pneumological effects.

Sunitinib is an inhibitor of the tyrosine kinases PDGFR, VEGFR-1, VEGFR-2, c-KIT, and FLIT3 [108, 109]. The rationale for its use in the treatment of PNETs is the frequent overexpression of VEGF or VEGFR by these tumors. A phase III study comparing sunitinib to a placebo has shown a response rate of 9.3% and an increased PFS of 11.1 months in the group treated with sunitinib (versus PFS of 5.5 months in the placebo group) [110]. Side effects of sunitinib include diarrhea, nausea, vomiting, asthenia, fatigue, hypertension, and neutropenia. Raymond et al. reported a partial tumor response in 42% of patients and stable disease in 33% of patients after treatment with 37.5 mg/day of sunitinib [110].

Radiolabeled somatostatin analogs represent a new treatment option in patients with strong radiotrace uptake on SRS [111]. Peptide receptor radionuclide therapy (PRRT) with radiolabeled SSAs allows administration of targeted radiotherapy to the tumor tissue and its metastases [112]. The most used radiolabels are 90Yttrium, a high-energy beta-particle emitter, and 177Lutetium, which emits beta particles and gamma rays. Even if complete tumor response is rare with this treatment (0–6%), results are encouraging, with partial tumor regression in 7–37% of patients and stabilization in 42–86% using 90Yttrium-labeled SSAs [112–114]. 177Lutetium octreotate was used on 510 patients, 40% of whom had PNETs, and partial response was observed in 28% of cases, with stabilization of the disease in 35% [115, 116]. PRRT is a promising therapeutic option, even if still investigational.

Conclusions

Therapeutic options for patients with liver metastases from pancreatic neuroendocrine tumors include surgery, loco-regional therapies, and medical therapies. Surgery represents the only potentially curative treatment and should be proposed for resectable patients, even if relapse rates are high. Efficacy of medical treatment has increased with advances in targeted therapies, such as everolimus and sunitinib, and with the introduction of radiolabeled somatostatin analogs. Several techniques for loco-regional control of metastases are available, including chemo- or radioembolization. Treatment of patients with pancreatic neuroendocrine metastases should be multidisciplinary, must be personalized according to the

features of individual patients and tumors, and should take into account all possible options in order to provide the best possible results in terms of survival and quality of life.

Abbreviations
5-FU: 5-Fluororacil; PFS: Progression-free survival; PNET: Pancreatic neuroendocrine tumor; PRRT: Peptide receptor radionuclide therapy; RFA: Radiofrequency ablation; SSAs: Somatostatin analogs; SSTR: Somatostatin receptor; TACE: Transarterial chemoembolization; TAE: Transarterial embolization; SIRT: Selective internal radiotherapy; OLT: Orthotropic liver transplantation

Authors' contributions
GN, NP, TD, and GR made substantial contribution to the conception and design, acquisition of data, and analysis and interpretation of data and have been involved in drafting the manuscript and revising it critically for important intellectual content. LM, AC, GM, RP, and PA made substantial contribution to the acquisition of data and have been involved in revising the manuscript critically for important intellectual content. GN, NP, TD, GR, LM, AC, GM, RP, and PA give final approval of the version to be published, take public responsibility for appropriate portions of the content, and agree to be accountable for all aspects of the work in ensuring that questions related to the accuracy or integrity of any part of the work are appropriately investigated and resolved. All authors read and approved the final manuscript.

Competing interests
The authors declare that they have no competing interests.

Author details
[1]Department of Medical and Surgical Science and Translational Medicine, St. Andrea Hospital Rome, Sapienza University of Rome, Via di Grottarossa 1035, 00189 Rome, Italy. [2]Digestive Surgery, Hepatobiliopancreatic Surgery and Liver Transplantation, UPEC University, Henri Mondor Hospital, Creteil, France. [3]Department of Digestive Surgery and Liver Transplantation, Nice University Hospital, Nice, France.

References
1. Frilling A, Modlin IM, Kidd M, Russell C, Breitenstein S, Salem R, Kwekkeboom D, et al. Recommendations for management of patients with neuroendocrine liver metastases. Lancet Oncol. 2014;15:e8–21.
2. Lawrence B, Gustafsson BI, Chan A, Svejda B, Kidd M, Modlin IM. The epidemiology of gastroenteropancreatic neuroendocrine tumors. Endocrinol Metab Clin N Am. 2011;40:1–18.
3. Sandvik OM, Soreide K, Gudlaugsson E, Kvaloy JT, Soreide JA. Epidemiology and classification of gastroenteropancreatic neuroendocrine neoplasms using current coding criteria. Br J Surg. 2016;103:226–32.
4. Vagefi PA, Razo O, Deshpande V, McGrath DJ, Lauwers GY, Thayer SP, et al. Evolving patterns in the detection and outcomes of pancreatic neuroendocrine neoplasms: the Massachusetts General Hospital experience from 1977 to 2005. Arch Surg. 2007;142:347–54.
5. Rindi G, Capella C, Solcia E. Introduction to a revised clinicopathological classification of neuroendocrine tumors of the gastroenteropancreatic tract. Q J Nucl Med. 2000;44:13–21.
6. Cheslyn-Curtis S, Sitaram V, Williamson RC. Management of non-functioning neuroendocrine tumours of the pancreas. Br J Surg. 1993;80:625–7.
7. Eriksson B, Oberg K. Neuroendocrine tumours of the pancreas. Br J Surg. 2000;87:129–31.
8. Mazzaferro V, Pulvirenti A, Coppa J. Neuroendocrine tumors metastatic to the liver: how to select patients for liver transplantation? J Hepatol. 2007;47:460–6.

9. Norton JA. Endocrine tumours of the gastrointestinal tract. Surgical treatment of neuroendocrine metastases. Best Pract Res Clin Gastroenterol. 2005;19:577–83.

10. Madeira I, Terris B, Voss M, Denys A, Sauvanet A, Flejou JF, et al. Prognostic factors in patients with endocrine tumours of the duodenopancreatic area. Gut. 1998;43:422–7.

11. Yu F, Venzon DJ, Serrano J, Goebel SU, Doppman JL, Gibril F, et al. Prospective study of the clinical course, prognostic factors, causes of death, and survival in patients with long-standing Zollinger-Ellison syndrome. J Clin Oncol. 1999;17:615–30.

12. Que FG, Nagorney DM, Batts KP, Linz LJ, Kvols LK. Hepatic resection for metastatic neuroendocrine carcinomas. Am J Surg. 1995;10:36–43.

13. Maithel SK, Fong Y. Hepatic ablation for neuroendocrine tumor metastases. J Surg Oncol. 2009;100:635–8.

14. Frilling A, Sotiropoulos GC, Li J, Kornasiewicz O, Plöckinger U. Multimodal management of neuroendocrine liver metastases. HPB (Oxford). 2010;12:361–79.

15. Rossi RE, Massironi S, Conte D, Peracchi M. Therapy for metastatic pancreatic neuroendocrine tumors. Ann Transl Med. 2014;2:8.

16. Singh S, Law C. Chromogranin A: a sensitive biomarker for the detection and post-treatment monitoring of gastroenteropancreatic neuroendocrine tumors. Expert Rev Gastroenterol Hepatol. 2012;6:313–34.

17. Kanakis G, Kaltsas G. Biochemical markers for gastroenteropancreatic neuroendocrine tumours (GEP-NETs). Best Pract Res Clin Gastroenterol. 2012;26:791–802.

18. Ardill JE, Erikkson B. The importance of the measurement of circulating markers in patients with neuroendocrine tumours of the pancreas and gut. Endocr Relat Cancer. 2003;10:459–62.

19. Ro C, Chai W, Yu VE, Yu R. Pancreatic neuroendocrine tumors: biology, diagnosis, and treatment. Chin J Cancer. 2013;32:312–24.

20. O'Grady HL, Conlon KC. Pancreatic neuroendocrine tumours. Eur J Surg Oncol. 2008;34:324–32.

21. Xiang G, Liu X, Tan C, Zhang H, Mai G, Zheng Z. Diagnosis and treatment of VIPoma: a case report and literature review in China. Pancreas. 2012;41:806–7.

22. Diakatou E, Alexandraki KI, Tsolakis AV, Kontogeorgos G, Chatzellis E, Leonti A, et al. Somatostatin and dopamine receptor expression in neuroendocrin neoplasms: correlation of immunohistochemical findings with somatostatin receptor scintigraphy visual scores. Clin Endocrinol. 2015;83:420–8.

23. Tan TH, Lee BN, Hassan SZ. Diagnostic value of (68)Ga-DOTATATE PET/CT in liver metastases of neuroendocrine tumours of unknown origin. Nucl Med Mol Imaging. 2014;48:212–5.

24. Ng CS, Hobbs BP, Chandler AG, Anderson EF, Herron DH, Charnsangavej C, et al. Metastases to the liver from neuroendocrine tumors: effect of duration of scan acquisition on CT perfusion values. Radiology. 2013;269:758–67.

25. Ambrosini V, Morigi JJ, Nanni C, Castellucci P, Fanti S. Current status of PET imaging of neuroendocrine tumors ([18F]FDOPA, [68Ga]tracers, [11C]/[18F]-HTP). Q J Nucl Med Mol Imaging. 2015;59:58–69.

26. Armbruster M, Zech CJ, Sourbron S, Ceelen F, Auernhammer CJ, Rist C, et al. Diagnostic accuracy of dynamic gadoxetic-acid-enhanced MRI and PET/CT compared in patients with liver metastases from neuroendocrine neoplasms. J Magn Reson Imaging. 2014;40:457–66.

27. Klimsta DS, Arnold R, Capella C, et al. Neuroendocrine neoplasms of the pancreas. In: Bosman F, Carneiro F, Hruban RH, et al., editors. WHO classification of tumours of the digestive system. Lyon: IARC Press; 2010. p. 322–6.

28. Rindi G, Kloppel G, Alhman H, Caplin M, Couvelard A, de Herder WW, et al. TNM staging of foregut (neuro)endocrine tumors: a consensus proposal including a grading system. Virchows Arch. 2006;449:395–401.

29. Exocrine and Endocrine Pancreas. AJCC Cancer Staging Manual. New York: Springer; 2010. p. 241–9.

30. Jia Z, Paz-Fumagalli R, Frey G, Sella DM, McKinney JM, Wang W. Single-institution experience of radioembolization with yttrium-90 microspheres for unresectable metastatic neuroendocrine liver tumors. J Gastroenterol Hepatol. 2017;32:1617–23.

31. Hodul PJ, Strosberg JR, Kvols LK. Aggressive surgical resection in the management of pancreatic neuroendocrine tumors: when is it indicated? Cancer Control. 2008;15:314–21.

32. Frilling A, Li J, Malamutmann E, Schmid KW, Schmid KW, Bockisch A, Broelsch CE. Treatment of liver metastases from neuroendocrine tumours in relation to the extent of hepatic disease. Br J Surg. 2009;96:175–84.

33. Alagusundaramoorthy SS, Gedaly R. Role of surgery and transplantation in the treatment of hepatic metastases from neuroendocrine tumor. World J Gastroenterol. 2014;20:14348–58.

34. Chen X, Ren H, Chi Y, He S, Huang Z, Hu X, Zhao H. Resection of postoperative liver metastasis from pancreatic neuroendocrine tumors: report of one case. Transl Gastroenterol Hepatol. 2016;1:47.

35. Gomez D, Malik HZ, Al-Mukthar A, Menon KV, Toogood GJ, Lodge JP, et al. Hepatic resection for metastatic gastrointestinal and pancreatic neuroendocrine tumours: outcome and prognostic predictors. HPB (Oxford). 2007;9:345–51.

36. Mayo SC, de Jong MC, Pulitano C, Clary BM, Reddy SK, Gamblin TC, et al. Surgical management of hepatic neuroendocrine tumor metastasis: results from an international multi-institutional analysis. Ann Surg Oncol. 2010;17:3129–36.

37. Eriksson J, Stålberg P, Nilsson A, Krause J, Lundberg C, Skogseid B, et al. Surgery and radiofrequency ablation for treatment of liver metastases from midgut and foregut carcinoids and endocrine pancreatic tumors. World J Surg. 2008;32:930–8.

38. Elias D, Goéré D, Leroux G, Dromain C, Leboulleux S, de Baere T, et al. Combined liver surgery and RFA for patients with gastroenteropancreatic endocrine tumors presenting with more than 15 metastases to the liver. Eur J Surg Oncol. 2009;35:1092–7.

39. Abood GJ, Go A, Malhotra D, Shoup M. The surgical and systemic management of neuroendocrine tumors of the pancreas. Surg Clin North Am. 2009;89:249–66.

40. Musunuru S, Chen H, Rajpal S, Stephani N, McDermott JC, Holen K, et al. Metastatic neuroendocrine hepatic tumors: resection improves survival. Arch Surg. 2006;141:1000–4.

41. Elias D, Lasser P, Ducreux M, Duvillard P, Ouellet JF, Dromain C, et al. Liver resection (and associated extrahepatic resections) for metastatic well-differentiated endocrine tumors: a 15-year single center prospective study. Surgery. 2003;133:375–82.

42. Sarmiento JM, Que FG, Grant CS, Thompson GB, Farnell MB, Nagorney DM. Concurrent resections of pancreatic islet cell cancers with synchronous hepatic metastases: outcomes of an aggressive approach. Surgery. 2002;132:976–82.

43. Chamberlain RS, Canes D, Brown KT, Saltz L, Jarnagin W, Fong Y, et al. Hepatic neuroendocrine metastases: does intervention alter outcomes? J Am Coll Surg. 2000;190:432–45.

44. Chen H, Hardacre JM, Uzar A, Cameron JL, Choti MA. Isolated liver metastases from neuroendocrine tumors: does resection prolong survival? J Am Coll Surg. 1998;187:88–93.

45. Nave H, Mossinger E, Feist H, Lang H, Raab H. Surgery as primary treatment in patients with liver metastases from carcinoid tumors: a retrospective, unicentric study over 13 years. Surgery. 2001;129:170–5.

46. Jaeck D, Oussoultzoglou E, Bachellier P, Lemarque P, Weber JC, Nakano H, et al. Hepatic metastases of gastroenteropancreatic neuroendocrine tumors: safe hepatic surgery. World J Surg. 2001;25:689–92.

47. Norton JA, Warren RS, Kelly MG, Zuraek MB, Jensen RT. Aggressive surgery for metastatic liver neuroendocrine tumors. Surgery. 2003;134:1057–65.

48. Bonney GK, Gomez D, Rahman SH, Verbeke CS, Prasad KR, Toogood GJ, et al. Results following surgical resection for malignant pancreatic neuroendocrine tumours. A single institutional experience. JOP. 2008;9:19–25.

49. Tao L, Xiu D, Sadula A, Ye C, Chen Q, Wang H, et al. Surgical resection of primary tumor improves survival of pancreatic neuroendocrine tumor with liver metastases. Oncotarget. 2017;8:79785–92.

50. Watzka FM, Fottner C, Miederer M, Schad A, Weber MM, Otto G, et al. Surgical therapy of neuroendocrine neoplasm with hepatic metastasis: patient selection and prognosis. Langenbecks Arch Surg. 2015;400:349–58.

51. Genc CG, Klümpen HJ, van Oijen MGH, van Eijck CHJ, Nieveen van Dijkum EJM. A nationwide population-based study on the survival of patients with pancreatic neuroendocrine tumors in the Netherlands. World J Surg. 2018;42:490–7.

52. Du S, Wang Z, Sang X, Lu X, Zheng Y, Xu H, et al. Surgical resection improves the outcome of the patients with neuroendocrine tumor liver metastases: large data from Asia. Medicine (Baltimore). 2015;94:e388.

53. Gurusamy KS, Ramamoorthy R, Sharma D, Davidson BR. Liver resection versus other treatments for neuroendocrine tumours in patients with resectableliver metastases. Cochrane Database Syst Rev. 2009;(2):CD007060.

54. Chung MH, Pisegna J, Spirt M, Giuliano AE, Ye W, Ramming KP, et al. Hepatic cytoreduction followed by a novel long-acting somatostatin analog: a paradigm for intractable neuroendocrine tumors metastatic to the liver. Surgery. 2001;130:954–62.

55. Morgan RE, Pommier SJ, Pommier RF. Expanded criteria for debulking of liver metastasis also apply to pancreatic neuroendocrine tumors. Surgery. 2018;163:218–25.

56. Sarmiento JM, Heywood G, Rubin J, Ilstrup DM, Nagorney DM, Que FG. Surgical treatment of neuroendocrine metastases to the liver: a plea for resection to increase survival. J Am Coll Surg. 2003;197:29–37.

57. Carty SE, Jensen RT, Norton JA. Prospective study of aggressive resection of metastatic pancreatic endocrine tumors. Surgery. 1992;112:1024–32.

58. Wong KP, Tsang JS, Lang BH. Role of surgery in pancreatic neuroendocrine tumor. Gland Surg. 2018;7:36–41.

59. Öberg K. Management of functional neuroendocrine tumors of the pancreas. Gland Surg. 2018;7:20–7.

60. Jin K, Xu J, Chen J, Chen M, Chen R, Chen Y, et al. Surgical management for non-functional pancreatic neuroendocrine neoplasms with synchronous liver metastasis: a consensus from the Chinese Study Group for Neuroendocrine Tumors (CSNET). Int J Oncol. 2016;49:1991–2000.

61. Moris D, Tsilimigras DI, Ntanasis-Stathopoulos I, Beal EW, Felekouras E, Vernadakis S, et al. Liver transplantation in patients with liver metastases from neuroendocrine tumors: a systematic review. Surgery. 2017;162:525–36.

62. Lehnert T. Liver transplantation for metastatic neuroendocrine carcinoma: an analysis of 103 patients. Transplantation. 1998;27:1307–12.

63. Sposito C, Droz Dit Busset M, Citterio D, Bongini M, Mazzaferro V. The place of liver transplantation in the treatment of hepatic metastases from neuroendocrine tumors: pros and cons. Rev Endocr Metab Disord. 2017;18:473–83.

64. Shimata K, Sugawara Y, Hibi T. Liver transplantation for unresectable pancreatic neuroendocrine tumors with liver metastases in an era of transplant oncology. Gland Surg. 2018;7:42–6.

65. Le Treut YP, Delpero JR, Dousset B, Cherqui D, Segol P, Mantion G, et al. Results of liver transplantation in the treatment of metastatic neuroendocrine tumors. A 31-case French multicentric report. Ann Surg. 1997;4:355–64.

66. Fernández JA, Robles R, Marín C, Hernández Q, Sánchez Bueno F, Ramírez P, et al. Role of liver transplantation in the management of metastatic neuroendocrine tumors. Transplant Proc. 2003;35:1832–3.

67. Olausson M, Friman S, Cahlin C, Nilsson O, Jansson S, Wängberg B, et al. Indications and results of liver transplantation in patients with neuroendocrine tumors. World J Surg. 2002;26:998–1004.

68. Rossi RE, Burroughs AK, Caplin ME. Liver transplantation for unresectable neuroendocrine tumor liver metastases. Ann Surg Oncol. 2014;21:2398–405.

69. NCCN Clinical Practice Guidelines in Oncology. Neuroendocrine tumors. https://www.nccn.org/professionals/physician_gls/pdf/neuroendocrine.pdf. Accessed May 14, 2018.

70. Lin C, Dai H, Hong X, Pang H, Wang X, Xu P, et al. The prognostic impact of primary tumor resection in pancreatic neuroendocrine tumors with synchronous multifocal liver metastases. Pancreatology. 2018. [Epub ahead of print]

71. Zhou B, Zhan C, Ding Y, Yan S, Zheng S. Role of palliative resection of the primary pancreatic neuroendocrine tumor in patients with unresectable metastatic liver disease: a systematic review and meta-analysis. Onco Targets Ther. 2018;11:975–82.

72. deBaere T, Deschamps F, Tselikas L, Ducreux M, Planchard D, Pearson E, et al. GEP-NETS UPDATE: interventional radiology: role in the treatment of liver metastases from GEP-NETs. Eur J Endocrinol. 2015;172:R151–66.

73. Karabulut K, Akyildiz HY, Lance C, Aucejo F, McLennan G, Agcaoglu O, et al. Multimodality treatment of neuroendocrine liver metastases. Surgery. 2011;150:316–25.

74. Cozzi PJ, Englund R, Morris DL. Cryotherapy treatment of patients with hepatic metastases from neuroendocrine tumors. Cancer. 1995;76:501–9.

75. Christante D, Pommier S, Givi B, Pommier R. Hepatic artery chemoinfusion with chemoembolization for neuroendocrine cancer with progressive hepatic metastases despite octreotide therapy. Surgery. 2008;144:885–93.

76. Akahori T, Sho M, Tanaka T, Nishiofuku H, Kinoshita S, Nagai M, et al. Significant efficacy of new transcatheter arterial chemoembolization technique for hepatic metastases of pancreatic neuroendocrine tumors. Anticancer Res. 2013;33:3355–8.

77. Fiore F, Del Prete M, Franco R, Marotta V, Ramundo V, Marciello F, et al. Transarterial embolization (TAE) is equally effective and slightly safer than transarterial chemoembolization (TACE) to manage liver metastases in neuroendocrine tumors. Endocrine. 2014;47:177–82.

78. Kennedy A, Bester L, Salem R, Sharma RA, Parks RW, Ruszniewski P. Role of hepatic intra-arterial therapies in metastatic neuroendocrine tumours (NET): guidelines from the NET-Liver-Metastases Consensus Conference. HPB (Oxford). 2015;17:29–37.

79. Gupta S. Intra-arterial liver-directed therapies for neuroendocrine hepatic metastases. Semin Intervent Radiol. 2013;30:28–38.

80. Grozinsky-Glasberg S, Kaltsas G, Kaltsatou M, Lev-Cohain N, Klimov A, Vergadis V, et al. Hepatic intra-arterial therapies in metastatic neuroendocrine tumors: lessons from clinical practice. Endocrine. 2018;60:499–509.

81. Okuyama H, Ikeda M, Takahashi H, Ohno I, Hashimoto Y, Mitsunaga S, et al. Transarterial (chemo)embolization for liver metastases in patients with neuroendocrine tumors. Oncology. 2017;92:353–9.

82. Gordon AC, Uddin OM, Riaz A, Salem R, Lewandowski RJ. Making the case: intra-arterial therapy for less common metastases. Semin Intervent Radiol. 2017;34:132–9.

83. Pelage JP, Fohlen A, Mitry E, Lagrange C, Beauchet A, Rougier P. Chemoembolization of neuroendocrine liver metastases using streptozocin and tris-acryl microspheres: Embozar (EMBOsphere + ZAnosaR) study. Cardiovasc Intervent Radiol. 2017;40:394–400.

84. Jia Z, Wang W. Yttrium-90 radioembolization for unresectable metastatic neuroendocrine liver tumor: a systematic review. Eur J Radiol. 2018;100:23–9.

85. Devcic Z, Rosenberg J, Braat AJ, Techasith T, Banerjee A, Sze DY, et al. The efficacy of hepatic 90Y resin radioembolization for metastatic neuroendocrine tumors: a meta-analysis. J Nucl Med. 2014;55:1404–10.

86. Turkmen C, Ucar A, Poyanli A, Vatankulu B, Ozkan G, Basaran M, et al. Initial outcome after selective intraarterial radionuclide therapy with yttrium-90 microspheres as salvage therapy for unresectable metastatic liver disease. Cancer Biother Radiopharm. 2013;28:534–40.

87. Kucuk ON, Soydal C, Lacin S, Ozkan E, Bilgic S. Selective intraarterial radionuclide therapy with Yttrium-90 (Y-90) microspheres for unresectable primary and metastatic liver tumors. World J Surg Oncol. 2011;9:86.

88. Alexander RA, Jensen RT. Pancreatic endocrine tumors. In: DeVita VT, Hellman S, Rosenberg SA, editors. Cancer: principles and practice of oncology. Philadelphia, PA: Lippincott Williams and Wilkins; 2001. p. 1788–813.

89. Valle JW, Eatock M, Clueit B, Gabriel Z, Ferdinand R, Mitchell S. A systematic review of non-surgical treatments for pancreatic neuroendocrine tumours. Cancer Treat Rev. 2014;40:376–89.

90. Appetecchia M, Baldelli R. Somatostatin analogues in the treatment of gastroenteropancreatic neuroendocrine tumours, current aspects and new perspectives. J Exp Clin Cancer Res. 2010;29:19.

91. Strosberg J, Kvols L. Antiproliferative effect of somatostatin analogs in gastroenteropancreatic neuroendocrine tumors. World J Gastroenterol. 2010;16:2963–70.

92. Rinke A, Müller HH, Schade-Brittinger C, Klose KJ, Barth P, Wied M, et al. Placebo controlled, double-blind, prospective, randomized study on the effect of octreotide LAR in the control of tumor growth in patients with metastatic neuroendocrine midgut tumors: a report from the PROMID Study Group. J Clin Oncol. 2009;27:4656–63.

93. Delavault P, Caplin ME, Liyange N, Blumberg J. The CLARINET study: assessing the effect of lanreotide autogel on tumor progression-free survival in patients with nonfunctioning gastroenteropancreatic neuroendocrine tumors. J Clin Oncol. 2012;30:abstr TPS4153.

94. Caplin ME, Pavel M, Ćwikła JB, Phan AT, Raderer M, Sedláčková E, et al. Lanreotide in metastatic enteropancreatic neuroendocrine tumors. N Engl J Med. 2014;371:224–33.

95. Jann H, Denecke T, Koch M, Pape UF, Wiedenmann B, Pavel M. Impact of octreotide long-acting release on tumour growth control as a first-line treatment in neuroendocrine tumours of pancreatic origin. Neuroendocrinology. 2013;98:137–43.

96. Wolin EM. The expanding role of somatostatin analogs in the management of neuroendocrine tumors. Gastrointest Cancer Res. 2012;5:161–8.

97. Ferolla P, Faggiano A, Grimaldi F, Ferone D, Scarpelli G, Ramundo V, et al. Shortened interval of long-acting octreotide administration is effective in patients with well-differentiated neuroendocrine carcinomas in progression on standard doses. J Endocrinol Investig. 2012;35:326–31.

98. Fazio N, de Braud F, Delle Fave G, Oberg K. Interferon-alpha and somatostatin analog in patients with gastroenteropancreaticneuroendocrine carcinoma: single agent or combination? Ann Oncol. 2007;18:13–9.

99. Sorscher S. Metastatic pancreatic poorly differentiated neuroendocrine carcinoma: current treatment considerations. Clin Adv Hematol Oncol. 2013;11:804–5.

100. Toumpanakis C, Meyer T, Caplin ME. Cytotoxic treatment including embolization/chemoembolization for neuroendocrine tumours. Best Pract Res Clin Endocrinol Metab. 2007;21:131–44.

101. Kouvaraki MA, Ajani JA, Hoff P, Wolff R, Evans DB, Lozano R, et al. Fluorouracil, doxorubicin, and streptozocin in the treatment of patients with locally

advanced and metastatic pancreatic endocrine carcinomas. J Clin Oncol. 2004; 22:4762–71.

102. Strosberg JR, Fine RL, Choi J, Nasir A, Coppola D, Chen DT, et al. First-line chemotherapy with capecitabine and temozolomide in patients with metastatic pancreatic endocrine carcinomas. Cancer. 2011;117:268–75.

103. Yamaguchi T, Machida N, Morizane C, Kasuga A, Takahashi H, Sudo K, et al. Multicenter retrospective analysis of systemic chemotherapy for advanced neuroendocrine carcinoma of the digestive system. Cancer Sci. 2014;105:1176–81.

104. Saif MW, Kaley K, Brennan M, Garcon MC, Rodriguez G, Rodriguez T. A retrospective study of capecitabine/temozolomide (CAPTEM) regimen in the treatment of metastatic pancreatic neuroendocrine tumors (pNETs) after failing previous therapy. JOP. 2013;14:498–501.

105. Shi C, Klimstra DS. Pancreatic neuroendocrine tumors: pathologic and molecular characteristics. Semin Diagn Pathol. 2014;31:498–511.

106. Wolin EM. Long-term everolimus treatment of patients with pancreatic neuroendocrine tumors. Chemotherapy. 2015;60:143–50.

107. Yao JC, Shah MH, Ito T, Bohas CL, Wolin EM, Van Cutsem E, et al. Everolimus for advanced pancreatic neuroendocrine tumors. N Engl J Med. 2011;364:514–23.

108. Capurso G, Archibugi L, Delle FG. Molecular pathogenesis and targeted therapy of sporadic pancreatic neuroendocrine tumors. J Hepatobiliary Pancreat Sci. 2015;22:594–601.

109. Leung R, Lang B, Wong H, Chiu J, Yat WK, Shek T, et al. Advances in the systemic treatment of neuroendocrine tumors in the era of molecular therapy. Anti Cancer Agents Med Chem. 2013;13:382–8.

110. Raymond E, Dahan L, Raoul JL, Bang YJ, Borbath I, Lombard-Bohas C, et al. Sunitinib malate for the treatment of pancreatic neuroendocrine tumors. N Engl J Med. 2011;364:501–13.

111. Kennedy AS, Dezarn WA, McNeillie P, Coldwell D, Nutting C, Carter D, et al. Radioembolization for unresectable neuroendocrine hepatic metastases using resin 90Y-microspheres: early results in 148 patients. Am J Clin Oncol. 2008;31:271–9.

112. Filice A, Fraternali A, Frasoldati A, Asti M, Grassi E, Massi L, et al. Radiolabeled somatostatin analogues therapy in advanced neuroendocrine tumors: a single centre experience. J Oncol. 2012;2012:320198.

113. Rossi RE, Massironi S, Spampatti MP, Conte D, Ciafardini C, Cavalcoli F, et al. Treatment of liver metastases in patients with digestive neuroendocrine tumors. J Gastrointest Surg. 2012;16:1981–92.

114. Seregni E, Maccauro M, Coliva A, Castellani MR, Bajetta E, Aliberti G, et al. Treatment with tandem [(90)Y]DOTA-TATE and [(177)Lu] DOTA-TATE of neuroendocrine tumors refractory to conventional therapy: preliminary results. Q J Nucl Med Mol Imaging. 2010;54:84–91.

115. Kwekkeboom DJ, de Herder WW, Kam BL, van Eijck CH, van Essen M, Kooij PP, et al. Treatment with the radiolabeled somatostatin analog [177 Lu-DOTA 0,Tyr3]octreotate: toxicity, efficacy, and survival. J Clin Oncol. 2008;26:2124–30.

116. Kwekkeboom DJ, Teunissen JJ, Bakker WH, Kooij PP, de Herder WW, Feelders RA, et al. Radiolabeled somatostatin analog [177Lu-DOTA0,Tyr3] octreotate in patients with endocrine gastroenteropancreatic tumors. J Clin Oncol. 2005;23:2754–62.

17

Comparison of the prevalence of incidental and non-incidental papillary thyroid microcarcinoma during 2008–2016: a single-center experience

Krzysztof Kaliszewski[1]*, Agnieszka Zubkiewicz-Kucharska[2], Paweł Kiełb[1], Jerzy Maksymowicz[1], Aleksander Krawczyk[1] and Otto Krawiec[1]

Abstract

Background: The incidence of papillary thyroid microcarcinoma (PTMC) is increasing; however, it is not clear whether this reflects an increase in the incidence of incidental or in that of non-incidentally (presurgically) discovered PTMC (IPTMC vs. NIPTMC). We assessed the incidence of IPTMC and NIPTMC over the past 9 years, to discern whether the increase in PTMC incidence is due to improved diagnostics or to a real increase in the incidence.

Methods: We performed a retrospective chart review of 4327 patients who were consecutively admitted to and surgically treated for thyroid pathology at a single institution. As a main presurgical diagnostic test, all patients underwent ultrasound-guided fine-needle aspiration biopsy (UG-FNAB). The analyzed time frame was divided into three equal periods (I: 2008–2010, II: 2011–2013, III: 2014–2016), and IPTMCs and NIPTMCs were assessed and compared in each period.

Results: We evaluated 393 (9.08%) patients with thyroid malignancy, of which 156 (3.60% of all thyroid tumors [TTs]; 39.69% of all thyroid cancers [TCs]) were diagnosed as PTMC. The prevalence of NIPTMC among all TCs increased from 16.66% in 2008 to 33.75% in 2016, while that of IPTMC decreased from 20.83% in 2008 to 13.75% in 2016. The incidence rates of NIPTMC and IPTMC in period III differed statistically significantly ($p < 0.0001$). The prevalence rate of NIPTMC in period III was higher than that in period II, yet comparable to that in period I ($p = 0.0014$; $p = 0.2804$, respectively).

Conclusions: The prevalence of NIPTMC, rather than that of IPTMC, is escalating; this may be due to better presurgical diagnosis.

Keywords: Incidental, Non-incidental, Papillary thyroid microcarcinoma

Background

Thyroid carcinoma (TC) is the most common malignant tumor of the endocrine system [1]. It constitutes approximately 1% of all human malignancies and is the main cause of death among endocrine tumor-related deaths [2]. In 2010, Jemal et al. reported 44,700 new cases of thyroid cancers per year, worldwide, and 1700 deaths due to this condition occurred annually [3]. An annual increase of 5.3% in TC incidence was reported by Magreni et al. in 2015 [4].

Papillary thyroid cancer (PTC), which is the main type of TC, accounts for 80% of all thyroid malignancies [5]. The prognosis of PTC is generally favorable; however, for some subtypes, prognosis may depend on the cancer stage at the time of diagnosis. For early stages, the 10-year survival rate reaches 90%, whereas for later stages, the 10-year survival rate is not as high [5].

A clinically important type of PTC is a tumor with a small size (diameter ≤ 1.0 cm), regardless of whether

* Correspondence: krzysztofkali@wp.pl
[1]First Department and Clinic of General, Gastroenterological, and Endocrine Surgery, Wroclaw Medical University, 66 Maria Skłodowska-Curie Street, 50-369 Wrocaw, Poland
Full list of author information is available at the end of the article

lymph node and local invasion, as well as distant metastases, has occurred. The World Health Organization (WHO) defines these tumors as a papillary thyroid microcarcinoma (PTMC) [6]. PTMCs account for approximately 30% of all PTCs [7]. Some authors have described PTMCs as tumors with low malignancy, which are slow-growing, minimally invasive, and associated with low mortality [8]. Based on autopsy studies, Solares et al. have confirmed that up to 36% of PTMCs had low aggressiveness [9]. Other reports have also described these tumors as common and typical findings, with a favorable prognosis [10]. However, very aggressive forms of PTMC have also been described [11]. Therefore, Gao et al. stated that PTCs with a small size (≤ 1.0 cm in diameters) do not always behave as indolent tumors [12].

To date, the diagnosis of PTMC has been highly reliant on a high-frequency ultrasonography examination and ultrasound-guided fine-needle aspiration biopsy (UG-F-NAB), which remains the standard diagnostic procedure for the evaluation of thyroid nodules. The main purpose of UG-FNAB is to distinguish between malignant and benign tumors and to identify patients requiring surgical treatment [13].

The accuracy of diagnostic procedures for thyroid nodules has improved over the last few years, and the ease of access to such diagnostic modalities may be the reason for the higher prevalence of thyroid tumors. However, the exact cause of this increase is still debated. As we have observed a continuous increase in the PTMC incidence over a number of years, we have contemplated various reasons for this phenomenon. Although improvements in the imaging tools, availability of UG-FNAB, and easier access to diagnostic thyroid pathology may play a role, some changes in the environment may also have caused a real increase in the morbidity rate.

The purpose of this study was to assess and compare the incidence of PTMC over the last 9 years and to identify whether there is a difference in the number of presurgically discovered (non-incidental) and non-discovered (incidental) PTMCs, to determine whether the increased incidence in PTMC is due to improved diagnostics (mainly UG-FNAB).

Methods

We performed a retrospective chart review of 4327 patients who were consecutively admitted to and surgically treated for thyroid pathology at a single institution, from January 1, 2008, to December 31, 2016. The analyzed time frame was divided into three equal periods (period I: 2008–2010, period II: 2011–2013, period III: 2014–2016). Next, we assessed and compared the incidence rates of incidental PTMCs (IPTMCs) and non-incidental PTMCs (NIPTMCs) in these three periods. All of the ultrasound examinations were performed by the same team of radiologists experienced in thyroid sonography.

All patients underwent UG-FNAB as the main presurgical diagnostic test. The same equipment and ultrasonography set in all biopsies were used. A 10-MHz linear probe of ultrasonography set has been applied. The UG-FNAB was performed using 0.5-mm gauge needles and 10-cc syringes for each procedure. Clinical and pathological classification was performed according to the TNM classification criteria (7th Edition, 2015) by the American Joint Committee on Cancer (AJCC) [14]. All of the patients underwent total thyroidectomy by the same team of surgeons experienced in thyroid surgery, and all histopathological specimens were examined by the same two pathologists, who were both experienced in diagnosing thyroid malignancy.

Statistical analysis

Statistical analysis was conducted with the use of Statistica vs. 12 (StatSoft, Inc., Tulsa, OK, USA; 2014). The following statistical measures were used: arithmetical mean (x), median and standard deviation (SD), and ranges of determined parameters in study groups.

The Shapiro-Wilk test was used to confirm the normality of data distribution. As data demonstrated a normal distribution, t tests were used to assess the significance of differences. Intergroup frequency assessment was performed using a chi-squared test. Yate's correction was applied when the expected frequency was less than 5 or the total count was less than 50.

P values < 0.05 were taken as indicating statistically significant differences, while p values from 0.05 to < 0.10 were considered as indicating borderline statistical significance.

Results

From 4327 patients diagnosed for thyroid pathology at our institute during the study period, we evaluated 393 (9.08%) patients with thyroid malignancy, of whom 156 (3.60% of total thyroid pathology; 39.69% of TC patients) were diagnosed with PTMC. In this homogenous group, there were 52 (33.33%) patients with IPTMC and 104 (66.67%) with NIPTMC. There were 45 (89.18%) females and 7 (10.82%) males in the IPTMC group and 98 (95%) females and 6 (5%) males in the NIPTMC group ($p = 0.1013$). The mean age of all patients with PTMC was 48.6 (± 14.6), and 44.6 (± 15.9) and 49.0 (± 14.5) for males and females, respectively ($p = 0.1390$; Table 1).

The prevalence of PTMC increased over the 9-year period, from 37.5% in 2008 to 47.5% in 2016 ($p = 0.0414$). The prevalence of NIPTMC increased from 16.66% of all TCs in 2008 to 33.75% in 2016, but IPTMC decreased from 20.83% in 2008 to 13.75% in 2016 (Table 2). In the years 2009, 2015, and 2016, we observed more patients with NIPTM than with IPTMC (Table 3; Fig. 1a, b and c). Moreover, we noticed a

Table 1 Demographic characteristics of patients with a diagnosis of papillary thyroid microcarcinoma (PTMC)

Parameter	PTMC (n = 156)
Gender	
Male	13 (8.3%)
Female	143 (91.7%)
Age (years)	
All patients	48.6 ± 14.6
Male	44.6 ± 15.9
Female	49.0 ± 14.5

Descriptive data are presented as numbers (n), percentage (%) and mean ± standard deviation (± SD)

Table 3 The prevalence of incidental and non-incidental papillary thyroid microcarcinoma in each year

	Incidental	Non-incidental	Total	p
2008	5 (1.03%)	4 (0.83%)	9 (1.86%)	0.7115
2009	3 (0.79%)	10 (2.62%)	13 (3.40%)	*0.0261*
2010	3 (0.71%)	9 (2.13%)	12 (2.84%)	0.0578
2011	4 (0.83%)	5 (1.04%)	9 (1.86%)	0.7169
2012	9 (1.66%)	9 (1.66%)	18 (3.31%)	1
2013	7 (1.24%)	9 (1.59%)	16 (2.83%)	0.5874
2014	4 (1.06%)	6 (1.60%)	10 (2.66%)	0.4911
2015	6 (1.01%)	25 (4.21%)	31 (5.22%)	*0.0001*
2016	11 (2.31%)	27 (5.66%)	38 (7.97%)	*0.003*

Statistically significant differences are shown in italics

statistically significant predominance of NIPTMC over IPTMC in periods I (2008–2010) and III (2014–2016), but not in period II (2011–2013), (p = 0.0216; p < 0.0001; p = 0.6176. respectively; Table 4, Fig. 1d, e, and f). Furthermore, there was an increase in the prevalence of NIPTMC in period III as compared to period II (p = 0.0014), but not as compared to period I (p = 0.2804) (Table 5).

Discussion

The incidence of PTMC has been increasing worldwide. In our study, we observed that the prevalence of this tumor has increased more than four times, from 1.86% of all thyroid tumors in 2008 to 7.97% in 2016. Although it is typically minimally invasive, Gao et al. described PTMC as a public health concern because of its tremendous increase in the past few decades [12]. Additionally, it has been suggested that if any additional factors, such as extrathyroidal invasion, lymph node metastases, or the *BRAF* V600E mutation, are found, PTMC should be treated as a "larger" papillary thyroid cancer [15].

Postoperatively, PTMC is often found in multinodular goiter (MNG) and it is then diagnosed as IPTMC [16]. In our study, the prevalence of IPTMC increased from 1.03% of all thyroid tumors in 2008 to 2.31% in 2016, together with the increase of all PTMCs (from 1.86% in 2008 to 7.97% in 2016). In terms of total PTMC, the prevalence of IPTMC has decreased approximately by half: from 20.83% in 2008 to 13.75% in 2016. Li et al. reported that IPTMC is undetectable before surgery, due to its coexistence with MNG, its small size, and its deep localization within thyroid gland [17]. For that reason, in MNG, every nodule should be assessed by ultrasound examination to determine the risk of cancer. In our previous study, we revealed that the assistance of a radiologist in UG-FNAB procedures increases the value of the procedure [18].

It was suggested that pre-operative diagnosis of PTMC is difficult and therefore rare, because of its slow growth rate, absence of specific symptoms, clinical characteristics, and potential co-occurrence with benign thyroid

Table 2 The prevalence of incidental and non-incidental papillary thyroid microcarcinoma (IPTMC and NIPTMC) according to all thyroid tumors and all thyroid cancers in years 2008–2016

	2008	2009	2010	2011	2012	2013	2014	2015	2016
For all thyroid tumors									
IPTMC	5 (1.03%)	3 (0.79%)	3 (0.71%)	4 (0.83%)	9 (1.66%)	7 (1.24%)	4 (1.06%)	6 (1.01%)	11 (2.31%)
NIPTMC	4 (0.83%)	10 (2.62%)	9 (2.13%)	5 (1.04%)	9 (1.66%)	9 (1.59%)	6 (1.60%)	25 (4.21%)	27 (5.66%)
PTMC	9 (1.86%)	13 (3.40%)	12 (2.84%)	9 (1.86%)	18 (3.31%)	16 (2.83%)	10 (2.66%)	31 (5.22%)	38 (7.97%)
All thyroid cancers	24 (4.96%)	26 (6.81%)	36 (8.51%)	29 (6.00%)	51 (9.39%)	53 (9.38%)	32 (8.51%)	62 (10.44%)	80 (16.77%)
All thyroid tumors	484 (100%)	382 (100%)	423 (100%)	483 (100%)	543 (100%)	565 (100%)	376 (100%)	594 (100%)	477 (100%)
For all thyroid cancers									
IPTMC	5 (20.83%)	3 (11.53%)	3 (8.33%)	4 (13.79%)	9 (17.64%)	7 (13.20%)	4 (12.5%)	6 (9.67%)	11 (13.75%)
NIPTMC	4 (16.66%)	10 (38.46%)	9 (25%)	5 (17.24%)	9 (17.64%)	9 (16.98%)	6 (18.75%)	25 (40.32%)	27 (33.75%)
PTMC	9 (37.5%)	13 (50%)	12 (33.33%)	9 (31.03%)	18 (35.29%)	16 (30.18%)	10 (31.25%)	31 (50%)	38 (47.5%)
All thyroid cancers	24 (100%)	26 (100%)	36 (100%)	29 (100%)	51 (100%)	53 (100%)	32 (100%)	62 (100%)	80 (100%)

IPTMC incidental papillary thyroid microcarcinoma, *NIPTMC* non-incidental papillary thyroid microcarcinoma, *PTMC* papillary thyroid microcarcinoma

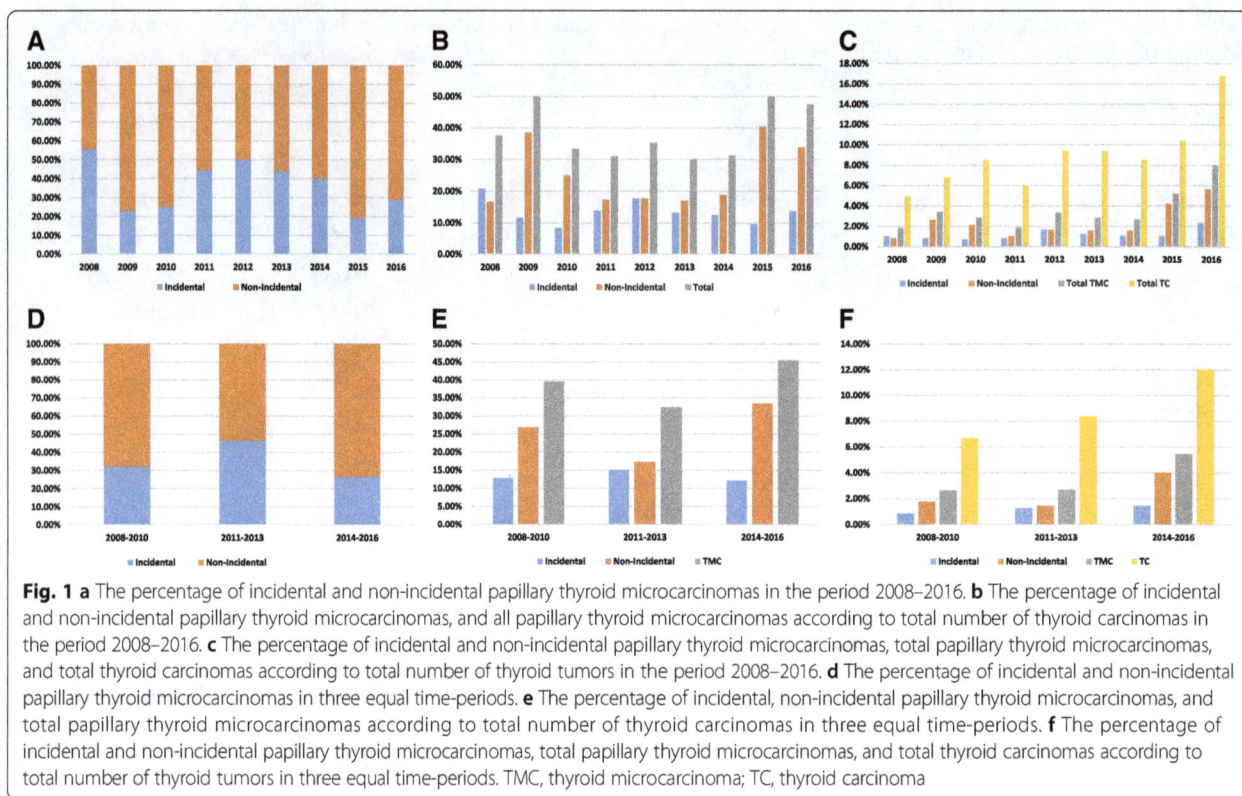

Fig. 1 a The percentage of incidental and non-incidental papillary thyroid microcarcinomas in the period 2008–2016. **b** The percentage of incidental and non-incidental papillary thyroid microcarcinomas, and all papillary thyroid microcarcinomas according to total number of thyroid carcinomas in the period 2008–2016. **c** The percentage of incidental and non-incidental papillary thyroid microcarcinomas, total papillary thyroid microcarcinomas, and total thyroid carcinomas according to total number of thyroid tumors in the period 2008–2016. **d** The percentage of incidental and non-incidental papillary thyroid microcarcinomas in three equal time-periods. **e** The percentage of incidental, non-incidental papillary thyroid microcarcinomas, and total papillary thyroid microcarcinomas according to total number of thyroid carcinomas in three equal time-periods. **f** The percentage of incidental and non-incidental papillary thyroid microcarcinomas, total papillary thyroid microcarcinomas, and total thyroid carcinomas according to total number of thyroid tumors in three equal time-periods. TMC, thyroid microcarcinoma; TC, thyroid carcinoma

nodules [19]. Some authors have stated that the increasing rate of the prevalence of non-incidental thyroid microcarcinoma (NIPTMC) during the past few decades may have been due to the extensive development of high-frequency ultrasonography and the UG-FNAB technique [20]. These observations are in accordance with the results of our study. At the beginning of this trial, in 2008, only 0.83% of all thyroid tumors were NIPTMC, whereas this figure was 5.66% in 2016.

The mortality rate of PTMC has remained unchanged over the last few decades, which additionally supports the hypothesis of increased NIPTMC diagnoses and treatment [21]. At present, even tumors with a 3-mm diameter can be detected by ultrasonography and subsequently qualify for UG-FNAB [15]. For this reason, a large number of very small malignant tumors are found, thus increasing the rate of NIPTMC. Chen et al. suggested that even nodules with a dimension of

Table 4 Patients with incidental and non-incidental papillary thyroid microcarcinoma, all thyroid cancers and all papillary thyroid microcarcinoma cases in three equal time-periods

NIPTMC	52 (33.3%)		
IPTMC	104 (66.7%)		
	Period I (2008–2010)	Period II (2011–2013)	Period III (2014–2016)
Number of cases in each period [n]			
NIPTMC	23	23	58
IPTMC	11	20	21
TC	86	133	174
Percentage of PTMC in all TC cases in each period [%]			
NIPTMC	26.74%	17.29%	33.33%
IPTMC	12.79%	15.04%	12.07%
PTMC	39.53%	32.33%	45.40%
p	*0.0216*	0.6176	*< 0.0001*

Statistically significant differences are shown in italics
IPTMC incidental papillary thyroid microcarcinoma, *NIPTMC* non-incidental papillary thyroid microcarcinoma, *PTMC* papillary thyroid microcarcinoma, *TC* all thyroid cancers

Table 5 Comparison of the three equal periods of time according to incidence of non-incidental and incidental papillary thyroid microcarcinoma

	p		
	Period I (2008–2010)	Period II (2011–2013)	Period III (2014–2016)
Period I (2008–2010)	–	0.0882	0.2804
Period II (2011–2013)	0.0882	–	*0.0014*
Period III (2014–2016)	0.2804	*0.0014*	–

Statistically significant differences are shown in italics

2–3 mm can be detected with the use of a high-resolution transducer [19]. Comparing the rates of NIPTMC to those of IPTMC in the equally divided time-periods of our study, we noticed a statistically significant increase of NIPTMC rate in the last period. In those years, even very small tumors with suspicions of malignancy qualified for UG-FNAB, followed by early radical surgery [16]; consequently, the "wait and see" approach until the tumor had increased in size was rejected [22, 23]. We propose that this is the reason for the continuous and significant increase in NIPTMC diagnoses. All of the patients admitted to our clinic for thyroid tumors, who subsequently underwent surgical treatment, also underwent UG-FNAB. This diagnostic method was widely used to distinguish PTMC from benign tumors. Nevertheless, not every PTMC diagnosed postoperatively had been biopsied before surgical treatment; thus, not every "suspicious" tumor was selected for biopsy. This observation explains the fact that, even in period III (2014–2016), in which high-quality UG-FNAB was available, we still observed 12.07% of IPTMC. This phenomenon may also be explained by the observation of Brito et al. [21], who noticed that increasing rates of thyroid operations were coupled with more radical surgical treatment. We used a more radical treatment strategy, and it may justify the high incidence rate of IPTMC [21]. Castro et al. [24] concluded that the major reason for the increasing incidence of NIPTMC is the detection of subclinical, indolent tumors, thus, overdiagnosis. Regarding the indolent type of NIPTMC, it has been suggested to change the term "carcinoma" to "small papillary lesions." [24] This might be more suitable for patients in terms of the overdiagnosis and overtreatment phenomenon.

Our study has certain limitations. Firstly, this was a retrospective study and included patients who underwent UG-FNAB and thyroid surgery during a relatively not very long time. Secondly, we could not perform lymph nodes status analysis, because of retrospective study design. Patients with IPTMC did not received central lymph node dissection, because the cancer diagnosis was established postsurgery. And finally, the study included a relatively small number of patients. Unfortunately, surgery still not only represents a treatment option but also is a diagnostic tool in thyroid pathology.

Microscopic evaluation of the surgical specimen still represents the gold standard for the diagnosis of thyroid nodules. In regards to overdiagnosis and overtreatment, further studies are necessary to resolve these issues.

Conclusions

The proportion of IPTMC and NIPTMC of all thyroid tumors is relatively high and is increasing. However, in terms of total TCs, only the prevalence of NIPTMC, but not that of IPTMC, is increasing; this may be explained by better presurgical diagnostic processes.

Abbreviations
IPTMC: Incidental papillary thyroid microcarcinoma; MNG: Multinodular goiter; NIPTMC: Non-incidental papillary thyroid microcarcinoma; PTC: Papillary thyroid cancer; PTMC: Papillary thyroid microcarcinoma; TC: Thyroid cancer; TT: Thyroid tumor; UG-FNAB: Ultrasound-guided fine-needle aspiration biopsy

Authors' contributions
KK is responsible for the conceptualization, investigation, methodology, project administration, resources, writing the original draft, and reviewing and editing the manuscript. KK, PK, JM, AK, and OK obtained the data. KK and AZK did the formal analysis, supervision, and validation. All authors read and approved the final manuscript.

Competing interests
The authors declare that they have no competing interest.

Author details
[1]First Department and Clinic of General, Gastroenterological, and Endocrine Surgery, Wroclaw Medical University, 66 Maria Skłodowska-Curie Street, 50-369 Wrocaw, Poland. [2]Department of Endocrinology and Diabetology for Children and Adolescents, Wroclaw Medical University, Wroclaw, Poland.

References
1. Hu D, Zhou J, He W, et al. Risk factors of lateral lymph node metastasis in cN0 papillary thyroid carcinoma. World J Surg Oncol. 2018;16:30.
2. Are C, Shaha AR. Anaplastic thyroid carcinoma: biology, pathogenesis, prognostic factors, and treatment approaches. Ann Surg Oncol. 2006;13:453–64.
3. Jemal A, Siegel R, Xu J, Ward E. Cancer statistics, 2010. CA Cancer J Clin. 2010;60:277–300.
4. Magreni A, Bann DV, Schubart JR, Goldenberg D. The effects of race and ethnicity on thyroid cancer incidence. JAMA Otolaryngol Head Neck Surg. 2015;141:319–23.
5. Lu J, Hu S, Miccoli P, et al. Non-invasive diagnosis of papillary thyroid microcarcinoma: a NMR-based metabolomics approach. Oncotarget. 2016;7: 81768–77.
6. Hedinger C, Williams ED, Sobin LH. The WHO histological classification of thyroid tumors: a commentary on the second edition. Cancer. 1989; 63:908–11.
7. Zhao Q, Ming J, Liu C, et al. Multifocality and total tumor diameter predict central neck lymph node metastases in papillary thyroid microcarcinoma. Ann Surg Oncol. 2013;20:746–52.

8. Mehanna H, Al-Maqbili T, Carter B, et al. Differences in the recurrence and mortality outcomes rates of incidental and nonincidental papillary thyroid microcarcinoma: a systematic review and meta-analysis of 21 329 person-years of follow-up. J Clin Endocrinol Metab. 2014;99:2834–43.
9. Solares CA, Penalonzo MA, Xu M, Orellana E. Occult papillary thyroid carcinoma in postmortem species: prevalence at autopsy. Am J Otolaryngol. 2005;26:87–90.
10. Harach HR, Franssila KO, Wasenius VM. Occult papillary carcinoma of the thyroid. A "normal" finding in Finland. A systematic autopsy study. Cancer. 1985;56:531–8.
11. Chow SM, Law SC, Chan JK, Au SK, Yau S, Lau WH. Papillary microcarcinoma of the thyroid - prognostic significance of lymph node metastasis and multifocality. Cancer. 2003;98:31–40.
12. Gao X, Zhang X, Zhang Y, Hua W, Maimaiti Y, Gao Z. Is papillary thyroid microcarcinoma an indolent tumor?: a retrospective study on 280 cases treated with radioiodine. Medicine (Baltimore). 2016;95:e5067.
13. Nikiforov YE, Steward DL, Robinson-Smith TM, et al. Molecular testing for mutations in improving the fine-needle aspiration diagnosis of thyroid nodules. J Clin Endocrinol Metab. 2009;94:2092–8.
14. Haugen BR, Alexander EK, Bible KC, et al. 2015 American Thyroid Association Management Guidelines for adult patients with thyroid nodules and differentiated thyroid cancer: the American Thyroid Association Guidelines Task Force on Thyroid Nodules and Differentiated Thyroid Cancer. Thyroid. 2016;26:1–133.
15. Shi C, Guo Y, Lv Y, et al. Clinicopathological features and prognosis of papillary thyroid microcarcinoma for surgery and relationships with the BRAFV600E mutational status and expression of angiogenic factors. PLoS One. 2016;11:e0167414.
16. Kaliszewski K, Wojtczak B, Strutyńska-Karpińska M, Łukieńczuk T, Forkasiewicz Z, Domosławski P. Incidental and non-incidental thyroid microcarcinoma. Oncol Lett. 2016;12:734–40.
17. Li B, Zhang Y, Yin P, Zhou J, Jiang T. Ultrasonic features of papillary thyroid microcarcinoma coexisting with a thyroid abnormality. Oncol Lett. 2016;12: 2451–6.
18. Kaliszewski K, Zubkiewicz-Kucharska A, Wojtczak B, Strutyńska-Karpińska M, Zaleska-Dorobisz U, Leśków E. Ultrasound guided fine-needle aspiration biopsy of thyroid nodules: does radiologist assistance decrease the rate of unsatisfactory biopsies? Adv Clin Exp Med. 2016;25:93–100.
19. Chen HY, Liu WY, Zhu H, et al. Diagnostic value of contrast-enhanced ultrasound in papillary thyroid microcarcinoma. Exp Ther Med. 2016;11:1555–62.
20. Yoon JH, Lee HS, Kim EK, et al. Short-term follow-up US leads to higher false-positive results without detection of structural recurrences in PTMC. Medicine (Baltimore). 2016;9:e2435.
21. Brito JP, Davies L. Is there really an increased incidence of thyroid cancer? Curr Opin Endocrinol Diabetes Obes. 2014;21:405–8.
22. Ito Y, Miyauchi A, Inoue H, et al. An observational trial for papillary thyroid microcarcinoma in Japanese patients. World J Surg. 2010;34:28–35.
23. Kim HY, Park WY, Lee KE, et al. Comparative analysis of gene expression profiles of papillary thyroid microcarcinoma and papillary thyroid carcinoma. J Cancer Res Ther. 2010;6:452–7.
24. Castro MR, Morris JC, Ryder M, Brito JP, Hay ID. Most patients with a small papillary thyroid carcinoma enjoy an excellent prognosis and may be managed with minimally invasive therapy or active surveillance. Cancer. 2015;121:3364–5.

18

Identification of hub genes with diagnostic values in pancreatic cancer by bioinformatics analyses and supervised learning methods

Chunyang Li[1,2], Xiaoxi Zeng[1,2], Haopeng Yu[1,2], Yonghong Gu[1,2] and Wei Zhang[1,2*]

Abstract

Background: Pancreatic cancer is one of the most lethal tumors with poor prognosis, and lacks of effective biomarkers in diagnosis and treatment. The aim of this investigation was to identify hub genes in pancreatic cancer, which would serve as potential biomarkers for cancer diagnosis and therapy in the future.

Methods: Combination of two expression profiles of GSE16515 and GSE22780 from Gene Expression Omnibus (GEO) database was served as training set. Differentially expressed genes (DEGs) with top 25% variance followed by protein-protein interaction (PPI) network were performed to find candidate genes. Then, hub genes were further screened by survival and cox analyses in The Cancer Genome Atlas (TCGA) database. Finally, hub genes were validated in GSE15471 dataset from GEO by supervised learning methods k-nearest neighbor (kNN) and random forest algorithms.

Results: After quality control and batch effect elimination of training set, 181 DEGs bearing top 25% variance were identified as candidate genes. Then, two hub genes, *MMP7* and *ITGA2*, correlating with diagnosis and prognosis of pancreatic cancer were screened as hub genes according to above-mentioned bioinformatics methods. Finally, hub genes were demonstrated to successfully differ tumor samples from normal tissues with predictive accuracies reached to 93.59 and 81.31% by using kNN and random forest algorithms, respectively.

Conclusions: All the hub genes were associated with the regulation of tumor microenvironment, which implicated in tumor proliferation, progression, migration, and metastasis. Our results provide a novel prospect for diagnosis and treatment of pancreatic cancer, which may have a further application in clinical.

Keywords: Pancreatic cancer, Bioinformatics analysis, Differentially expressed genes, Hub genes, Diagnosis

Background

Pancreatic cancer is one of the most lethal tumors due to the poor prognosis, and now it is the fourth or fifth most common causes of cancer mortality in developed countries [1]. And it is estimated that by the year 2020, pancreatic cancer would move to the second leading cause of death [2]. Although some advances in understanding the molecular mechanisms of pancreatic cancer have been achieved, there still exist difficulties in early diagnosis due to non-specific symptoms and lacking

effective testing identification, making it usually found in its late stage [3]. Until now, 1-year survival in pancreatic cancer patients is still not significantly improved [4], and the 5-year survival is less than 10% [5].

Numerous studies have focused on the investigation of biomarkers and molecular mechanisms of pancreatic cancers, and it is demonstrated that accumulated mutations in genes like oncogene *Kras*, and tumor-suppressor genes including *P16* as well as *TP53* resulted in the occurrence of pancreatic cancer [4]. One study performed the whole-genome sequencing and copy number variation (CNV) analyses showed that several genes including *TP53*, *SMAD4*, *CDKN2A*, *ARID1A*, *ROBO2*, *PREX2*, and *KDM6A* were disrupt

---

* Correspondence: weizhang005@126.com
[1]West China Biomedical Big Data Center, West China Hospital, Sichuan University, Chengdu, China
[2]Medical Big Data Center, Sichuan University, Chengdu, China

resulting from chromosomal rearrangements in pancreatic ductal adenocarcinomas patients [6]. Molecular mechanisms researches demonstrated that overexpression of protein-coupled receptor GPR87 enhanced pancreatic cancer aggressiveness by activating NF-κB signaling pathway [7]. Moreover, Zhong and colleges have found that functional P38 MAPK activity contributed to overall survival through suppressing JNK signaling in pancreatic cancer [8]. In addition, aberrant expressions of some microRNAs have emerged as an important hallmark of cancer recently [9]. It was reported that microRNA-21 was overexpressed in pancreatic cancer, and could serve as a potential predictor of survival [10]. One study has found that miR-506 facilitated pancreatic cancer progression and chemoresistance via SPHK1/Akt/NF-κB signaling pathway [11]. Another study demonstrated that suppressing microRNA-34 expression downregulated Bcl-2 and Notch1/2 in pancreatic cancer cells, as well as significantly inhibited cell growth and invasion, induced apoptosis and G1 and G2/M arrest in cell cycle, and sensitized the cells to chemotherapy and radiation [12].

However, traditional experimental methods as mentioned above could only identify single gene or a few genes at once, which limits large-scale investigation of hub genes and pathways in the systematic biology level. Development of microarray and sequencing technologies provides better methods for biomarker screening and molecular mechanism discovery in cancer research. Recent years with the accessibility of multi-omics database like Gene Expression Omnibus (GEO) [13] as well as The Cancer Genome Atlas (TCGA) [14] and so on, it is now possible to acquire multi-sample data and compare cancer profiles with normal profiles in multiple omics dimensions. On one hand, omics data in multiple dimensions leading to the system biology- and/or network-based approach, which could better understand the dysregulated molecular mechanisms in cancer development and progression [15]. On the other hand, biology- and/or network-based method can not only identify critical genes but also can detect corresponding pathways and/or interactive network, which may provide better insights into molecular mechanisms investigation than dysregulated gene analysis individually [16]. For example, Kras was proved to be the most frequently mutated gene in pancreatic ductal adenocarcinoma [17], and the mutation of Kras was a hallmark of pancreatic cancer [18]. However, inhibitors targeting Kras gene were largely unsuccessful, while some omics-based strategies targeting Kras correlated pathways and interactive genes were proved to bear better therapeutic effects than targeting Kras individually [19].

To date, diagnosis of pancreatic cancer is mainly based on clinical signs and pathology confirmation. However, the specific symptoms and pathological imagines may only be detected unambiguously at the late stage of pancreatic cancer, which may lead to a limited therapies and poor prognosis. This raises an urgent need for the development of reliable biomarkers which can effectively differ tumor from normal tissues based on analyses of gene expression profiles. Herein, in order to identify novel diagnostic predictors and molecular markers, we integrated two microarray datasets from GEO database, and 11 candidate genes significantly differentially expressed between tumor and normal samples were screened by bioinformatics analyses. Then two hub genes, matrix metallopeptidase 7 (MMP7) and integrin, alpha 2 (ITGA2), were further identified by survival and cox analyses in TCGA database. These two hub genes were validated in another expression profile from GEO database, demonstrating that these hub genes can successfully differ normal tissues from tumor samples. The predictive accuracies of k-nearest neighbor (kNN) and random forest algorithms were almost 94% and almost 82%, respectively. Results in our study may provide an auxiliary evidence of pancreatic cancer diagnosis and therapy in the future.

Methods

Data collection and preprocessing

A workflow of this study was shown in Fig. 1. Datasets in our study were firstly searched in GEO database (http://www.ncbi.nlm.nih.gov/geo/) by using these keywords "pancreatic/pancreas" + "tumor/cancer" + "normal" + "GPL570," and 165 datasets were obtained until June 20th, 2018. Then these datasets were further screened as following criteria: (1) Samples were from human pancreatic tissues. (2) Samples were not interfered with any other treatments. Finally, three datasets, GSE16515 [20], GSE22780, and GSE15471 [21], were included in our study for further analysis.

All the datasets were performed by Affymetrix Human Genome U133 Plus 2.0 Array (Affymetrix, Santa Clara, CA, USA). GSE16515 dataset included 36 malignant pancreatic samples and 16 normal pancreatic samples, while the corresponding numbers in GSE22780 dataset were 8 and 8. In order to obtain sample balance, combination of GSE16515 and GSE22780 was used as training set to determine hub genes. Besides, raw expression data of GSE15471 was downloaded from GEO, also performed by Affymetrix Human Genome U133 Plus 2.0 Array. It composed of 39 normal and 39 malignant pancreatic samples, and served as testing set.

Firstly, the quality of all the datasets were detected with "affyPLM" package in R, herein FitPLM weight, residual, relative log expression (RLE), normalized unscaled standard errors (NUSE), and RNA degradation images were evaluated. Then robust multiarray averaging (RMA) with

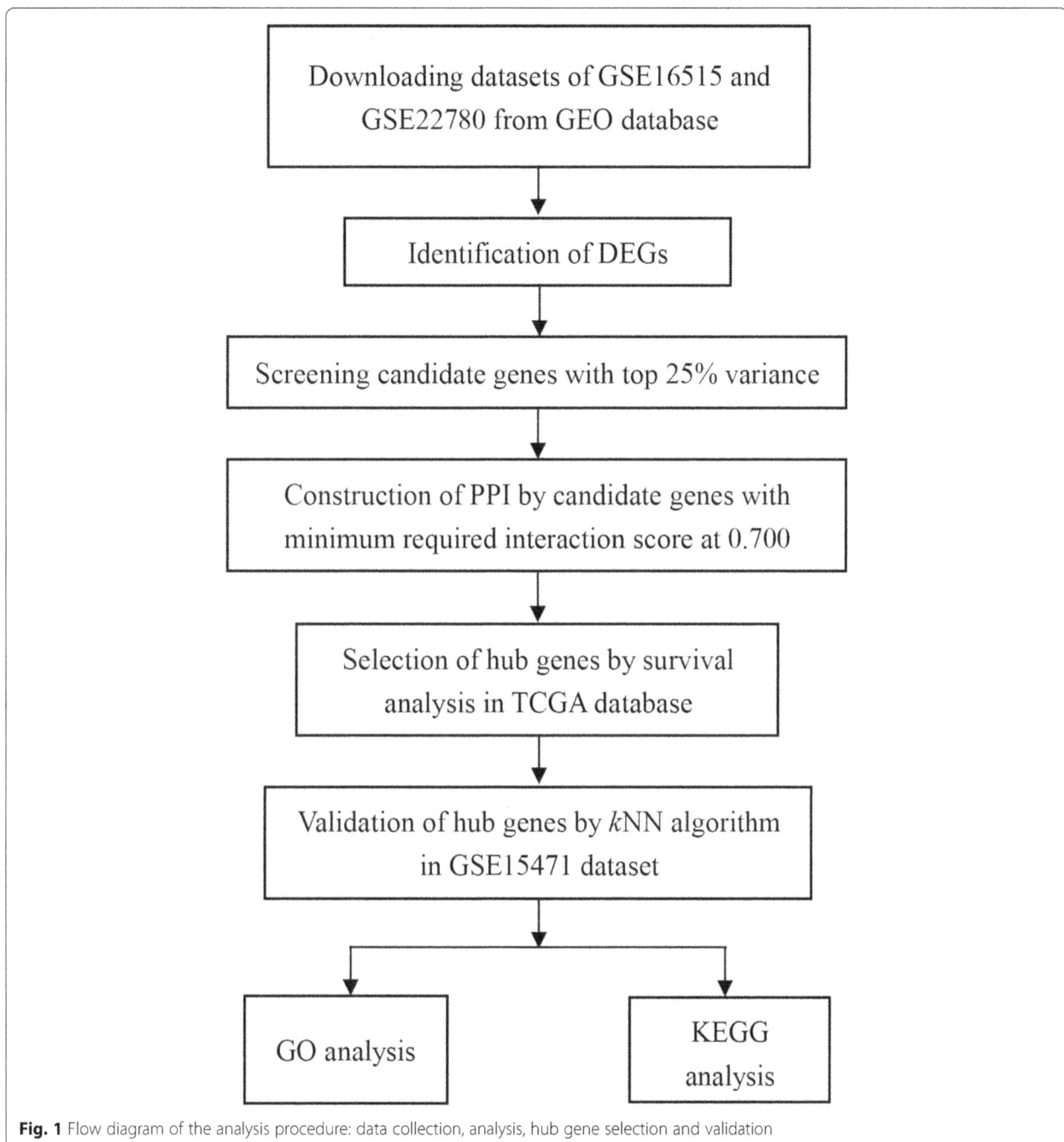

Fig. 1 Flow diagram of the analysis procedure: data collection, analysis, hub gene selection and validation

"affy" package was used to do the background correction and normalization. Before subsequent hub gene selection in training set, empirical Bayes framework with "sva" package in R was used to adjust the batch effects between these two datasets.

In addition, we also downloaded RNA-sequencing data of pancreatic cancer from The Cancer Genome Atlas (TCGA) database (https://cancergenome.nih.gov/), and all the raw data were also converted into gene symbol expression matrix by R software and Perl software.

Differentially expressed genes screening

Herein, "limma" package was used to detect differentially expressed genes (DEGs) between malignant pancreatic samples and normal samples in training set with the threshold of adj.P value < 0.01 and absolute log2-based fold change > 1.

Candidate gene selection

Variance of every DEGs in different samples were calculated and sorted by descending order, and the top 25%

results were selected. Then, 181 genes bearing top 25% variance were uploaded in Search Tool for the Retrieval of Interacting Genes (STRING) database (https://string-db.org/), and PPI network was constructed [22] by setting minimum required interaction score at 0.700. Then a plug-in Cytohubba in Cytoscape [23] was used to further screen candidate genes. Herein, degree algorithm was applied and the screening criterion was degree > 5.

Hub gene screening by survival and cox regression analyses in TCGA
Candidate genes were further screened by survival analysis and cox regression analysis in TCGA database with "survival" package. Genes with P value less than 0.05 both in survival analysis and cox analysis were further screened as hub genes.

Gene ontology annotation and pathway analyses of candidate genes
In order to depict the biological function of candidate genes, gene ontology (GO) biological process enrichments were performed through Database for Annotation, Visualization and Integrated Discovery (DAVID) (https://david.ncifcrf.gov/) [24, 25]. And the visualization of GO results was performed by "GOplot" package in R.

Validation of hub genes by supervised learning methods
In order to verify whether these hub genes were "real hub genes" to discriminate tumor and normal samples,

kNN algorithm in "class" package and random forest algorithm in "randomForest" package were performed. The accuracy was used to evaluate the predictive results. Herein, random forest algorithm was rerun for 100 times, and the mean value of the accuracies was calculated finally.

Results
Identification of DEGs
After the quality control of GSE16515 and GSE22780 datasets, these two profiles were suitable for subsequent analyses. And all the raw probe expression data were converted into gene expression data finally. The heat map of all the gene expressions in training set was shown in Fig. 2a. After background correction and normalization as well as batch effects adjustment, 724 DEGs were determined with the threshold of adj.P value < 0.01 and absolute log2-based fold change > 1 (Additional file 1). Among all the DEGs, there were 591 upregulated genes and 133 downregulated genes, and the volcano map for DEGs selection was shown in Fig. 2b.

Determination of candidate genes
Variance analyses of 724 DEGs were further performed in all the 68 different samples, and 181 candidate genes with top 25% variance were screened (shown in Additional file 2). Subsequently, all the 181 candidate genes were uploaded to STRING database, and PPI network was

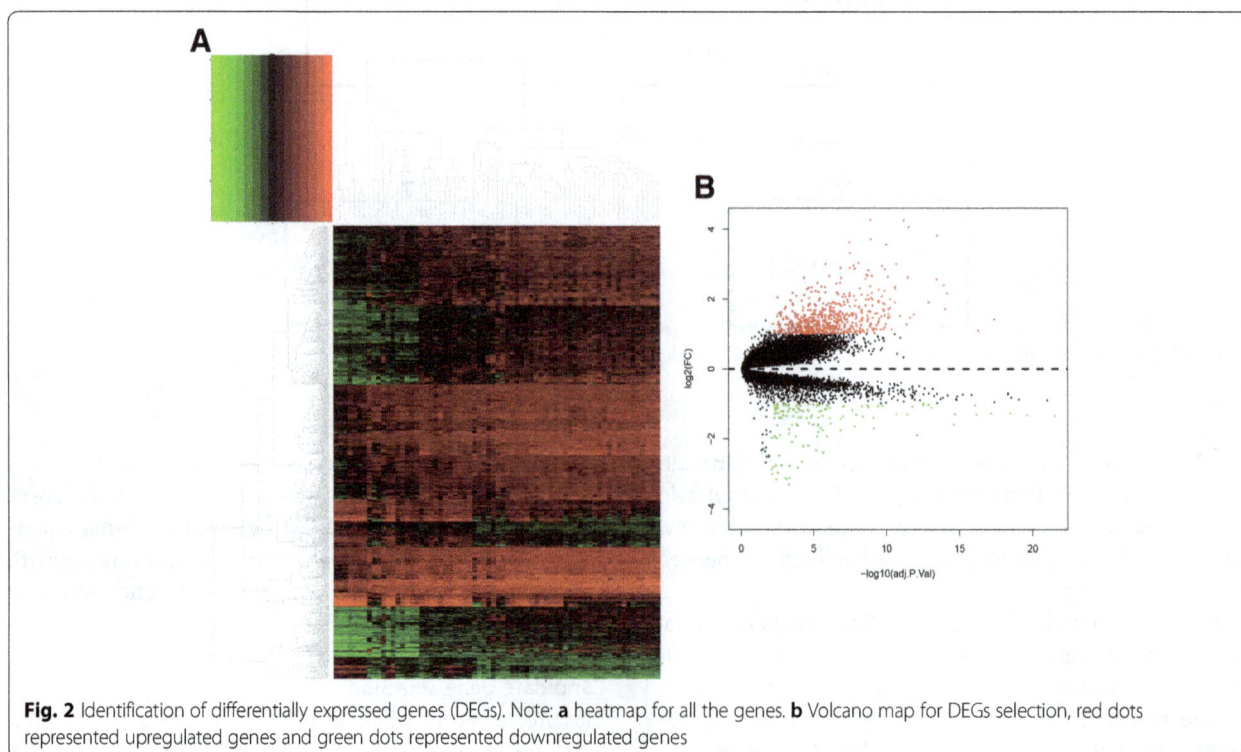

Fig. 2 Identification of differentially expressed genes (DEGs). Note: **a** heatmap for all the genes. **b** Volcano map for DEGs selection, red dots represented upregulated genes and green dots represented downregulated genes

constructed with minimum required interaction score at 0.700. After elimination of disconnected node in the network, there were 175 nodes and 102 edges in this PPI network (Fig. 3). Finally, 11 genes (*ALB*, *EGF*, *FN1*, *ITGA2*, *COL1A2*, *SPARC*, *COL3A1*, *TIMP1*, *COL5A1*, *COL11A1*, and *MMP7*) with degree > 5 were screened as candidate genes.

Selection of hub genes by survival and cox analyses

There were 178 pancreatic cancer samples and 4 normal samples in TCGA database. In survival analysis, two groups were defined, one is high expression group (expressions greater than mean expression of the gene) and the other one is low expression group (expressions lower than mean expression of the gene). After survival analyses of 11 candidate genes, 3 genes (*MMP7*, *COL1A2*, and *ITGA2*) had significant difference of survival time between these two groups (Fig. 4). As for cox regression analysis, two genes (*MMP7* and *ITGA2*) bear significant

difference between alive and death patients. Therefore, *MMP7* and *ITGA2* were further screened as hub genes for further analysis.

Functional annotation and pathway enrichment

GO enrichment results showed that 181 genes were participated in 75 different biological process, and genes in GO:0030198 implicated in extracellular matrix organization exhibited the most significantly upregulated expressions (Fig. 5a). In Fig. 5b, the biological processes of top 5 GO terms enriched the most genes were shown, of which GO:0007165 enriched 22 genes ranked as the first with the biological process of signal transduction. GO enrichment of two hub genes demonstrated that these hub genes mainly participated in the regulation of cell adhesion, transforming growth factor beta receptor signaling pathway and extracellular matrix organization or disassembly (Table 1).

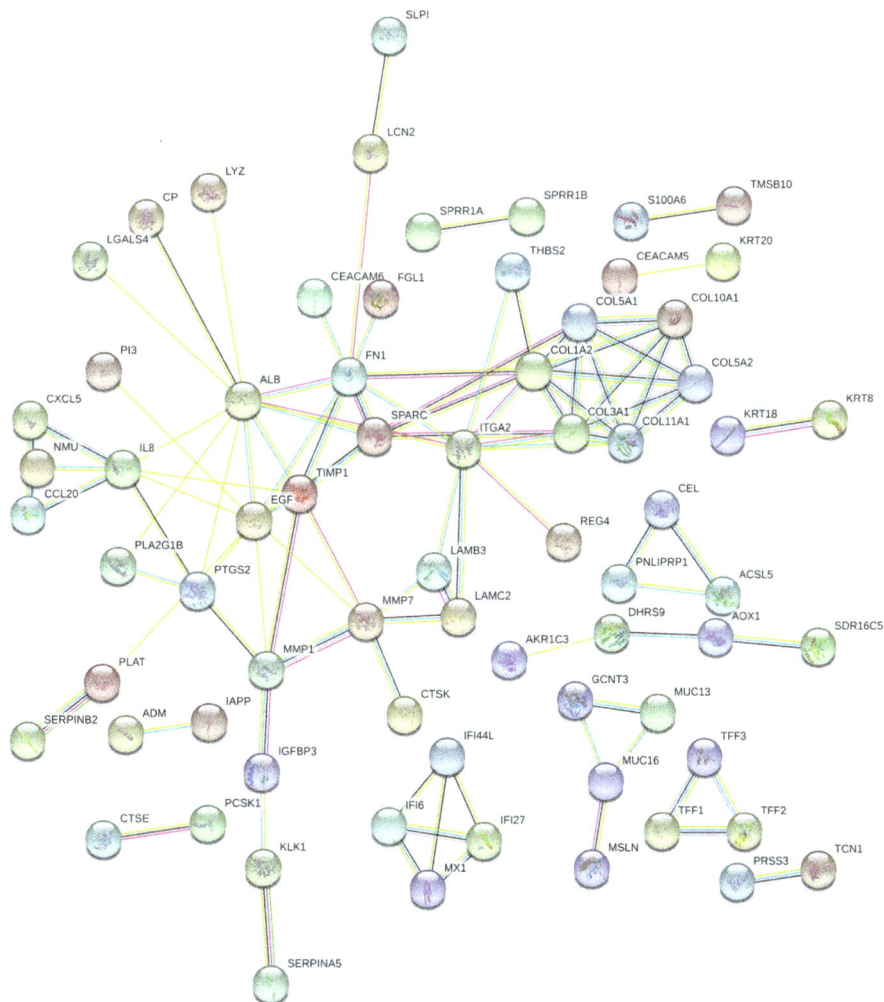

Fig. 3 PPI network constructed by 181 candidate genes with minimum required interaction score at 0.700

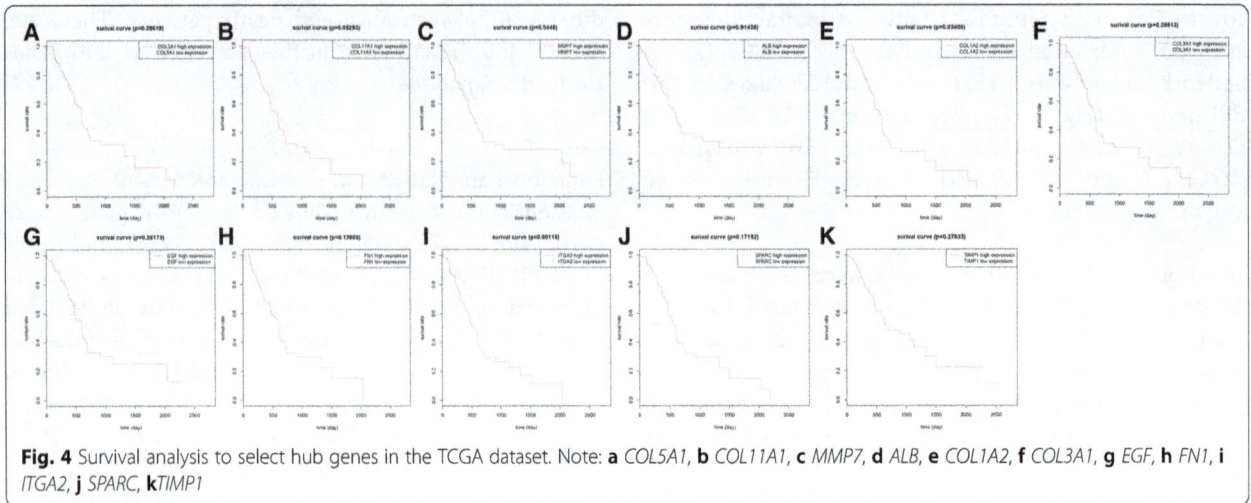

Fig. 4 Survival analysis to select hub genes in the TCGA dataset. Note: **a** *COL5A1*, **b** *COL11A1*, **c** *MMP7*, **d** *ALB*, **e** *COL1A2*, **f** *COL3A1*, **g** *EGF*, **h** *FN1*, **i** *ITGA2*, **j** *SPARC*, **k** *TIMP1*

Prediction of pancreatic cancer by hub genes

Herein, *k*NN and random forest algorithms were applied to detect whether these two hub genes could correctly distinguish malignant samples from normal samples. We can see from Table 2 that hub genes selected by method 1 (the method performed in this study) bear the highest predictive accuracy, which reached to almost 93.59% by using *k*NN method. As for random forest algorithm, the mean predictive accuracy was 81.31% after rerunning the method for 100 times. Furthermore, predictive

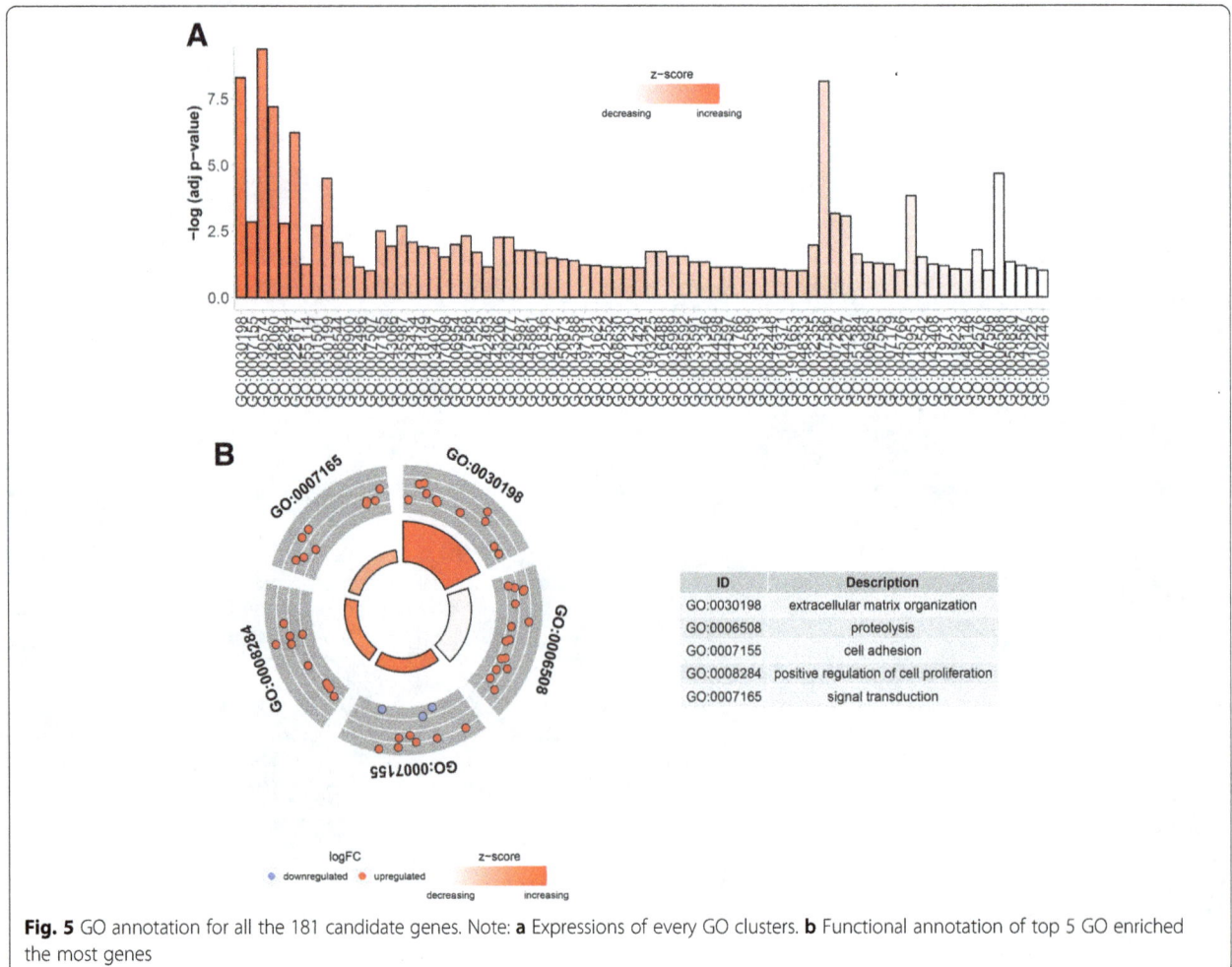

Fig. 5 GO annotation for all the 181 candidate genes. Note: **a** Expressions of every GO clusters. **b** Functional annotation of top 5 GO enriched the most genes

Table 1 Functional annotation of two hub genes *ITGA2* and *MMP7*

Genes	GO number	Biological process
ITGA2	GO:0045987	Positive regulation of smooth muscle contraction
	GO:0033591	Response to L-ascorbic acid
	GO:0031346	Positive regulation of cell projection organization
	GO:0043589	Skin morphogenesis
	GO:0048333	Mesodermal cell differentiation
	GO:0030198	Extracellular matrix organization
	GO:0007155	Cell adhesion
	GO:0042493	Response to drug
	GO:0007596	Blood coagulation
	GO:0007565	Female pregnancy
MMP7	GO:0006508	Proteolysis
	GO:0030574	Collagen catabolic process
	GO:0022617	Extracellular matrix disassembly
	GO:0007568	Aging

accuracies of different hub genes selected by other methods were compared, and the results were listed in Table 2. Conclusion could be drawn from Table 2 that method 1 as proposed in this study had highly predictive accuracies in both *k*NN and random forest algorithms.

Discussion

Compared with other cancers, the occurrence of pancreatic cancer is relatively rare; however, it is still a lethal disease with poor prognosis. Until now, there still lacks effective therapies against pancreatic cancer, and many novel therapies are in the experimental stage. Therefore, it is important to find some potential hub genes playing crucial roles in regulating cancer occurrence and progression, which may become key targets in the treatment of pancreatic cancer in the future. In addition, these hub genes effectively differing cancer tissues from normal samples may provide novel auxiliary evidence in pancreatic cancer diagnosis. It is demonstrated that pancreatic cancer results from the accumulation of acquired mutations, which may lead to the upregulation of some oncogenes and downregulation of some tumor-suppressing genes and genomic maintenance genes [4]. Therefore, there might exist some DEGs between normal and tumor samples, and these DEGs may play important roles in regulating tumor occurrence, development, and progression. In the present study, two genes *ITGA2* and *MMP7* were screened from DEGs as hub genes by using a series of bioinformatics methods, and they could discriminate normal samples and tumor samples.

The matrix metalloproteinase (MMPs) is a family of enzymes, bearing the capability to cleave extracellular matrix substrates [26], as well as promotes the release of

pro-TNF-α, Fas ligand, and some cytokines in various cancers cells [27]. One previous study has experimentally demonstrated that genes in matrix metallopeptidase family, collagen family, and integrin family were upregulated in pancreatic cancer, and they may correlate with cancer activity and poor prognosis [28]. MMPs also involved in proliferative, migrating, and differentiated processes in cells [29]. The interaction between MMPs and extracellular ligand induced a series of signaling cascade, and thus led to the functional regulation of intracellular and extracellular activities. The expression of MMP7 has been reported to be upregulated in several kinds of cancer, including colon cancer [27], pancreatic cancer [30], breast cancer [31], gastric cancer [32], and esophageal cancer [33]. One study has demonstrated that multiplex detection of pancreatic biomarkers CA19-9, MMP7, and MUC4 in sera samples were of high sensitivity, which may act as the critical biomarker in diagnosis of pancreatic cancer [34]. Another study compared tumor tissues with healthy control samples revealed that MMP7 was highly predictive for advanced stage of pancreatic cancer, which strongly associated with N1 status, T3/T4 stage, moderate/poor differentiation, and perineural invasion [35]. It has been reported that Stat3 was a critical factor to facilitate precursor formation and enforced MMP7 expression in pancreatic cancer cells, while MMP7 level was correlated with metastasis and survival in pancreatic cancer patients [36].

ITGA2 encoding by *ITGA2* gene is the alpha subunit of the transmembrane receptor integrin, and it mainly exerts the adhesive roles in cell-cell interaction, also promotes the generation and adhesion of newly synthesized extracellular matrix [37, 38]. The polymorphisms of *ITGA2* gene was related to the poor survival of nasopharyngeal carcinoma [39]. *ITGA2* gene was reported to play migrating roles in colon cancer cells [40], and it expressed in colorectal cancer with liver metastasis tissues but absent in normal tissue [41]. In addition, epigenetic modifications such as DNA methylation were also important in tumorigenesis, and hypomethylation of *ITGA2* with high gene expression was associated with poor survival in pancreatic cancer patients [42]. One research has found that ITGA2 was overexpressed in a variety of gastric cancer patients mainly playing pro-survival roles, and the blockage of ITGA2 could induce apoptosis and inhibit cell migration in gastric cancer [43]. Another research in gastric cancer revealed that HMGA2, FOXL2, and ITGA2 were increased in metastatic lymph nodes and distant metastases in gastric cancer, and suppressing the HMGA2-FOXL2-ITGA2 pathway could serve as a new strategy in further treatment in gastric cancer [44]. The transcriptional co-activators yes-associated protein (YAP) was considered as oncogene in many types of cancer; ITGA2 stimulating

Table 2 Comparison of predictive accuracy resulted from different screening methods

Minimum required interaction score	Methods	Hub genes	k	Accuracy of kNN algorithm	Mean accuracy of random forest algorithm (rerun 100 times)
0.700	Method 1: 724 DGEs-181 candidate genes-genes bearing top 10 degrees in PPI-2 hub genes by survival analysis and cox analysis	MMP7, ITGA2	2	78.21%	81.31%
			5	84.62%	
			10	87.18%	
			23	92.31%	
			27	93.59%	
	Method 2: 724 DGEs-181 candidate genes-genes bearing top 10 degrees in PPI	ALB, EGF, FN1, ITGA2, COL1A2, SPARC, COL3A1, TIMP1, COL5A1, COL11A1, MMP7	2	79.49%	83.54%
			4	70.51%	
			6	76.92%	
			9	78.20%	
			13	80.77%	
			15	88.46%	
			18	83.33%	
	Method 3: 724 DGEs-genes bearing top 10 degrees in PPI-2 hub genes by survival analysis and cox analysis	TOP2A, MAD2L1	2	65.38%	69.82%
			5	69.23%	
			8	65.38%	
			12	66.67%	
			23	67.95%	
	Method 4: 724 DGEs-genes bearing top 10 degrees in PPI	CCNB1, CCNA2, MAD2L1, TOP2A, UBE2C, CDC20, TTK, MELK, BUB1B, NDC80	2	70.51%	74.81%
			5	71.80%	
			8	76.92%	
			13	75.64%	
			23	74.36%	
0.400	Method 5: 724 DGEs-181 candidate genes-genes bearing top 10 degrees in PPI-1 hub genes by survival analysis and cox analysis	ITGA2	2	74.36%	69.23%
			5	80.77%	
			10	80.77%	
			14	80.77%	
			18	82.05%	
			22	85.90%	
	Method 6: 724 DGEs-181 candidate genes-genes bearing top 10 degrees in PPI	ALB, EGF, ITGA2, FN1, COL1A2, TIMP1, MMP1, COL3A1, PTGS2, CEL	2	82.05%	83.72%
			4	71.80%	
			6	79.49%	

Table 2 Comparison of predictive accuracy resulted from different screening methods (Continued)

Minimum required interaction score	Methods	Hub genes	k	Accuracy of kNN algorithm	Mean accuracy of random forest algorithm (rerun 100 times)
			10	75.64%	
			13	74.36%	
			18	73.08%	
	Method7:724 DGEs-genes bearing top10 degrees in PPI-2 hub genes by survival analysis and cox analysis	TOP2A, MAD2L1	2	65.38%	69.82%
			5	69.23%	
			8	65.38%	
			12	66.67%	
			23	67.95%	
	Method8:724 DGEs-genes bearing top 10 degrees in PPI	ALB, GAPDH, EGF, TOP2A, CCNB1, NDC80, CCNA2, CDC20, UBE2C, BUB1B, MAD2L1, TTK, OIP5, KIF11	2	71.79%	73.05%
			6	73.08%	
			11	69.23%	
			15	70.51%	
			22	73.08%	

Method 1: Identification of DEGs → screening candidate genes with top 25% variance → construction of PPI by candidate genes with minimum required interaction score at 0.700, and further screen candidate genes with top 10 degrees in PPI → Selection of hub genes by survival and cox analyses in TCGA database

Method 2: Identification of DEGs → screening candidate genes with top 25% variance → construction of PPI by candidate genes with minimum required interaction score at 0.700, and further identification of hub genes bearing top 10 degrees in PPI

Method 3: Identification of DEGs → construction of PPI by candidate genes with minimum required interaction score at 0.700, and further screen candidate genes with top 10 degrees in PPI → selection of hub genes by survival and cox analyses in TCGA database

Method 4: Identification of DEGs → construction of PPI by candidate genes with minimum required interaction score at 0.700, and further identification of hub genes bearing top 10 degrees in PPI

Method 5: Identification of DEGs → screening candidate genes with top 25% variance → construction of PPI by candidate genes with minimum required interaction score at 0.400, and further screen candidate genes with top 10 degrees in PPI → selection of hub genes by survival and cox analyses in TCGA database

Method 6: Identification of DEGs → screening candidate genes with top 25% variance → construction of PPI by candidate genes with minimum required interaction score at 0.400, and further identification of hub genes bearing top 10 degrees in PPI

Method 7: Identification of DEGs → construction of PPI by candidate genes with minimum required interaction score at 0.400, and further screen candidate genes with top 10 degrees in PPI → selection of hub genes by survival and cox analyses in TCGA database

Method 8: Identification of DEGs → construction of PPI by candidate genes with minimum required interaction score at 0.400, and further identification of hub genes bearing top 10 degrees in PPI

YAP activity was associated with unfavorable survival of pancreatic cancer patients [45].

In order to validate whether these genes were real hub genes, another mRNA expression profile GSE15471 from GEO database was utilized as testing set. Herein, kNN and random forest algorithms were performed to detect whether these hub genes could successfully distinguish tumor tissues from normal samples. We can see from Table 2 that hub genes selected by method 1 in this study represented the highest accuracy reaching to 94% approximately with 2.56% false negative and 3.84% false positive. In the cases of differing from tumor and normal samples, reduction of false negative results was more important than the reduction of false positive result. Since false negative results may lead to wrongly diagnose pancreatic cancer as normal condition, it may result in the delay of timely treatment, and further lead to more serious progression of disease as well as more waste of medical resources and costs. Bedsides, random forest algorithm also represented highly predictive accuracy of 81.31% after rerun for 100 times of method 1. Therefore, method 1 bear highly predictive accuracies in both of the two methods, and it could be inferred that these two hub genes were real hub genes, which could successfully discriminate normal and tumor samples. Another interesting result could be found in Table 2 that selection of genes with top 25% variance obviously increased the predictive accuracy from 70 to 94% (method 1 vs. method 3).

In addition, we can choose different minimum required interaction score when constructing PPI network. Minimum required interaction score is a threshold providing a score for each interactive pair, which is computed as the joint probability from different evidence (e.g., protein interaction, fusion, co-expression, text mining). Higher score may represent more confident interaction while lower score may lead to more false positives [22]. In order to elucidate whether setting different minimum required interaction score may have influence on hub gene selection, predictive accuracy was compared (shown in Table 2). It can be found that higher minimum required interaction score led to much higher predictive accuracies; method 5 bear the highest accuracy of 85% while the predictive accuracy of method 1 could reach to almost 95% by using kNN method.

Hub genes screened in this study were rational. Firstly, all the candidate genes and these two hub genes were closely correlated with the progression of tumor. As shown in GO enrichment, most of the candidate genes were implicated in the biological process of extracellular matrix, cell adhesion, cell proliferation, and signal transduction; they play important role in the progression of cancers. Moreover, both of the hub genes were implicated in the regulation of tumor microenvironment, including the regulation of tumor cells, stroma cells,

extracellular matrix (ECM), and some extracellular molecules like cytokines as well as chemokines. It has been demonstrated that microenvironment was usually dysregulated and disorganized in cancer cells. Thus, disordered microenvironment may be favorable to tumor proliferation, progression, invasion and metastasis, and exert drug-hampering roles [46, 47], and now some treatment strategies have focused on the regulation of tumor microenvironment. Since pancreatic cancer was featured as uncontrolled and malignant invasion and migration, therefore we can infer that these hub genes implicated in tumor microenvironment might be core mediators in pancreatic cancer diagnosis and therapy. Secondly, two supervised learning methods were performed, and both of the predictive results of these two hub genes were good with lower false negative in discriminating tumor samples from normal samples.

However, there also exist some limitations in our study. Firstly, the number of samples in our study is not too much. According to the dataset screening criteria, three datasets were included in our study. There were 146 samples totally, of which 68 were training set and 78 were testing set. In the future, with more and more investigations about pancreatic cancer would be performed, more samples should be included. Secondly, in this study, we mainly focused on the genes in the pancreatic tissue not the genes from circulating tumor cells (CTC) nor circulating tumor DNA (ctDNA) in peripheral blood, since the genes in tissue are more accurate to analyze the important biomarkers. Moreover, the datasets about peripheral blood in GEO database are not enough to do the same research. In the future, the microarray analysis of DNA in peripheral blood of pancreatic cancer patients should be further proposed. Thirdly, in our study, all the hub genes were screened and validated only by bioinformatics method, and further exploration of the biological functions and molecular mechanisms of these hub genes both in vitro and in vivo are needed to be fulfilled.

Conclusions

In summary, we conducted a series of bioinformatics methods to find DEGs, further screened and validated hub genes. These two hub genes, *ITGA2* and *MMP7*, may act as potential diagnostic and therapeutic biomarkers in pancreatic cancer patients. This study provides several useful hub genes for future in vitro and in vivo investigations of their molecular mechanisms in pancreatic cancer diagnosis and therapy. And profile data mining by bioinformatics analysis is an available method to find potential diagnostic and prognostic biomarkers systematically. Nevertheless, further molecular mechanisms investigations by biological experiments are still needed to be verified in pancreatic cancer cells.

Acknowledgements

We sincerely thank Professor Qiu Li and Doctor Pengfei Zhang (Department of Cancer Center, West China Hospital) for their good suggestions on pancreatic cancer diagnosis, treatment, and management.

Funding

This work was supported by Science & Technology Department of Sichuan Province funding project (No. 2016FZ0108), Health and Family Planning Commission of Sichuan Province project (No. 17PJ443), international cooperation project of Science and Technology Department of Sichuan Province (2016HH0069).

Authors' contributions

CL participated in study design, data preprocessing and analysis, as well as manuscript writing. XZ involved in data preprocessing, data analysis, and results double check. HY participated in supervised learning analysis, and manuscript writing. YG implicated in statistics analysis and language polishing. WZ designed the study and help to write the manuscript. All authors read and approved the final manuscript.

Competing interests

The authors declare that they have no competing interests.

References

1. Li C, Heidt DG, Dalerba P, Burant CF, Zhang L, Adsay V, Wicha M, Clarke MF, Simeone DM. Identification of pancreatic cancer stem cells. Cancer Res. 2007;67:1030–7.
2. Rahib L, Smith BD, Aizenberg R, Rosenzweig AB, Fleshman JM, Matrisian LM. Projecting cancer incidence and deaths to 2030: the unexpected burden of thyroid, liver, and pancreas cancers in the United States. Cancer Res. 2014; 74:2913–21.
3. Korc M. Pancreatic cancer-associated stroma production. Am J Surg. 2007; 194:S84–6.
4. Kleeff J, Korc M, Apte M, La Vecchia C, Johnson CD, Biankin AV, Neale RE, Tempero M, Tuveson DA, Hruban RH, Neoptolemos JP. Pancreatic cancer. Nat Rev Dis Primers. 2016;2:16022.
5. Neoptolemos JP, Palmer DH, Ghaneh P, Psarelli EE, Valle JW, Halloran CM, Faluyi O, O'Reilly DA, Cunningham D, Wadsley J, et al. Comparison of adjuvant gemcitabine and capecitabine with gemcitabine monotherapy in patients with resected pancreatic cancer (ESPAC-4): a multicentre, open-label, randomised, phase 3 trial. Lancet. 2017;389:1011–24.
6. Waddell N, Pajic M, Patch AM, Chang DK, Kassahn KS, Bailey P, Johns AL, Miller D, Nones K, Quek K, et al. Whole genomes redefine the mutational landscape of pancreatic cancer. Nature. 2015;518:495–501.
7. Wang L, Zhou W, Zhong Y, Huo Y, Fan P, Zhan S, Xiao J, Jin X, Gou S, Yin T, et al. Overexpression of G protein-coupled receptor GPR87 promotes pancreatic cancer aggressiveness and activates NF-kappaB signaling pathway. Mol Cancer. 2017;16:61.
8. Zhong Y, Naito Y, Cope L, Naranjo-Suarez S, Saunders T, Hong SM, Goggins MG, Herman JM, Wolfgang CL, Iacobuzio-Donahue CA. Functional p38 MAPK identified by biomarker profiling of pancreatic cancer restrains growth through JNK inhibition and correlates with improved survival. Clin Cancer Res. 2014;20:6200–11.
9. Khan MA, Zubair H, Srivastava SK, Singh S, Singh AP. Insights into the role of microRNAs in pancreatic cancer pathogenesis: potential for diagnosis, prognosis, and therapy. Adv Exp Med Biol. 2015;889:71–87.
10. Dillhoff M, Liu J, Frankel W, Croce C, Bloomston M. MicroRNA-21 is overexpressed in pancreatic cancer and a potential predictor of survival. J Gastrointest Surg. 2008;12:2171–6.
11. Li J, Wu H, Li W, Yin L, Guo S, Xu X, Ouyang Y, Zhao Z, Liu S, Tian Y, et al. Downregulated miR-506 expression facilitates pancreatic cancer progression and chemoresistance via SPHK1/Akt/NF-kappaB signaling. Oncogene. 2016; 35:5501–14.
12. Ji Q, Hao XB, Zhang M, Tang WH, Meng Y, Li L, Xiang DB, DeSano JT, Bommer GT, Fan DM, et al. MicroRNA miR-34 inhibits human pancreatic cancer tumor-initiating cells. PLoS One. 2009;4:e6816.
13. Edgar R, Domrachev M, Lash AE. Gene expression omnibus: NCBI gene expression and hybridization array data repository. Nucleic Acids Res. 2002; 30:207–10.
14. Cancer Genome Atlas Research N, Weinstein JN, Collisson EA, Mills GB, Shaw KR, Ozenberger BA, Ellrott K, Shmulevich I, Sander C, Stuart JM. The Cancer Genome Atlas Pan-Cancer analysis project. Nat Genet. 2013;45:1113–20.
15. Rajamani D, Bhasin MK. Identification of key regulators of pancreatic cancer progression through multidimensional systems-level analysis. Genome Medicine. 2016;8:38.
16. Chuang HY, Lee E, Liu YT, Lee D, Ideker T. Network-based classification of breast cancer metastasis. Mol Syst Biol. 2007;3:140.
17. Sivakumar S, de Santiago I, Chlon L, Markowetz F. Master regulators of oncogenic KRAS response in pancreatic cancer: an integrative network biology analysis. PLoS Medicine / Public Library of Science. 2017;14: e1002223.
18. Muzumdar MD, Chen PY, Dorans KJ, Chung KM, Bhutkar A, Hong E, Noll EM, Sprick MR, Trumpp A, Jacks T. Survival of pancreatic cancer cells lacking KRAS function. Nat Commun. 2017;8:1090.
19. Wolfgang CL, Herman JM, Laheru DA, Klein AP, Erdek MA, Fishman EK, Hruban RH. Recent progress in pancreatic cancer. CA Cancer J Clin. 2013;63: 318–48.
20. Pei H, Li L, Fridley BL, Jenkins GD, Kalari KR, Lingle W, Petersen G, Lou Z, Wang L. FKBP51 affects cancer cell response to chemotherapy by negatively regulating Akt. Cancer Cell. 2009;16:259–66.
21. Badea L, Herlea V, Dima SO, Dumitrascu T, Popescu I. Combined gene expression analysis of whole-tissue and microdissected pancreatic ductal adenocarcinoma identifies genes specifically overexpressed in tumor epithelia. Hepatogastroenterology. 2008;55:2016–27.
22. Szklarczyk D, Franceschini A, Wyder S, Forslund K, Heller D, Huerta-Cepas J, Simonovic M, Roth A, Santos A, Tsafou KP, et al. STRING v10: protein-protein interaction networks, integrated over the tree of life. Nucleic Acids Res. 2015;43:D447–52.
23. Chin CH, Chen SH, Wu HH, Ho CW, Ko MT, Lin CY. cytoHubba: identifying hub objects and sub-networks from complex interactome. BMC Syst Biol. 2014;8(Suppl 4):S11.
24. Ashburner M, Ball CA, Blake JA, Botstein D, Butler H, Cherry JM, Davis AP, Dolinski K, Dwight SS, Eppig JT, et al. Gene ontology: tool for the unification of biology. The gene ontology consortium. Nat Genet. 2000;25:25–9.
25. Dennis G Jr, Sherman BT, Hosack DA, Yang J, Gao W, Lane HC, Lempicki RA. DAVID: database for annotation, visualization, and integrated discovery. Genome Biol. 2003;4:P3.
26. Van Wart HE, Birkedal-Hansen H. The cysteine switch: a principle of regulation of metalloproteinase activity with potential applicability to the entire matrix metalloproteinase gene family. Proc Natl Acad Sci U S A. 1990; 87:5578–82.
27. Jang B, Jung H, Choi S, Lee YH, Lee S-T. Oh E-S: Syndecan-2 cytoplasmic domain up-regulates matrix metalloproteinase-7 expression via the protein kinase Cgamma-mediated FAK/ERK signaling pathway in colon cancer. J Biol Chem. 2017;292:16321–32.
28. Moffitt RA, Marayati R, Flate EL, Volmar KE, Loeza SG, Hoadley KA, Rashid NU, Williams LA, Eaton SC, Chung AH, et al. Virtual microdissection identifies distinct tumor- and stroma-specific subtypes of pancreatic ductal adenocarcinoma. Nat Genet. 2015;47:1168–78.
29. Malemud CJ. Matrix metalloproteinases (MMPs) in health and disease: an overview. Front Biosci. 2006;11:1696–701.
30. Chen SH, Hung WC, Wang P, Paul C, Konstantopoulos K. Mesothelin binding to CA125/MUC16 promotes pancreatic cancer cell motility and invasion via MMP-7 activation. Sci Rep. 2013;3:1870.
31. Lin HY, Sun SM, Lu XF, Chen PY, Chen CF, Liang WQ, Peng CY. CCR10 activation stimulates the invasion and migration of breast cancer cells through the ERK1/2/MMP-7 signaling pathway. Int Immunopharmacol. 2017; 51:124–30.
32. Xu J, E C, Yao Y, Ren S, Wang G, Jin H. Matrix metalloproteinase expression and molecular interaction network analysis in gastric cancer. Oncol Lett. 2016;12:2403–8.
33. Juchniewicz A, Kowalczuk O, Milewski R, Laudanski W, Dziegielewski P, Kozlowski M, Niklinski J. MMP-10, MMP-7, TIMP-1 and TIMP-2 mRNA expression in esophageal cancer. Acta Biochim Pol. 2017;64:295–9.
34. Banaei N, Foley A, Houghton JM, Sun YB, Kim B. Multiplex detection of pancreatic cancer biomarkers using a SERS-based immunoassay. Nanotechnology. 2017;28:455101.

35. Wang SC, Parekh JR, Porembka MR, Nathan H, D'Angelica MI, DeMatteo RP, Fong Y, Kingham TP, Jarnagin WR, Allen PJ. A pilot study evaluating serum MMP7 as a preoperative prognostic marker for pancreatic ductal adenocarcinoma patients. J Gastrointest Surg. 2016;20:899–904.

36. Fukuda A, Wang SC, JPt M, Folias AE, Liou A, Kim GE, Akira S, Boucher KM, Firpo MA, Mulvihill SJ, Hebrok M. Stat3 and MMP7 contribute to pancreatic ductal adenocarcinoma initiation and progression. Cancer Cell. 2011;19:441–55.

37. Bergelson JM, St John N, Kawaguchi S, Chan M, Stubdal H, Modlin J, Finberg RW. Infection by echoviruses 1 and 8 depends on the alpha 2 subunit of human VLA-2. J Virol. 1993;67:6847–52.

38. Graham KL, Halasz P, Tan Y, Hewish MJ, Takada Y, Mackow ER, Robinson MK, Coulson BS. Integrin-using rotaviruses bind alpha2beta1 integrin alpha2 I domain via VP4 DGE sequence and recognize alphaXbeta2 and alphaVbeta3 by using VP7 during cell entry. J Virol. 2003;77:9969–78.

39. Ban EZ, Lye MS, Chong PP, Yap YY, Lim SYC, Abdul Rahman H. Association of hOGG1 Ser326Cys, ITGA2 C807T, TNF-A -308G>a and XPD Lys751Gln polymorphisms with the survival of Malaysian NPC patients. PLoS One. 2018;13:e0198332.

40. Ferraro A, Boni T, Pintzas A. EZH2 regulates cofilin activity and colon cancer cell migration by targeting ITGA2 gene. PLoS ONE [electronic Resource]. 2014;9:e115276.

41. Yang Q, Bavi P, Wang JY, Roehrl MH. Immuno-proteomic discovery of tumor tissue autoantigens identifies olfactomedin 4, CD11b, and integrin alpha-2 as markers of colorectal cancer with liver metastases. J Proteome. 2017;168: 53–65.

42. Nones K, Waddell N, Song S, Patch AM, Miller D, Johns A, Wu J, Kassahn KS, Wood D, Bailey P, et al. Genome-wide DNA methylation patterns in pancreatic ductal adenocarcinoma reveal epigenetic deregulation of SLIT-ROBO, ITGA2 and MET signaling. Int J Cancer. 2014;135:1110–8.

43. Chuang YC, Wu HY, Lin YL, Tzou SC, Chuang CH, Jian TY, Chen PR, Chang YC, Lin CH, Huang TH, et al. Blockade of ITGA2 induces apoptosis and inhibits cell migration in gastric Cancer. Biol Proced Online. 2018;20:10.

44. Dong J, Wang R, Ren G, Li X, Wang J, Sun Y, Liang J, Nie Y, Wu K, Feng B, et al. HMGA2-FOXL2 Axis regulates metastases and epithelial-to-mesenchymal transition of chemoresistant gastric cancer. Clin Cancer Res. 2017;23:3461–73.

45. Rozengurt E, Sinnett-Smith J, Eibl G. Yes-associated protein (YAP) in pancreatic cancer: at the epicenter of a targetable signaling network associated with patient survival. Signal Transduct Target Ther. 2018;3:11.

46. Kessenbrock K, Plaks V, Werb Z. Matrix metalloproteinases: regulators of the tumor microenvironment. Cell. 2010;141:52–67.

47. Hanahan D, Coussens LM. Accessories to the crime: functions of cells recruited to the tumor microenvironment. Cancer Cell. 2012;21:309–22.

19

MiR-218 produces anti-tumor effects on cervical cancer cells in vitro

Li Zhu[1], Huaidong Tu[1], Yanmei Liang[1] and Dihong Tang[2*]

Abstract

Background: As indoleamine-2,3-dioxygenase 1 (IDO1) is critical in tumor immune escape, we determined to study the regulatory mechanism of miR-218 on IDO1 in cervical cancer.

Methods: Real-time PCR (RT-qPCR) was carried out to measure the expression of miR-218. RT-qPCR and Western blot were performed to detect the expression of IDO1 in cervical cancer. Dual-luciferase reporter assay was used to determine the binding of miR-218 on the IDO1 3'UTR. Cell viability, apoptosis, and related factors were determined using cell counting kit-8 (CCK-8), Annexin-V/PI (propidium) assay, enzyme-linked immunosorbnent assay (ELISA), RT-qPCR, and Western blot assays after miR-218 mimics has been transfected to HeLa cervical cancer cells.

Results: MiR-218 was downregulated in cervical cancer. The expression of miR-218 was negatively correlated with IDO1 in cervical cancer tissues and cells. IDO1 is a direct target of miR-218. MiR-218 overexpression was found to inhibit cell viability and promoted apoptosis via activating the expression of Cleaved-Caspase-3 and to inhibit the expression of Survivin, immune factors (TGF-β, VEGF, IL-6, PGE2, COX-2), and JAK2/STAT3 pathway.

Conclusion: MiR-218 inhibits immune escape of cervical cancer cells by direct downregulating IDO1.

Keywords: MiR-218, Immune escape, Cervical cancer, IDO1, JAK2/STAT3, Apoptosis

Background

Cervical cancer is one of the most common malignancies in the female reproductive system. Globally, the cancer has the second highest death rate among other cancer deaths among females [1, 2]. Advances in diagnostic technology allow many cervical cancer patients to be diagnosed and treated at an early stage [3, 4]. However, the mortality of cervical cancer is still high, accounting for approximately 50% [5, 6]. Studies have shown that tumor occurrence is closely related to the immune system, which has immune surveillance functions [7, 8]. The immune system can recognize and specifically eliminate "non-self" cells through immune mechanisms to resist the occurrence and development of tumors [9]. However, in some cases, via tumor immune escape process, malignant cells could result in occurrence, development, metastasis, and recurrence of tumors [10]. In addition, as the tumor grows, it can form a microenvironment that helps the tumor escape immune surveillance [11]. The tumor cells secrete immunosuppressive factors, to name a few, transforming growth factor-β(TGF-β). Interleukin-6 (IL-6), vascular endothelial growth factor (VEGF), prostaglandin 2 (PGE2), and cytochrome c oxidase subunit II (COX-2), etc., induce normal host cells to undergo immunosuppression, reduce immune function, and cause immune escape [12–15].

As a heme-containing enzyme, indoleamine-2,3-dioxygenase (IDO) is a negative immunoregulatory factor that not only decomposes tryptophan into multiple metabolites, therefore preventing an effective immune response of T cells, but also induces regulatory T cells (Tregs)-mediated immune escape [16, 17]. IDO was observed to be expressed in some primary tumors, for example, gastric cancer, colon cancer, and renal cell carcinoma [17, 18]. The expression of IDO1 in cervical cancer, breast cancer, ovarian cancer, endometrial cancer, colon cancer, and brain tumors predicts less satisfied clinical prognosis [19, 20]. In a study of non-small cell lung cancer, ovarian cancer and other tumor tissues, IDO1 was found to be associated with malignancy degrees of the tumors [21]. Studies have confirmed that IDO was overexpressed in primary myeloblasts, leading to

* Correspondence: dihongt_tangdh@163.com
[2]Department of Gynecologic Oncology, Hunan Cancer Hospital, No.283 Tongzipo Road, Yuelu District, Changsha 410006, Hunan Province, China
Full list of author information is available at the end of the article

a significant lack of tryptophan, and that IDO overexpression was also found to inhibit the proliferation of T cells, and this is because T cells in G1 phase are highly sensitive to tryptophan deficiency [19, 22]. On the other hand, the metabolites of tryptophan can cause apoptosis of T cells, leading to immune escape [23, 24]. Thus, inhibiting the proliferation of tumor cells by suppressing the function of IDO1 has drawn much research attention [25–27].

MicroRNA-218 (miR-218) is a tumor-suppressive miRNA in cancers. MiR-218 inhibits cell proliferation of glioma cells [28], osteogenic differentiation in synovial mesenchymal stem cells [29], and tumor angiogenesis in prostate cancer [30]. MiR-218 is downregulated in renal cell carcinoma (RCC) tissue, and cell proliferation is suppressed by miR-218 overexpression in RCC cells [31]. The bioinformatics analysis shows that IDO1 has binding targets of miR-218; we decided to study the mechanism of miR-218 functioning on IDO1 in the tumor immune escape of cervical cancer.

Therefore, we aimed to measure the effects of miR-218 on cervical cancer. This study will help to understand the principle of tumor development, to improve the immune status of the body, to reverse the tumor escape, and to design new treatment strategies.

Methods

Patients and tissues

Cervical cancer tissues were collected from The People's Hospital of Taojiang County during October 2014 to January 2016. Patients with primary cervical squamous cell carcinoma and complete clinical data and who received radical hysterectomy and pelvic lymphadenectomy were included. The average age of all patients was 42.1 years old (22–63 years old). All patients did not receive radiotherapy or chemotherapy prior to surgery. Tissues were divided into different stages with reference to the International Federation of Gynecology and Obstetrics (FIGO) criteria. Clinical pathological features of patients with cervical cancer were shown in Table 1. The normal control was isolated from the corresponding adjacent non-carcinoma tissues of the patients with

Table 1 Clinical pathological features of patients with cervical cancer

Factors		IDO1 levels		P values
		Higher	Lower	
Age (years)	< 50	11	5	0.893
	≥ 50	14	7	
FIGO stages	I, II	7	10	0.002**
	III, IV	18	2	
Histological grade	Well/middle differentiated	8	8	0.046**
	Low differentiated	17	4	

**P < 0.01, chi-square test

cervical cancer. The use of all tissue specimens was approved by the Ethics Committee of The People's Hospital of Taojiang County. Tissues obtained were frozen and preserved in liquid nitrogen for mRNA analyses of miR-218 and IDO1. Spearman nonparametric correlation test was used to analyze correlation between miR-218 and IDO1.

Cell culture and transfection

Human cervical epithelial cells (HcerEpic cells) and cervical cancer cells (HeLa, SiHa, C-33 and Caski cells) were purchased from Shanghai Institute of Cell Biology and cultured with Dulbecco's modified Eagle's medium (DMEM; Gibco, USA), which contained 10% fetal bovine serum (FBS; Gibco, USA), 1% penicillin, and streptomycin (Invitrogen, USA)with 5% CO_2 at 37 °C. The cells cultured to logarithm phase were used in following experiments. The expression levels of miR-218 and IDO1 were first detected in above cell lines. The MiR-218 mimics (Mimics group) and NC control sequence (NC group) were synthesized by GenePharm (Shanghai, China) and then respectively transfected to HeLa cervical cancer cells using lipofectamine 2000 (Invitrogen, USA) as a transfection reagent. Cells with non-treatment were treated as control (Cntl group). Next, the expression levels of miR-218 and IDO1 were detected in Cntl, NC, and Mimics groups.

Bioinformatics and dual-luciferase reporter assays

The potential target sequences of miR-218 in 3′-UTR fragment of IDO1 were predicted with reference to TargetScan website (http://www.targetscan.org/vert_72/). Next, a direct combination of miR-218 and IDO1 was verified by dual-luciferase reporter assay. Using the GeneTailor Site-Directed Mutagenesis System (Invitrogen, USA), the binding sequence of miR-218 on the 3′-UTR fragment of IDO1 was intentionally mutated. The IDO1-3′-UTR sequence or mutated IDO1-3′-UTR sequence (IDO1-3′-UTR mut) was then ligated to pmirGLO firefly and rinilla dual-luciferase reporter vector (Promega, USA). IDO1-3′-UTR or IDO1-3′-UTR mut recombinant luciferase reporter plasmid was co-transfected with miR-218 mimics. Finally, the luciferase activities were measured using the Dual-Glo™ Luciferase Reporter Assay System (Promega, USA) according to the manufacturer's protocols.

Cell counting kit-8 (CCK-8) assay

The effect of miR-218 mimics transfection on cell viability of HeLa cells was determined by CCK-8 assay (Beyotime, China). Cells in the Cntl, NC, and Mimics groups were respectively seeded into 96-well plates at a density of 5×10^3 cells/well, with each experiments being repeated five times. After being incubated at 37 °C for 24 h, 20 μL CCK-8 reagent was added into each well for another 1 h of incubation at 37 °C. Next, optical density

(OD) values were read at 450 nm using a microplate reader (Thermo, USA).

Annexin-V/PI (propidium) assay

The effect of miR-218 mimics transfection on apoptosis of HeLa cells was determined by Annexin-V/PI assay (Roche, USA) according to the protocols of the manufacturer. Cells in Cntl, NC, and Mimics groups were respectively seeded in 6-well plates (5×10^4 cells/well) and then put into reaction with 5 µl Annexin-V and 5 µl PI in the dark at 37 °Cfor 5 min. The apoptosis rates were analyzed using a flow cytometer (BD, USA) and Cell Quest software.

Enzyme-linked immunosorbnent assay (ELISA)

The quantities of TGF-β, VEGF, IL-6, and PGE2 in the Cntl, NC, and Mimics groups were determined by ELISA kits (R&D, Minneapolis, USA) according to the manufacturer's instructions. Samples were added into 96-well plate and incubated at 37 °C for 90 min, and bio-tinylated antibodies were then added into the plate and incubated for another 60 min. Next, avidin peroxidase complex (ABC) was added and incubated for 30 min prior to TMB (tetramethylbenzidine) coloration. Finally, OD values were read at 450 nm by a microplate reader (Thermo, USA), and the quantities were calculated by standard curve.

Real-time-qPCR (RT-qPCR)

The mRNA levels of miR-218 and IDO1 were detected in cervical cancer tissues and cervical cancer cells (HeLa, SiHa, C-33, and Caski cells). In addition, the mRNA levels of miR-218, IDO1, Survivin, TGF-β, VEGF, IL-6, and COX-2 were detected in the Cntl, NC, and Mimics groups. The primers used were listed in Table 2. U6 (for miR-218) and GAPDH (for others) were used as internal control. Total RNA was extracted using Trizol reagent (Invitrogen, USA) and reversely transcribed to cDNA using Transcript-ase (Roche, USA). The PCR amplification process was then conducted using LightCycler® Multiplex Masters (Roche, USA) with LightCycler® 480II System (Roche, USA). The procedures for miR-218 amplification were at 95 °C, 10 s, 40 cycles (at 95 °C, 10 s; at 60 °C, 30 s). The procedures for other target genes was at 95 °C, 5 min, 40 cycles (at 95 °C, 30 s, at 60 °C, 30 s, at 72 °C, 30 s) and at 72 °C, 10 min. The results were calculated using $2^{-\Delta\Delta Cq}$ method.

Western blot

The protein levels of IDO1 were detected in cervical cancer tissues and cervical cancer cells (HeLa, SiHa, C-33, and Caski cells). In addition, the protein levels of IDO1, Survivin, Cleaved-caspase-3, Pro-caspase-3, TGF-β, VEGF, IL-6, COX-2, Janus kinase 2 (JAK2), phosphorylated-JAK2 (p-JAK2), signal transducers and activators of transcription 3 (STAT3), and phosphorylated-STAT3 (p-STAT3)

Table 2 The primer sequences applied in the study

Name	Type	Sequence (5'-3')
GAPDH	Forward	CCATCTTCCAGGAGCGAGAT
	Reverse	TGCTGATGATCTTGAGGCTG
IDO1	Forward	GGGCTTTGCTCTACCACATCCACT
	Reverse	ACATCGTCATCCCCTCGGTTCC
Survivin	Forward	GGACCACCGCATCTCTACAT
	Reverse	TTGGTTTCCTTTGCATGGGG
TGF-β	Forward	TACAGCAACAATTCCTGGCG
	Reverse	GTGAACCCGTTGATGTCCAC
VEGF	Forward	CGGTATAAGTCCTGGAGCGT
	Reverse	TTTAACTCAAGCTGCCTCGC
IL-6	Forward	AGACAGCCACTCACCTCTTC
	Reverse	TTTCACCAGGCAAGTCTCCT
COX-2	Forward	ACCGTCTGAACTATCCTGCC
	Reverse	AGATTAGTCCGCCGTAGTCG
miR-218	Forward	TTGCGGATGGTTCCGTCA AGCA
	Reverse	ATCCAGTGCAGGGTCCGAGG
U6	Forward	AGAGAAGATTAGCATGGCCCCTG
	Reverse	ATCCAGTGCAGGGTC CGAGG

were detected in the Cntl, NC, and Mimics groups. The proteins were first extracted by RIPA and quantified by BCA (Pierce, USA). Twelve percent of sodium dodecyl sulfate-polyacrylamide gel electrophoresis (SDS-PAGE) was used to isolate the proteins, which were then transferred to polyvinylidene fluoride (PVDF) membranes (ThermoFisher, USA). Next, the membranes were blocked in 5% non-fat dry milk for 1 h at 37 °C and incubated first with specific primary antibodies (Abcam, USA) overnight at 4 °C and then with secondary antibodies conjugated with horseradish peroxidase (CST, 7074, 1:5000, USA) at 37 °C for 1 h. GAPDH was used as loading control. The proteins were detected by enhanced chemiluminescense (ECL; Pierce, USA) and analyzed by Bio-Rad ChemiDoc XRS densitometry with Image Lab™ Software version 4.1 (Bio-Rad, USA).

Statistical analysis

SPSS 18.0 statistical package with mean ± standard deviations (mean ± SD) was used to conduct statistical analysis. One-way analysis of variance (ANOVA) followed with Dunnett's test was used to compare the differences. $P < 0.05$ was considered as significantly different.

Results

MiR-218 was downregulated and negatively correlated with IDO1 in cervical cancer tissues and cells

RT-qPCR was used to detect the expression levels of miR-218 and IDO1 in 37 cervical cancer tissues. The results demonstrated that miR-218 levels were largely downregulated in cervical cancer tissues and that the survival rate of patients in the miR-218 low-expression group was lower than that in the miR-218 high-expression group within 2 years (Fig. 1a, b). Meanwhile, IDO1 levels were mostly upregulated in cervical cancer specimens, and the survival rate of patients in the IDO1 high-expression group was lower than that in the IDO1 low-expression group within 2 years (Fig. 1c, d). According to Spearman nonparametric correlation test ($P = 0.0268$, Fig. 1e), miR-218, and IDO1 were found to negatively correlate in cervical cancer tissues. The clinical pathological features were determined, and our results indicated that high IDO1 levels were correlated to advanced FIGO stages and low differentiated histological features of cervical cancer; however, it was not correlated with ages (Table 1).

Subsequently, we detected the mRNA expression levels of IDO1 and miR-218 in several cervical cancer cells such as HeLa, SiHa, C-33, and Caski cells. RT-qPCR results showed that the mRNA levels of IDO1 significantly increased, while miR-218 remarkably decreased in HeLa, SiHa, C-33, and Caski cervical cells, compared with cervical epithelial HcerEpic cells ($P < 0.05$, Fig. 1f, g). The protein levels of IDO1 were detected by Western blot, and the results showed similar pattern to that of the mRNA assay ($P < 0.05$, Fig. 1h, i).Expression changes of IDO1 and miR-218 were the greatest in HeLa cells among others. Therefore, HeLa cell line was used for miR-218 mimics transfection.

MiR-218 directly targets the 3'-UTR fragment of IDO1

Using bioinformatics analysis of TargetScan, we found potential target sequences of miR-218 in the 3'-UTR fragment of IDO1 (Fig. 1j). Three bases in the target sequence were then mutated to obtain mutated 3'-UTR sequence of IDO1. Luciferase activity assay was used to observe the effect of miR-218 on the firefly luciferase activity of pmirGLO-UTR. The results showed that the co-transfection of miR-218 and IDO1-3'-UTR resulted in a significant downregulation of the luciferase activity of the reporter vector, and a statistically significant difference was identified compared to Cntl+IDO1-3'-UTR group ($P < 0.01$, Fig. 1k). However, no significant change in luciferase activity was found in the miR-218 +IDO1-3'-UTR mut co-transfection group. The interaction between miR-218 and IDO1-3'-UTR affected the expression level of the reporter gene, suggesting that miR-218 might act on the 3'-UTR region of the IDO1 gene, regulating the expression of IDO1.

MiR-218 overexpression inhibited cell viability and promoted cell apoptosis of cervical cancer cells

By performing RT-qPCR and Western blot assays ($P < 0.05$, Fig. 2a–d), we found that after miR-218 mimics has been transfected into cervical cancer HeLa cells, the

mRNA levels of miR-218 were found to be sharply upregulated and that the mRNA and protein levels of IDO1 were markedly downregulated in the Mimics group, compared with the Cntl and NC groups. CCK-8 and Annexin-V/PI assays results showed that cell viability was significantly inhibited and that apoptosis was dramatically promoted in Mimics group, compared with the Cntl and NC groups ($P < 0.05$, Fig. 2e, f).

MiR-218 overexpression inhibited cell viability and promoted cell apoptosis of cervical cancer cells by regulating apoptosis-related factors

As apoptosis is a mechanism that is characterized by some factors, we detected the expression levels of Survivin and Caspase-3. RT-qPCR showed that the mRNA expression levels of Survivin were downregulated, while the protein levels of Cleaved-Caspase-3 were upregulated and Pro-Caspase-3 was downregulated in the Mimics group, compared with the Cntl and NC groups ($P < 0.05$, Fig. 3).

MiR-218 overexpression inhibited cell viability and promoted cell apoptosis of cervical cancer cells by regulating immune escape-related factors

Tumor immune escape can be characterized by levels of immune escape-related factors. In our study, RT-qPCR and Western blot were used to analyze the mRNA and protein levels of immune escape-related factors, for example, TGF-β, VEGF, IL-6, and COX-2, and they significantly decreased in the Mimics group ($P < 0.05$, Fig. 4a–f). ELISA was used to detect relative contents of TGF-β, VEGF, IL-6, and PGE2 to further verify the phenomenon, and the results showed significantly decreased levels of them ($P < 0.05$, Fig. 4g).

MiR-218 overexpression inhibited cell viability and promoted cell apoptosis of cervical cancer cells via JAK2/ STAT3 pathway

Western blot was performed to detect the activation status of JAK2 and STAT3. Our results observed less p-JAK2 and p-STAT3 in the Mimics group, compared with the Cntl and NC groups ($P < 0.01$, Fig. 5).

Discussion

In tumor immune escape, IDO1 is a critically negative immunoregulatory factor, which induces the development, metastasis, and recurrence of tumors [32]. In this study, we adopted bioinformatics method and dual-luciferase reporter assay to confirm the direct targeting of miR-218 on the 3'-UTR of IDO1. Thus, miR-218 might have critical regulatory functions on the molecular mechanism of IDO1 in cervical cancer. Thirty-seven cervical cancer tissues were collected and detected, and we found that miR-218 was upregulated, while IDO1 was downregulated

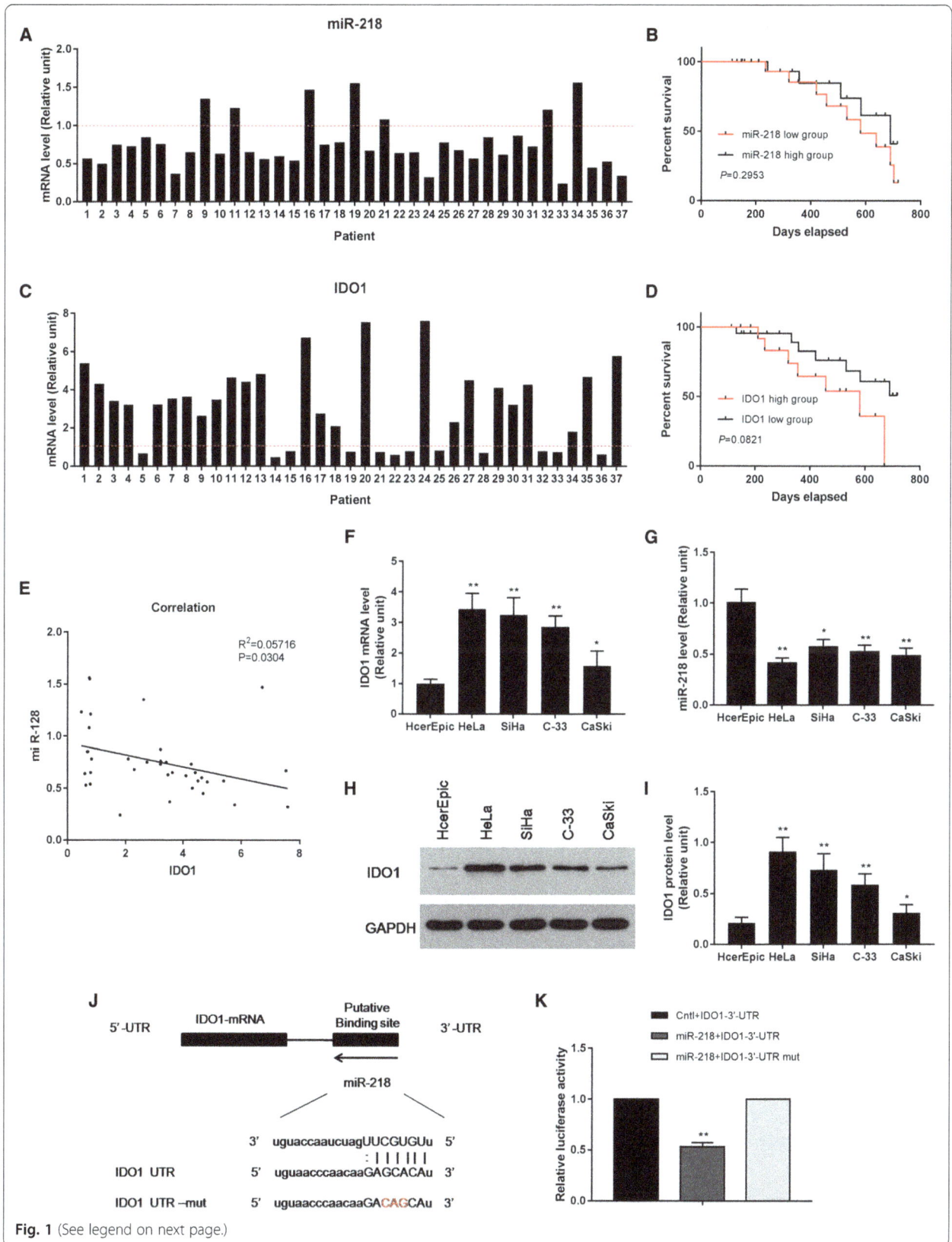

Fig. 1 (See legend on next page.)

(See figure on previous page.)
Fig. 1 MiR-218 was upregulated and negatively correlated with IDO1 by direct targeting on IDO1 in cervical cancer tissues and cells. **a** The mRNA levels of miR-218 were downregulated in cervical cancer specimens. **b** The survival rate of miR-218 low group was lower than that in miR-218 high group. **c** The mRNA levels of IDO1 were upregulated in cervical cancer specimens. **d** The survival rate of IDO1 high group was lower than that in miR-218 high group. **e** MiR-218 and IDO1 were well negatively correlated in cervical cancer tissues. **f, g** The mRNA levels of IDO1 (**f**) increased, while miR-218 decreased (**g**) in HeLa, SiHa, C-33, and Caski cervical cells. **h, i** The protein levels of IDO1 increased in HeLa, SiHa, C-33, and Caski cervical cells. **j** The target sequences of miR-218 in the 3′-UTR fragment of IDO1 were identified by TargetScan bioinformatics analysis. **k** The co-transfection of miR-218 and IDO1-3′-UTR resulted in a significant downregulation of the luciferase activity. *$P < 0.05$ and **$P < 0.01$ vs. cervical epithelial HcerEpic cells in **f–i**. **$P < 0.01$ vs. Cntl+IDO1-3′-UTR group in **k**

and that the two were negatively correlated with each other. In addition, high-level IDO1 and low-level miR-218 were correlated to advanced FIGO stages and low differentiated histological features of cervical cancers, as well as low survival rates in 2 years. Therefore, we studied the expression of miR-218 and IDO1 in some commonly used cervical cancer cells (HeLa, SiHa, C-33, and Caski cells), and the results showed the miR-218 was inhibited and the IDO1 levels were promoted. By transfecting miR-218 mimics into HeLa cervical cancer cells, we observed that

the overexpression of miR-218 significantly suppressed the expression of IDO1, inhibited cell viability, and promoted apoptosis of cervical cancer cells.

Subsequently, variations of critical effectors in apoptosis caused by miR-218 overexpression were measured. Caspase-3, the direct execution factor to initiate apoptosis, is a cysteine protease protein specifically cleaving peptide bonds after aspartic acid residues. Caspase-3 usually acts as pro-caspase-3 in normal conditions; however, it will be phosphorylated and activated when

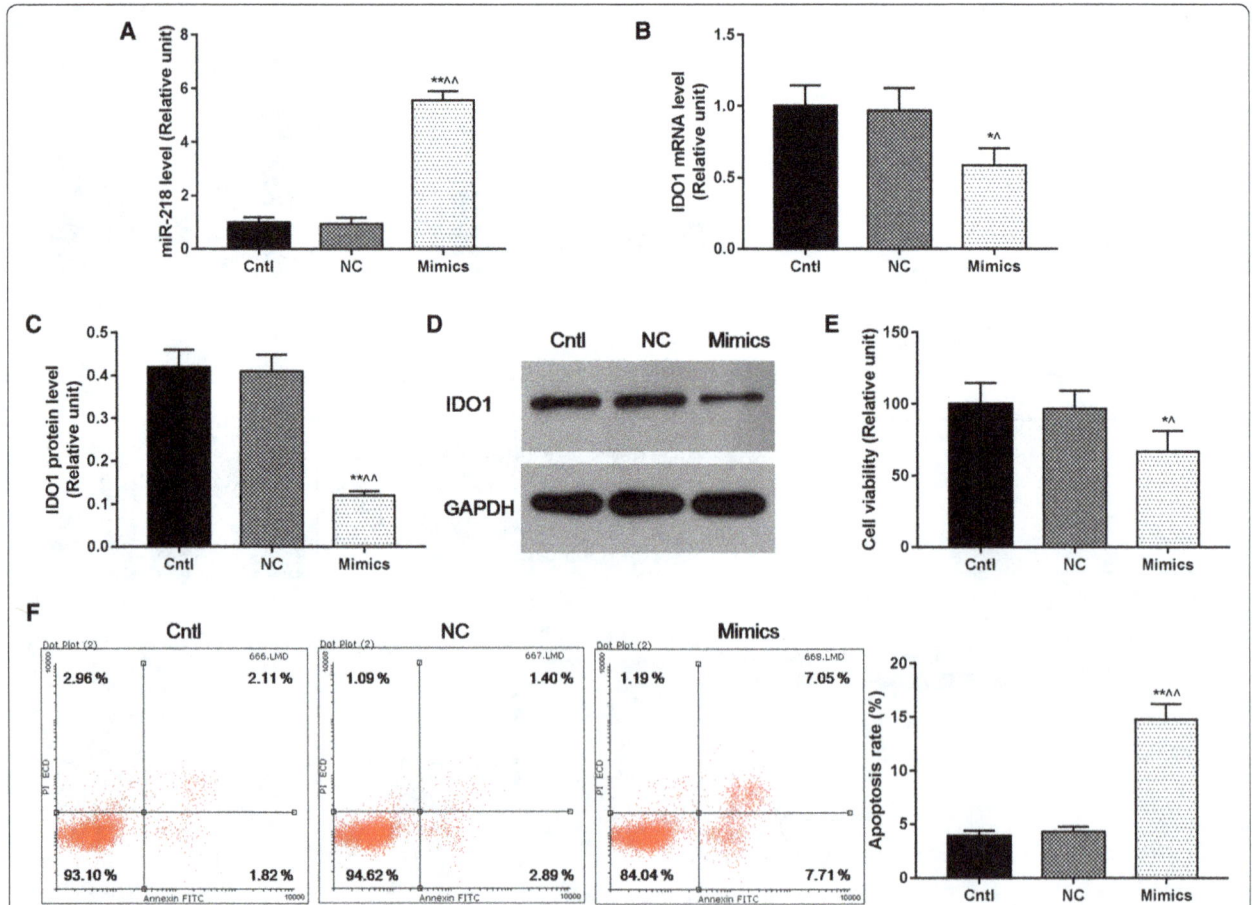

Fig. 2 MiR-218 overexpression inhibited cell viability and promoted cell apoptosis of cervical cancer cells. **a** The mRNA levels of miR-218 were upregulated, in the Mimics group. **b–d** The mRNA (**b**) and protein (**c, d**) levels of IDO1 were downregulated in the Mimics group. **e, f** Cell viability (**e**) was inhibited, and apoptosis (**f**) was promoted in the Mimics group. *$P < 0.05$ and **$P < 0.01$ vs. the Cntl group, ^$P < 0.05$ and ^^$P < 0.01$ vs. the NC group

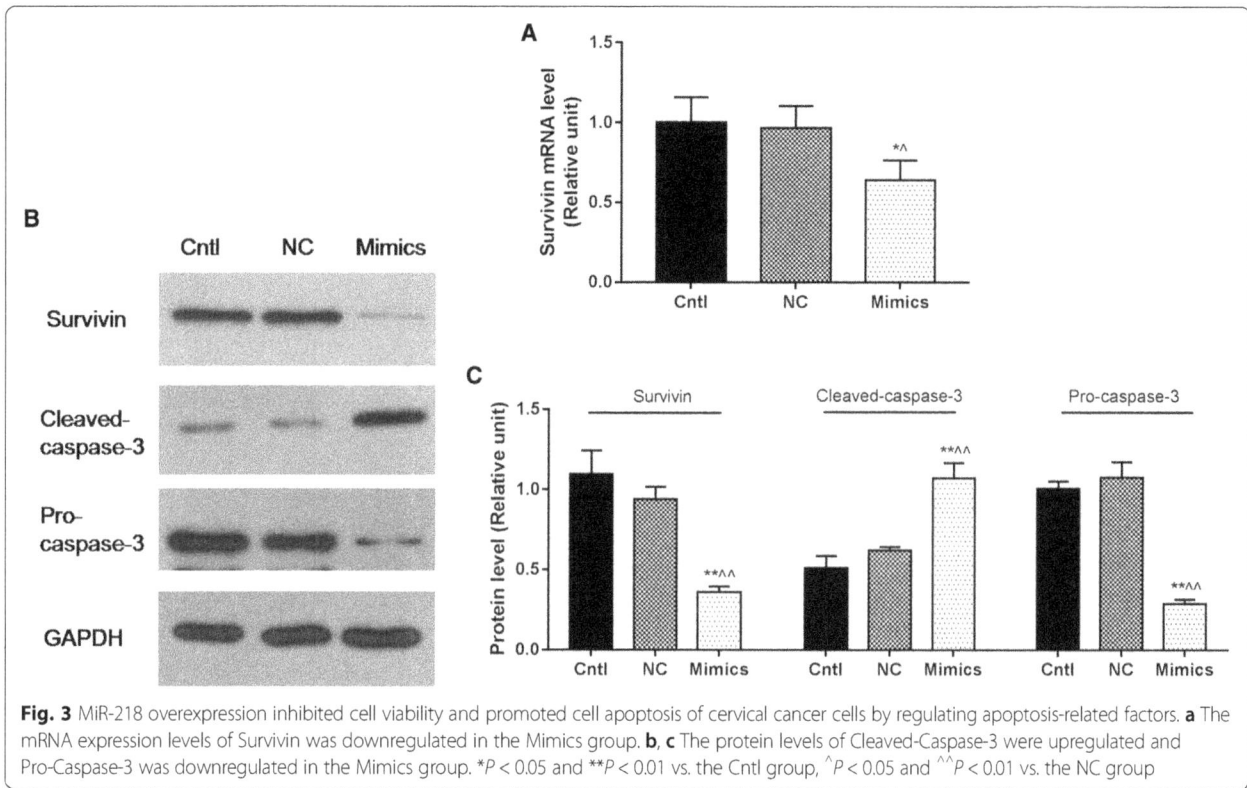

Fig. 3 MiR-218 overexpression inhibited cell viability and promoted cell apoptosis of cervical cancer cells by regulating apoptosis-related factors. **a** The mRNA expression levels of Survivin was downregulated in the Mimics group. **b**, **c** The protein levels of Cleaved-Caspase-3 were upregulated and Pro-Caspase-3 was downregulated in the Mimics group. *$P < 0.05$ and **$P < 0.01$ vs. the Cntl group, ^$P < 0.05$ and ^^$P < 0.01$ vs. the NC group

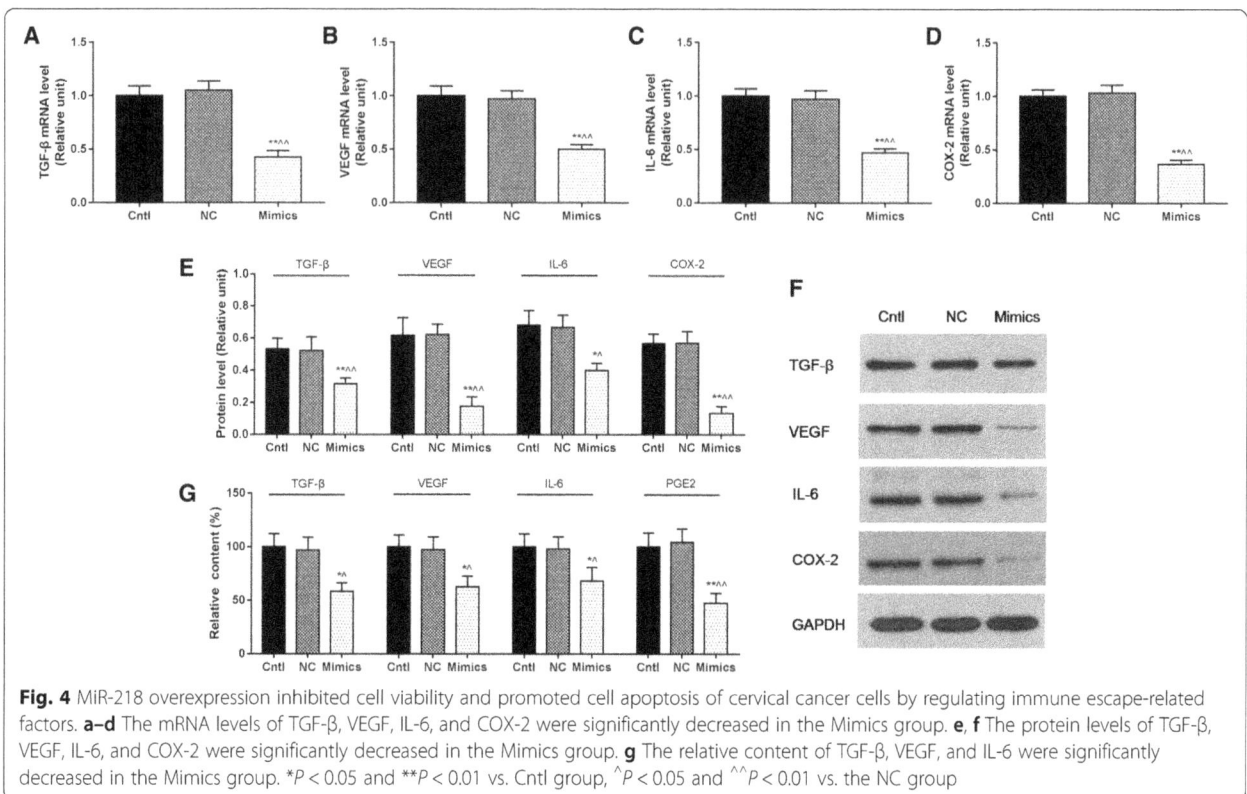

Fig. 4 MiR-218 overexpression inhibited cell viability and promoted cell apoptosis of cervical cancer cells by regulating immune escape-related factors. **a–d** The mRNA levels of TGF-β, VEGF, IL-6, and COX-2 were significantly decreased in the Mimics group. **e**, **f** The protein levels of TGF-β, VEGF, IL-6, and COX-2 were significantly decreased in the Mimics group. **g** The relative content of TGF-β, VEGF, and IL-6 were significantly decreased in the Mimics group. *$P < 0.05$ and **$P < 0.01$ vs. Cntl group, ^$P < 0.05$ and ^^$P < 0.01$ vs. the NC group

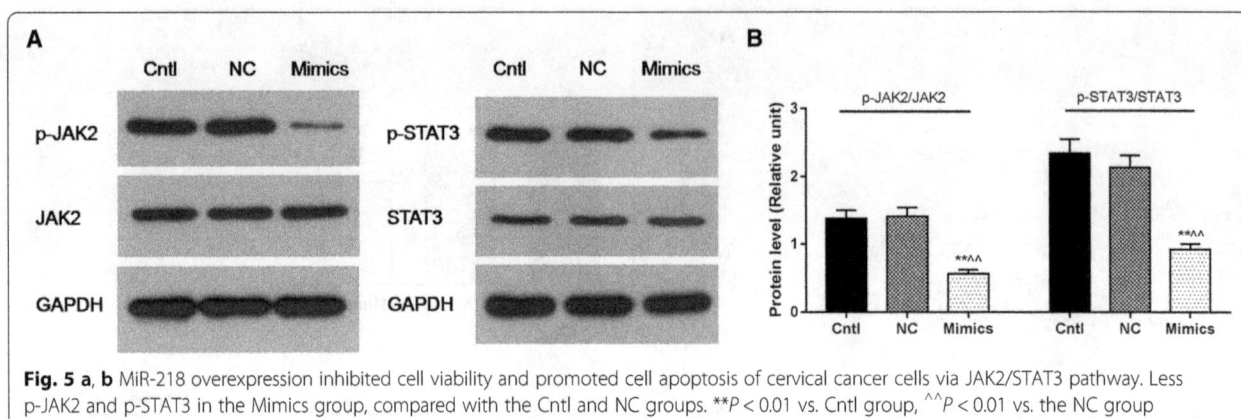

Fig. 5 a, b MiR-218 overexpression inhibited cell viability and promoted cell apoptosis of cervical cancer cells via JAK2/STAT3 pathway. Less p-JAK2 and p-STAT3 in the Mimics group, compared with the Cntl and NC groups. **$P < 0.01$ vs. Cntl group, $^{\wedge\wedge}P < 0.01$ vs. the NC group

apoptosis occurs. Survivin is a new member of the apoptotic inhibitor protein family, and it is also a tumor-specific apoptosis inhibitor that is expressed only in tumors and embryonic tissues. Survivin directly acts on Caspase by mainly inhibiting the activity of Caspase-3. In our study, miR-218 overexpression was observed to inhibit the expression of Survivin and promoted the activity of Caspase-3.

Researchers found that the body's immune suppression was associated with a variety of cytokines [33]. TGF-β inhibits the immune system so as to protect tumor cells from being killed by immune cells [34]. The increase of VEGF levels in tumors reduces the immune function and promotes the formation of tumor interstitial blood vessels, allowing the tumors to grow rapidly [35, 36]. IL-6 stimulates the proliferation, differentiation, and function of cells involved in the immune response [37]. PGE2 is an important cell growth and regulation factor that can dilate blood vessels and can produce both immunosuppressive and anti-inflammatory effects. Under normal physiological conditions [38, 39], COX-2 is not expressed. However, in pathological conditions such as inflammation and tumors, COX-2 expression will be increased after being induced by pro-inflammatory mediators, for example, inflammatory stimulators, injuries, and carcinogens, participating in various pathological and physiological processes [40–42]. During our research, miR-218 overexpression inhibited the expression and function of these inflammatory factors TGF-β, VEGF, IL-6, PGE2, and COX-2 in cervical cancer cells.

JAK2/STAT3 signaling pathway and immune escape signaling pathway are important pathways of inflammatory response [43]. Many cytokines transfer from the outside to the nucleus via JAK2/STAT3 pathway and mediate the response of cells under the corresponding conditions [44]. STAT3 can mediate the onset of inflammatory reactions via IL-6/JAK pathway [45]. In addition, STATs can also modulate inflammatory/immune responses by regulating COX-2 and IDO, becoming intermediate bridges linking

tumors and inflammatory responses [46]. In our study, the activation of JAK2 and STAT3 were significantly inhibited by miR-218 overexpression.

Conclusions

The expression of miR-218 was negatively correlated with IDO1 in cervical cancer. IDO1 is a direct target of miR-218. Overexpression of miR-218 exerted anti-tumor effects on cervical cancer through promoting apoptosis and inhibiting the expression of inflammatory factors. The inhibition of JAK2/STAT3 signaling pathway contributed to the anti-tumor effect produced by miR-218. This study will provide effective solutions for biological treatment of cervical cancer and other tumors.

Authors' contributions
LZ and HT provided substantial contributions to the conception and design. YL and DT contributed to the data acquisition, data analysis, and its interpretation. YL is responsible for drafting the article or critically revising it for important intellectual content. All authors gave their final approval of the version to be published. DT agreed to be accountable for all aspects of the work in ensuring that questions related to the accuracy or integrity of the work are appropriately investigated and resolved.

Competing interests
The authors declare that they have no competing interests.

Author details
[1]Department of Gynecologic Oncology, The People's Hospital of Taojiang County, Taojiang, China. [2]Department of Gynecologic Oncology, Hunan Cancer Hospital, No.283 Tongzipo Road, Yuelu District, Changsha 410006, Hunan Province, China.

References
1. Flanagan MB. Primary high-risk human papillomavirus testing for cervical cancer screening in the United States: is it time? Arch Pathol Lab Med. 2018;142:688–92.
2. Feng C, Dong J, Chang W, Cui M, Xu T. The progress of methylation regulation in gene expression of cervical cancer. Int J Genomics. 2018;2018:8260652.
3. Tzafetas M, Mitra A, Kalliala I, Lever S, Fotopoulou C, Farthing A, Smith JR, Martin-Hirsch P, Paraskevaidis E, Kyrgiou M. Fertility-sparing surgery for presumed early-stage invasive cervical cancer: a survey of practice in the United Kingdom. Anticancer Res. 2018;38:3641–6.

4. He X, Li JP, Liu XH, Zhang JP, Zeng QY, Chen H, Chen SL. Prognostic value of C-reactive protein/albumin ratio in predicting overall survival of Chinese cervical cancer patients overall survival: comparison among various inflammation based factors. J Cancer. 2018;9:1877–84.

5. Lee KB, Shim SH, Lee JM. Comparison between adjuvant chemotherapy and adjuvant radiotherapy/chemoradiotherapy after radical surgery in patients with cervical cancer: a meta-analysis. J Gynecol Oncol. 2018;29:e62.

6. Vazquez-Sanchez AY, Hinojosa LM, Parraguirre-Martinez S, Gonzalez A, Morales F, Montalvo G, Vera E, Hernandez-Gallegos E, Camacho J. Expression of KATP channels in human cervical cancer: potential tools for diagnosis and therapy. Oncol Lett. 2018;15:6302–8.

7. Zhu M, Feng M, He F, Han B, Ma K, Zeng X, Liu Z, Liu X, Li J, Cao H, et al. Pretreatment neutrophil-lymphocyte and platelet-lymphocyte ratio predict clinical outcome and prognosis for cervical cancer. Clin Chim Acta. 2018; 483:296–302.

8. Fahey LM, Raff AB, Da Silva DM, Kast WM. A major role for the minor capsid protein of human papillomavirus type 16 in immune escape. J Immunol. 2009;183:6151–6.

9. Song H, Park H, Park G, Kim YS, Lee HK, Jin DH, Kang HS, Cho DH, Hur D. Corticotropin-releasing factor induces immune escape of cervical cancer cells by downregulation of NKG2D. Oncol Rep. 2014;32:425–30.

10. Zhang H, Zhang S. The expression of Foxp3 and TLR4 in cervical cancer: association with immune escape and clinical pathology. Arch Gynecol Obstet. 2017;295:705–12.

11. Wang N, Wang Z, Xu Z, Chen X, Zhu G. A cisplatin-loaded immunochemotherapeutic nanohybrid bearing immune checkpoint inhibitors for enhanced cervical cancer therapy. Angew Chem Int Ed Engl. 2018;57:3426–30.

12. Niebler M, Qian X, Hofler D, Kogosov V, Kaewprag J, Kaufmann AM, Ly R, Bohmer G, Zawatzky R, Rosl F, Rincon-Orozco B. Post-translational control of IL-1beta via the human papillomavirus type 16 E6 oncoprotein: a novel mechanism of innate immune escape mediated by the E3-ubiquitin ligase E6-AP and p53. PLoS Pathog. 2013;9:e1003536.

13. Conesa-Zamora P. Immune responses against virus and tumor in cervical carcinogenesis: treatment strategies for avoiding the HPV-induced immune escape. Gynecol Oncol. 2013;131:480–8.

14. Fausch SC, Da Silva DM, Rudolf MP, Kast WM. Human papillomavirus virus-like particles do not activate Langerhans cells: a possible immune escape mechanism used by human papillomaviruses. J Immunol. 2002;169:3242–9.

15. Medema JP, de Jong J, Peltenburg LT, Verdegaal EM, Gorter A, Bres SA, Franken KL, Hahne M, Albar JP, Melief CJ, Offringa R. Blockade of the granzyme B/perforin pathway through overexpression of the serine protease inhibitor PI-9/SPI-6 constitutes a mechanism for immune escape by tumors. Proc Natl Acad Sci U S A. 2001;98:11515–20.

16. Williams DK, Markwalder JA, Balog AJ, Chen B, Chen L, Donnell J, Haque L, Hart AC, Mandal SK, Nation A, et al. Development of a series of novel o-phenylenediamine-based indoleamine 2,3-dioxygenase 1 (IDO1) inhibitors. Bioorg Med Chem Lett. 2018;28:732–6.

17. Cheong JE, Sun L. Targeting the IDO1/TDO2-KYN-AhR pathway for cancer immunotherapy - challenges and opportunities. Trends Pharmacol Sci. 2018;39:307–25.

18. Zou Y, Wang Y, Wang F, Luo M, Li Y, Liu W, Huang Z, Zhang Y, Guo W, Xu Q, Lai Y. Discovery of potent IDO1 inhibitors derived from tryptophan using scaffold-hopping and structure-based design approaches. Eur J Med Chem. 2017;138:199–211.

19. Davar D, Bahary N. Modulating tumor immunology by inhibiting indoleamine 2,3-dioxygenase (IDO): recent developments and first clinical experiences. Target Oncol. 2018;13:125–40.

20. Folgiero V, Cifaldi L, Li Pira G, Goffredo BM, Vinti L, Locatelli F. TIM-3/Gal-9 interaction induces IFNgamma-dependent IDO1 expression in acute myeloid leukemia blast cells. J Hematol Oncol. 2015;8:36.

21. Pan K, Wang H, Chen MS, Zhang HK, Weng DS, Zhou J, Huang W, Li JJ, Song HF, Xia JC. Expression and prognosis role of indoleamine 2,3-dioxygenase in hepatocellular carcinoma. J Cancer Res Clin Oncol. 2008;134:1247–53.

22. ?>Folgiero V, Miele E, Carai A, Ferretti E, Alfano V, Po A, Bertaina V, Goffredo BM, Benedetti MC, Camassei FD, et al. IDO1 involvement in mTOR pathway: a molecular mechanism of resistance to mTOR targeting in medulloblastoma. Oncotarget. 2016;7:52900–11.

23. Moretti S, Menicali E, Voce P, Morelli S, Cantarelli S, Sponziello M, Colella R, Fallarino F, Orabona C, Alunno A, et al. Indoleamine 2,3-dioxygenase 1 (IDO1) is up-regulated in thyroid carcinoma and drives the development of an immunosuppressant tumor microenvironment. J Clin Endocrinol Metab. 2014;99:E832–40.

24. Boscke R, Vladar EK, Konnecke M, Husing B, Linke R, Pries R, Reiling N, Axelrod JD, Nayak JV, Wollenberg B. Wnt signaling in chronic rhinosinusitis with nasal polyps. Am J Respir Cell Mol Biol. 2017;56(5):575–84.

25. Hascitha J, Priya R, Jayavelu S, Dhandapani H, Selvaluxmy G, Sunder Singh S, Rajkumar T. Analysis of kynurenine/tryptophan ratio and expression of IDO1 and 2 mRNA in tumour tissue of cervical cancer patients. Clin Biochem. 2016;49:919–24.

26. Mittal D, Kassianos AJ, Tran LS, Bergot AS, Gosmann C, Hofmann J, Blumenthal A, Leggatt GR, Frazer IH. Indoleamine 2,3-dioxygenase activity contributes to local immune suppression in the skin expressing human papillomavirus oncoprotein e7. J Invest Dermatol. 2013;133:2686–94.

27. Punt S, Houwing-Duistermaat JJ, Schulkens IA, Thijssen VL, Osse EM, de Kroon CD, Griffioen AW, Fleuren GJ, Gorter A, Jordanova ES. Correlations between immune response and vascularization qRT-PCR gene expression clusters in squamous cervical cancer. Mol Cancer. 2015;14:71.

28. Gao Y, Sun L, Wu Z, Xuan C, Zhang J, You Y, Chen X. miR218 inhibits the proliferation of human glioma cells through downregulation of Yin Yang 1. Mol Med Rep. 2018;17:1926–32.

29. Cong R, Tao K, Fu P, Lou L, Zhu Y, Chen S, Cai X, Mao L. MicroRNA218 promotes prostaglandin E2 to inhibit osteogenic differentiation in synovial mesenchymal stem cells by targeting 15hydroxyprostaglandin dehydrogenase [NAD(+)]. Mol Med Rep. 2017;16:9347–54.

30. Guan B, Wu K, Zeng J, Xu S, Mu L, Gao Y, Wang K, Ma Z, Tian J, Shi Q, et al. Tumor-suppressive microRNA-218 inhibits tumor angiogenesis via targeting the mTOR component RICTOR in prostate cancer. Oncotarget. 2017;8:8162–72.

31. Wang J, Ying Y, Bo S, Li G, Yuan F. Differentially expressed microRNA-218 modulates the viability of renal cell carcinoma by regulating BCL9. Mol Med Rep. 2016;14:1829–34.

32. Li F, Zhang R, Li S, Liu J. IDO1: an important immunotherapy target in cancer treatment. Int Immunopharmacol. 2017;47:70–7.

33. Li S, Gong X, Chen Q, Zheng F, Ji G, Liu Y. Threshold level of Riemerella anatipestifer crossing blood-brain barrier and expression profiles of immune-related proteins in blood and brain tissue from infected ducks. Vet Immunol Immunopathol. 2018;200:26–31.

34. Heldin, C.H. Development and possible clinical use of antagonists for PDGF and TGF-beta.Ups J Med Sci. 2004;109(3):165.

35. Yang J, Yan J, Liu B. Targeting VEGF/VEGFR to modulate antitumor immunity. Front Immunol. 2018;9:978.

36. Shibao S, Ueda R, Saito K, Kikuchi R, Nagashima H, Kojima A, Kagami H, Pareira ES, Sasaki H, Noji S, et al. A pilot study of peptide vaccines for VEGF receptor 1 and 2 in patients with recurrent/progressive high grade glioma. Oncotarget. 2018;9:21569–79.

37. Tanaka T, Narazaki M, Kishimoto T. IL-6 in inflammation, immunity, and disease. Cold Spring Harb Perspect Biol. 2014;6:a016295.

38. Yang HM, Song WJ, Li Q, Kim SY, Kim HJ, Ryu MO, Ahn JO, Youn HY. Canine mesenchymal stem cells treated with TNF-alpha and IFN-gamma enhance anti-inflammatory effects through the COX-2/PGE2 pathway. Res Vet Sci. 2018;119:19–26.

39. Trabanelli S, Lecciso M, Salvestrini V, Cavo M, Ocadlikova D, Lemoli RM, Curti A. PGE2-induced IDO1 inhibits the capacity of fully mature DCs to elicit an in vitro antileukemic immune response. J Immunol Res. 2015;2015:253191.

40. Carvalho MI, Bianchini R, Fazekas-Singer J, Herrmann I, Flickinger I, Thalhammer JG, Pires I, Jensen-Jarolim E, Queiroga FL. Bidirectional regulation of COX-2 expression between cancer cells and macrophages. Anticancer Res. 2018;38:2811–7.

41. Kim HG, Kim YR, Park JH, Khanal T, Choi JH, Do MT, Jin SW, Han EH, Chung YH, Jeong HG. Endosulfan induces COX-2 expression via NADPH oxidase and the ROS, MAPK, and Akt pathways. Arch Toxicol. 2015;89:2039–50.

42. Cesario A, Rocca B, Rutella S. The interplay between indoleamine 2,3-dioxygenase 1 (IDO1) and cyclooxygenase (COX)-2 in chronic inflammation and cancer. Curr Med Chem. 2011;18:2263–71.

43. Wu Y, et al. Study on the mechanism of JAK2/STAT3 signaling pathway-mediated inflammatory reaction after cerebral ischemia. Molecular Medicine Reports, 2018; 17(4).

44. Wang T, Chen D, Wang P, Xu Z, Li Y. miR-375 prevents nasal mucosa cells from apoptosis and ameliorates allergic rhinitis via inhibiting JAK2/STAT3 pathway. Biomed Pharmacother. 2018;103:621–7.

45. Wang Y, Wong CW, Yan M, Li L, Liu T, Mei-Yu Or P, Kwok-Wing Tsui S, Miu-Yee Waye M, Man-Lok Chan A. Differential regulation of the pro-inflammatory biomarker, YKL-40/CHI3L1, by PTEN/phosphoinositide 3-kinase and JAK2/STAT3 pathways in glioblastoma. Cancer Lett. 2018;429:54–65.

20

The risk factors for benign small bowel obstruction following curative resection in patients with rectal cancer

Liang Tang, Peng Zhao and Dalu Kong[*] (ID)

Abstract

Background: So far there have been limited studies about the risk factors for benign small bowel obstruction (SBO) after colorectal cancer surgery. This study aimed to determine the factors affecting the development of benign SBO following curative resection in patients with rectal cancer.

Methods: Patients (3472) receiving curative resection of rectal cancer at the Department of Colorectal Cancer, Tianjin Medical University Cancer Institute and Hospital, between January 2003 and December 2012 were retrospectively studied. The incidence of benign SBO and its risk factors were then determined.

Results: The incidence of benign SBO was 7.3% (253/3472) in follow-up studies with an average time of 68 months. Further, 27% (68/253) of the patients received operative treatment because of the signs of strangulation or the lack of clinical improvement with conservative management. Open surgery and radiotherapy were defined as the risk factors for benign SBO after curative resection in patients with rectal cancer ($P < 0.001$).

Conclusion: Open surgery plus radiotherapy led to an increased risk of benign SBO in rectal cancer patients receiving curative resection.

Keywords: Risk factor, Small bowel obstruction (SBO), Rectal cancer, Open surgery, Radiotherapy, Resection

Background

Previously, abdominal surgery is the leading cause of adhesive small bowel obstruction (SBO) [1, 2]. Patients receiving colorectal surgeries are at higher risk of postoperative SBO, which might be resulting from the dissection in the peritoneal cavity [3–5]. It has been shown that the incidence of SBO requiring hospitalization following colorectal resection was 3.6% 3 years after surgery [6] and that SBO was found in ~9% patients with colorectal procedures [7]. However, the said findings were obtained based on information from various colorectal surgeries, such as anorectal procedures, or different diseases like carcinomatosis. Therefore, these findings cannot demonstrate the accurate incidence of benign SBO following curative resection in rectal cancer patients.

To date, there have been limited studies about the risk factors of benign SBO following colorectal cancer surgery [6, 8–12]. In the present study, we determined the incidence of benign SBO and its risk factors following curative resection for rectal cancer, providing guidance for operative treatment of rectal cancer patients.

Methods

Patients and the diagnosis of benign SBO

This retrospective research was approved by the Ethics Committee of Tianjin Medical University Cancer Institute and Hospital. Written informed consent for publication of the patient's information was obtained from all patients.

In total, 3472 consecutive patients undergoing rectal cancer surgery at the Department of Colorectal Cancer, Tianjin Medical University Cancer Institute and Hospital, between January 2003 and December 2012 were enrolled. The clinicopathological data were extracted from patient files. The patients' information was collected, such as age, gender, type of primary surgery, surgery duration, and

* Correspondence: kongdalutjmuch@163.com
Department of Colorectal Cancer, Tianjin Medical University Cancer Institute and Hospital, Key Laboratory of Cancer Prevention and Therapy, National Clinical Research Center of Cancer, Huanhuxi Road, Hexi District, Tianjin, People's Republic of China

hospitalized days. The patients were followed up with an average time of 68 (7–89) months.

The diagnosis criteria of benign SBO were as follows: patients showing clinical symptoms as below, including ventosity, constipation, colicky abdominal pain, nausea, and hyperactive bowel sounds. The patients with SBO were further confirmed when fluid levels in dilated loops were shown by the plain abdominal X-ray. The contents of serum carcinoembryonic antigen in patients were also measured. Besides, the possible tumor recurrence or carcinomatosis in patients was determined by the imaging procedures of computed tomography (CT) and positron emission tomography (PET).

The exclusion criteria were as follows: patients with distant metastasis (e.g., liver, lung, brain, or peritoneal carcinomatosis), patients died 30 days after surgery, patients with SBO resulting from cancer recurrence or peritoneal carcinomatosis, and patients without complete follow-up data.

Statistical analysis

The SPSS 13.0 software (SPSS, Chicago, IL, USA) was used for statistical analysis. The correlation of benign SBO and clinicopathological factors was evaluated by a chi-square (χ^2) test or Fisher's exact test. Risk factors for benign SBO following curative resection in rectal cancer patients were analyzed by univariate and multivariate logistic regression analysis. $P < 0.05$ was taken as statistically significant.

Results

Two hundred and fifty-three patients (7.3%, 253/3472) hospitalized were diagnosed with benign SBO. Among these patients, 247 cases (97.6%, 247/253) were first subjected to conservative treatment. The conservative treatment included venous transfusion, total parenteral nutrition, gastric tube insertion, coloclysis, and bowel rest. However, conservative treatment was ineffective for 95 patients, who were then subjected to surgeries. Additionally, six (2.4%) patients underwent laparotomy in the initial 12 h of hospitalization due to the possibility of small bowel strangulation indicated by imaging.

The categories of surgery included lysis of adhesions, small bowel resection, ileocecectomy, and colectomy. When comparing to the conservative treatment group, surgical treatment group possessed a lower incidence of

recurrent benign SBO, higher mortality, and longer hospital stay (Table 1). It was noteworthy that most patients undergoing operation received primary conservative

Table 1 The outcome of patients with small bowel obstruction (SBO) through different treatments (N = 253)

	Conservative treatment group (n = 152)	Surgical treatment group (n = 101)	P value
SBO recurrence	54 (35.5%)	15 (14.8%)	< 0.001
Mean hospital stay (days)	5.8	14.5	< 0.001
Mortality	2 (1.32%)	4 (3.96%)	0.176

Table 2 Risk factors for benign small bowel obstruction (SBO) by the univariate analysis

Variables	No. of patients	No. of SBO	OR	95% CI	P value
Age			0.82	0.62–1.07	0.14
≤ 60	1318	85			
> 60	2154	168			
Gender			0.87	0.67–1.12	0.267
Male	1805	123			
Female	1667	130			
Type of surgery			NA	NA	0.299
Anterior resection	2547	176			
Abdominoperineal resection	783	67			
Hartmann's operation	142	10			
Surgical approach			1.59	1.21–2.09	0.001
Open	2014	172			
Laparoscopic	1458	81			
Duration of surgery			0.78	0.59–1.01	0.062
≤ 3 h	2378	160			
> 3 h	1094	93			
Radiotherapy			2.49	1.92–3.23	< 0.001
Yes	901	113			
No	2571	140			
Chemotherapy			0.81	0.63–1.07	0.144
Yes	2341	160			
No	1131	93			
Antiadhesive materials			1.42	1.05–1.93	0.023
Yes	2489	197			
No	983	56			
Pelvic peritoneum sutured			1.48	1.12–1.96	0.007
Yes	2638	174			
No	834	79			
Blood loss			0.71	0.54–0.93	0.012
≤ 400	2513	166			
> 400	959	87			
Previous laparotomy			0.75	0.35–1.62	0.598
Yes	125	7			
No	3347	246			
Tumor stage (TNM)			NA	NA	0.043
I	512	35			
II	1295	78			
III	1665	140			

treatment; therefore, a careful determination of hospitalized days should be taken.

As shown in Table 2, multiple variables were likely correlated with benign SBO, including surgical approach, radiotherapy, antiadhesive materials, pelvic peritoneum sutured, blood loss, and tumor stage (TNM). Then the multivariate logistic regression analysis demonstrated that open surgery (OR, 8.25; 95% CI, 2.18–17.32; $P < 0.001$) and radiotherapy (OR, 6.13; 95% CI, 1.47–15.36; $P < 0.001$) were the independent risk factors of benign SBO in rectal cancer patients receiving curative resection (Table 3).

Discussion

SBO is a potentially life-threatening complication after primary rectal cancer surgery. Though the patients undergoing colorectal surgery are at high risk of SBO [3, 5], there have been limited studies about the accurate incidence of SBO following colorectal operation [4, 6, 7, 13–16]. It has been reported that the occurrence rate of SBO following colorectal resection varied between 1.5–12.5% [7, 15] and 24–32.6% [6, 14, 16]. In this study, the incidence of benign SBO following rectal cancer resection was 7.3% (253/3472), which was lower compared with previous studies [6, 7, 14–16]. This difference might be resulted from the technological innovation, especially after the wide application of laparoscopic surgery [6]. The incidence of adhesive SBO was shown to be 32.6% in a 10-year follow-up study [16]. However, the average follow-up period in our study was 68 months, possibly leading to the lower benign SBO incidence. It has been found that the average period between primary colorectal operation and SBO was 8.4 years [17]. Therefore, a long-range follow-up is required for determining the accurate incidence of SBO in rectal cancer patients receiving initial operation.

In our study, the results showed that open surgery was a risk factor for benign SBO following rectal cancer operation, concurring with a previous finding, increased incidence of SBO after laparotomy [18]. Studies have shown that the abdominal wall damage and intestinal operation increased inflammatory reactions [19], possibly resulting in the occurrence of SBO after an open rectectomy [8]. In contrast, multiple studies have demonstrated that laparoscopic proctectomy could reduce adhesion-related complications and produce better short-term outcome [20–22]. Besides, in this study, the

incidence of benign SBO following rectal cancer surgery in the laparoscopic group was much lower compared with the open surgical group. Taken together, the results demonstrated the advantages of laparoscopy, providing a theoretical basis for treating rectal cancer patients using laparoscopic surgery.

Owing to the advantages of adjuvant radiotherapy, an increasing number of rectal cancer patients choose this option. But the long-range effects of radiotherapy should be completely studied to avoid the undesired side effects. It is well established that bowel obstruction is a long-term post-irradiation complication, and the incidence of bowel obstruction is increased when large quantities of small bowel are exposed to irradiation, especially the doses more than 50–55 Gy [23]. In the long term, small bowel, affected by heavy quantities of irradiation could develop fibrosis and ischemia, might show as SBO. However, the incidence of post-irradiation SBO varies a lot, and no definite reasons could account for this variation. The fixed loops of small bowel in pelvis were observed in 65% of patients receiving postoperative irradiation relative to 18% of patients without operation [24]. As fixed bowel maintains location during the treatment, the fixed bowel is potentially exposed to a significantly higher amount of irradiation compared with mobile bowel. Therefore, caution should be taken in the application of radiotherapy. A previous study showed that no difference in the occurrence rate of SBO was observed between surgery group (11%) and surgery combined with short-term preoperative irradiation group (11%) during a 5.1-year follow-up, suggesting the superiority of short-term preoperative irradiation over postoperative irradiation [25]. However, in our study, most patients (683/901) undergoing radiotherapy were treated with postoperative irradiation. And we found that radiotherapy was the risk factor for SBO in rectal cancer patients subjected to radical resection, which was in line with previous findings [9]. Taken together, these results reinforced the superiority of preoperative radiotherapy to reduce the long-run risk of developing SBO.

Notably, a recent study examined the risk factors for SBO that occurred within 30 days following anterior resection for rectal cancer [10]. Patients with perioperative complications other than SBO and with simultaneous resection of other organs were excluded from the study. The univariate logistic regression was conducted to screen for the factors related to the occurrence of SBO; the identified factors were then used in a multivariate logistic model to evaluate the independent risk factors for SBO; they found D3 node dissection and defunctioning ileostomy formation were the independent risk factors for early postoperative SBO after anterior resection for rectal cancer. Therefore, basically, their research and our research are methodologically

Table 3 Independent risk factors for benign small bowel obstruction (SBO) by logistic regression analysis

Variables	χ^2	P value	OR	95% CI
Open surgery	15.07	< 0.001	8.25	2.18–17.32
Radiotherapy	11.69	< 0.001	6.13	1.47–15.36

consistent; the biggest difference lies in the subjects of interest. The subjects with a long-term follow-up (68 months) in our study might result in the finding of different risk factors for SBO from previous studies.

Conclusion

In conclusion, we found that open surgery and radiotherapy were the independent risk factors of benign SBO following curative resection in rectal cancer patients. Therefore, laparoscopic surgery was confirmed to be a useful countermeasure against the long-term risk of benign SBO.

Acknowledgements
The authors thank Lin Mei for his assistance in editing the manuscript.

Authors' contributions
LT collected the data and drafted the manuscript. PZ analyzed the data. DLK conceived of the study and participated in its design and coordination and helped to draft the manuscript. All authors read and approved the final manuscript.

Competing interests
All authors declare that they have no competing interests.

References
1. Brolin RE, Krasna MJ, Mast BA. Use of tubes and radiographs in the management of small bowel obstruction. Ann Surg. 1987;206(2):126–33.
2. Malangoni MA, et al. Admitting service influences the outcomes of patients with small bowel obstruction. Surgery. 2001;130(4):706–11 discussion 711-3.
3. Seror D, et al. How conservatively can postoperative small bowel obstruction be treated? Am J Surg. 1993;165(1):121–5 discussion 125-6.
4. Cox MR, et al. The operative aetiology and types of adhesions causing small bowel obstruction. Aust N Z J Surg. 1993;63(11):848–52.
5. Miller G, et al. Natural history of patients with adhesive small bowel obstruction. Br J Surg. 2000;87(9):1240–7.
6. Ryan MD, et al. Adhesional small bowel obstruction after colorectal surgery. ANZ J Surg. 2004;74(11):1010–2.
7. Edna TH, Bjerkeset T. Small bowel obstruction in patients previously operated on for colorectal cancer. Eur J Surg. 1998;164(8):587–92.
8. Nakajima J, et al. Risk factors for early postoperative small bowel obstruction after colectomy for colorectal cancer. World J Surg. 2010;34(5):1086–90.
9. Baxter NN, et al. Postoperative irradiation for rectal cancer increases the risk of small bowel obstruction after surgery. Ann Surg. 2007;245(4):553–9.
10. Suwa K, et al. Risk factors for early postoperative small bowel obstruction after anterior resection for rectal cancer. World J Surg. 2018;42(1):233–8.
11. Weng J, Wu H, Wang Z. Risk factors for early postoperative small bowel obstruction after anterior resection for rectal cancer: methodological issues. World J Surg. 2018;42(6):1907.
12. Mizushima T, et al. Risk factors of small bowel obstruction following total proctocolectomy and ileal pouch anal anastomosis with diverting loop-ileostomy for ulcerative colitis. Ann Gastroenterol Surg. 2017;1(2):122
13. Ellis CN, et al. Small bowel obstruction after colon resection for benign and malignant diseases. Dis Colon Rectum. 1991;34(5):367–71.
14. Parker MC, et al. Postoperative adhesions: ten-year follow-up of 12,584 patients undergoing lower abdominal surgery. Dis Colon Rectum. 2001; 44(6):822 9 discussion 829-30.   –8.
15. Brightwell NL, McFee AS, Aust JB. Bowel obstruction and the long tube stent. Arch Surg. 1977;112(4):505–11.
16. Ellis H, et al. Adhesion-related hospital readmissions after abdominal and pelvic surgery: a retrospective cohort study. Lancet. 1999;353(9163):1476
17. Williams SB, et al. Small bowel obstruction: conservative vs. surgical management. Dis Colon Rectum. 2005;48(6):1140–6.
18. Duepree HJ, et al. Does means of access affect the incidence of small bowel obstruction and ventral hernia after bowel resection? Laparoscopy versus laparotomy. J Am Coll Surg. 2003;197(2):177–81.   –80.
19. Kalff JC, et al. Surgically induced leukocytic infiltrates within the rat intestinal muscularis mediate postoperative ileus. Gastroenterology. 1999;117(2):378
20. Ng SS, et al. Long-term morbidity and oncologic outcomes of laparoscopic-assisted anterior resection for upper rectal cancer: ten-year results of a prospective, randomized trial. Dis Colon Rectum. 2009;52(4):558–66.
21. Gao F, Cao YF, Chen LS. Meta-analysis of short-term outcomes after laparoscopic resection for rectal cancer. Int J Color Dis. 2006;21(7):652 –87.
22. Aziz O, et al. Laparoscopic versus open surgery for rectal cancer: a meta-analysis. Ann Surg Oncol. 2006;13(3):413–24.
23. Coia LR, Myerson RJ, Tepper JE. Late effects of radiation therapy on the gastrointestinal tract. Int J Radiat Oncol Biol Phys. 1995;31(5):1213–
24. Green N. The avoidance of small intestine injury in gynecologic cancer.Int J Radiat Oncol Biol Phys. 1983;9(9):1385–90.
25. Peeters KC, et al. Late side effects of short-course preoperative radiotherapy combined with total mesorectal excision for rectal cancer: increased bowel dysfunction in irradiated patients--a Dutch colorectal cancer group study. J Clin Oncol. 2005;23(25):6199–206.

21

Progress in research on the role of circular RNAs in lung cancer

Yang Chen[2†], Shuzhen Wei[1†], Xiyong Wang[2], Xiaoli Zhu[1,2] and Shuhua Han[1,2*]

Abstract

Background: Circular RNA (circRNA), as a covalently closed circular RNA molecule, is widely present, which is recognized as a competing endogenous RNA. A large number of differentially expressed circRNAs have been identified and are recognized as potential biomarkers for the diagnosis of tumors.

Main body: CircRNAs play an important role in the regulation of cell signaling pathways. The main biological functions of circRNAs include acting as miRNA sponges, regulating the transcription of the parental genes, and acting as adapters to regulate the interactions between proteins and encoding proteins. Compared with normal tissues, there are differentially expressed circRNAs in lung cancer tissue, and the expression levels of circRNAs are correlated with clinicopathological features of lung cancer. Their roles in pathway regulation are described, and the diagnostic and prognostic values are further evaluated.

Conclusion: In lung cancer, circRNAs participate in the proliferation, migration, and invasion, acting as a competitive endogenous RNA. Differentially expressed circRNAs may serve as non-invasive diagnostic markers for lung cancers. Further investigation of the roles of circRNAs in the pathogenesis and regulatory pathways is conducive to the development of novel approaches for the diagnosis and accurate treatment of lung cancers.

Keywords: Lung cancer, Circular RNA, Endogenous regulation, Biological diagnosis, Biomarker

Background

In the 1970s, Sanger et al. examined viroids by electron microscopy and discovered that the viroids were single-stranded RNA molecules with a covalently closed circular structure and high thermal stability [1]. In the early days of the discovery of circRNAs, due to the limitation of the detection techniques, most circRNAs were expressed in only a few cell types and at low abundance. With the development of RNA sequencing and bioinformatics technologies in recent years, circular RNAs were found to be stable and prevalent in a variety of species and tissues, with cell phenotype specificity and tissue developmental stage specificity. Xu et al. analyzed six types of normal human tissues (colon, heart, kidney, liver, lung, and stomach tissues) based on RNA-seq data and detected at least 1000 circRNAs in each tissue [2]. Approximately 36.97–50.04% of the circRNAs exhibited tissue-specific expression. For example, 1224 circRNAs were identified in adult normal lung tissues, among which 452 were specifically expressed.

The regulatory mechanism of circular RNAs has been further explored. Some of the circRNAs play an endogenous regulatory role by acting as a sponge to adsorb microRNAs (miRNAs). These circRNAs affect the functions of target genes downstream of the miRNAs, thereby participating in tumor development and progression. To date, a large number of differentially expressed circRNAs have been identified in esophageal cancer, gastric cancer, and colon cancer and are recognized as potential biomarkers for diagnosis. Lung cancer is a malignancy with the highest mortality rate worldwide [3]. The diagnosis and treatment of lung cancer significantly influence patient prognosis. At present, the 5-year survival rate of lung cancer patients is merely 17.7% [4]. The survival rate is significantly increased in patients with early-stage lung cancer compared with patients with advanced lung cancer (the 5-year survival rate of patients with early-stage lung cancer was 55.6%, whereas the 5-year survival rate of patients with

* Correspondence: hanshuhua0922@126.com
†Yang Chen and Shuzhen Wei contributed equally to this work.
¹Department of Respiratory, Zhongda Hospital, Southeast University, Nanjing, China
²Medical School of Southeast University, Nanjing, China

advanced lung cancer was 4.5%) [5]. Therefore, early detection of lung cancer is crucial. The biological methods for efficient diagnosis of lung cancer is worthy of further exploration. Zhao et al. carried out a high-throughput circRNA microarray to investigate the expression profile of circRNAs in tumor tissues and adjacent normal tissues from four patients with early lung adenocarcinoma [6]. It was found that 356 circRNAs were differentially expressed. Two hundred four circRNAs were upregulated, and 152 circRNAs were downregulated in tumor samples. The discovery of lung cancer-related circRNAs has provided novel ideas for the diagnosis and treatment of lung cancer. By reviewing the biological functions and regulation mechanisms of circRNAs as well as the lung cancer-related pathways regulated by circRNAs, this paper further expounds the potential value of circRNAs as diagnostic and prognostic markers or therapeutic targets for lung cancer.

Main text
The functions of circRNAs
To date, numerous studies have assessed circRNAs. The biological functions of circRNAs have gradually been recognized by scholars. Currently, the known functions of circRNAs include acting as miRNA sponges, regulating the transcription of the parental genes, and acting as adapters to regulate the interactions between proteins and encoding proteins.

CircRNAs act as a miRNA sponge
CircRNAs could function as a miRNA sponge to regulate the gene expression. CDR1as is an antisense transcript of cerebellar degeneration-related protein 1 (CDR1) [7] that contains 63 conserved miR-7 binding sites. After binding to miR-7, CDR1as inhibits the function of miR-7 and exerts a negative regulatory effect. As a competitive endogenous RNA (ceRNA), circRNA can compete with miRNA. miRNA is usually combined with argonaute 2 (AGO2) protein to form RNA-induced silencing complex (RISC), thus regulating the expression of target genes. Because AGO2 can combine with circRNAs and miRNAs, the RNA-protein complex can be precipitated under the action of AGO2 protein antibody by RNA immunoprecipitation (RIP) experiment. Through sequencing RNAs combined with AGO2, the binding targets of miRNAs can be found. CircRNF13 [8] is a highly expressed circular RNA in lung cancer. The RIP experiment was used to explore the RNAs precipitated by AGO2 antibody and IgG antibody. It was found that circRNF13 and miR-93-5p were more obviously enriched in RNAs retrieved from the AGO2 antibody, which confirmed that circRNF13 and miR-93-5p could be directly combined, and circRNF13 could function as a sponge for miR-93-5p. However, Guo et al. found that circRNA-forming exons did not exhibit

higher argonaute 2 (AGO2)-binding ability [9]. Therefore, they hypothesized that only certain circRNAs were able to act as sponges to adsorb miRNAs, whereas the majority of circRNAs did not have such function.

CircRNAs regulate the transcription of parental genes
CircRNAs are capable of regulating the transcription of parental genes. Intronic circRNAs (ciRNAs), which are formed from introns, contain a small number of miRNA binding sites and are virtually incapable of acting as miRNA sponges. However, ciRNAs could positively regulate RNA polymerase II (RNA Pol II) and promote the expression of maternal genes [10]. Exon-intron circRNAs (EIciRNAs), which are formed from exons and introns, interact with U1 small nuclear RNA (snRNA) through RNA-RNA binding, forming the EIciRNA-U1 snRNP complex. The complex promotes the expression of parental genes by affecting RNA Pol II [11].

CircRNA functions as an adapter between proteins
CircRNAs may exert their regulatory effects by binding to proteins. For example, circRNA derived from forkhead box O3 (circ-Foxo3) is related to cell senescence. circ-Foxo3 is highly expressed in senescent cardiomyocytes and is capable of inhibiting cell proliferation and cell cycle progression. circ-Foxo3 binds to cyclin-dependent kinases 2 (CDK2) and cyclin-dependent kinase inhibitor p21, forming the circ-Foxo3-p21-CDK2 ternary complex. The formation of the ternary complex reduces CDK2 activity, thereby further inhibiting cell cycle progression [12]. Similarly, circ-Foxo3 interacts with the anti-aging protein ID-1 (inhibitor of DNA binding 1), the transcription factor E2F1, and the anti-stress proteins FAK (focal adhesion kinase) and HIF1α (hypoxia-inducible factor 1-alpha) [13]. Such interactions block the entry of circ-Foxo3 into the nucleus and suppress the anti-aging and anti-stress effects of circ-Foxo3, resulting in cell senescence. The interactions between circRNAs and proteins expand the regulatory functions of circRNAs.

CircRNAs have protein translation functions
CircRNAs can be translated into proteins via a rolling circle mechanism, which not only provides repeated polypeptide sequences but also enhances polypeptide yields per unit of time as ribosomes do not need to bind repeatedly to the RNA template [14]. Rice yellow mottle virus consists of a covalently closed circular (CCC) RNA that can be directly translated into a 16-kD protein. CCC RNA contains one internal ribosome entry site (IRES) and two to three open reading frames (ORFs), which play important roles in the translation process [15]. Circular RNAs are rich in IRES and ORF elements. Of the 32,914 human exonic circRNAs included in the circRNADb database, 16,328 circRNAs contain ORFs

that encode greater than 100 amino acids. Among the 16,328 circRNAs, 7170 contain IRES elements [16]. The presence of abundant IRES and ORF elements in circRNAs indicates that the translation of circRNAs may have a more general significance in human cells. CircRNAs participate in the regulation of tumors through translation into proteins. Yang et al. found that the circRNA derived from the F-box/WD repeat-containing protein 7 (FBXW7) gene (circ-FBXW7) encoded a 21-kDa protein FBXW7-185aa [17]. circ-FBXW7 and FBXW7-185aa were expressed at low levels in glioblastoma tissues, and a correlation between the expression level of circ-FBXW7 and the prognosis of patients with glioblastoma was noted. Functional studies revealed that upregulation of FBXW7-185aa in tumor cells inhibited cell proliferation and cell cycle progression, whereas knockdown of FBXW7-185aa promoted the malignant development of tumors. The translation of circRNAs and their regulatory role in tumor tissues may provide ideas for further research on circRNAs.

Circular RNAs and lung cancer

Lung cancer-related studies reveal that circRNAs play an endogenous regulatory role in the development and progression of lung cancers and have potential diagnostic values (Table 1).

The function and regulation mechanisms of circRNAs in lung cancer

CDR1as is an antisense transcript of CDR1 [7]. CDR1as contains 63 miR-7 binding sites. Once bound to miR-7, CDR1as inhibits miR-7 function and thus exerts a negative regulatory effect. Based on the role of CDR1as as a miR-7 "sponge," Hansen et al. hypothesized that the CDR1as/miR-7 axis might be potentially involved in tumorigenesis [18]. MiR-7 downregulates the expression of epidermal growth factor receptor (EGFR) mRNA and protein and participates in tumor regulation as a regulator of EGFR [19]. EGFR activates miR-7 through the Ras/extracellular signal-regulated kinase (ERK)/Myc pathway and inhibits ETS2 repressor factor (ERF, a transcriptional repressor of V-ets avian erythroblastosis virus E26 oncogene homolog 2 (Ets2)), thereby promoting cell growth and the occurrence of lung cancers [20]. A regulatory loop may exist between miR-7 and EGFR. The direction of the balance between miR-7 and EGFR determines whether a cell is benign or malignant [20]. In lung adenocarcinoma tissues with an EGFR mutation, the mutation enhances the expression of miR-7 through promoting EGFR phosphorylation. There is a loss of balance between EGFR and miR-7. EGFR expression levels are significantly positively correlated with miR-7 expression levels [20]. By virtue of its sponge-like adsorptive activity, CDR1as may participate in the regulation of

miR-7/EGFR and thus be involved in the development and progression of lung cancers.

As a circRNA, cir-ITCH and the three prime untranslated regions (3′-UTR) of E3 ubiquitin ligases (ITCH) share some common miRNA binding sites. Cir-ITCH acts as a sponge to absorb miR-7 and miR-214, thereby regulating the expression of ITCH [21]. ITCH participates in the ubiquitin-mediated degradation of a variety of proteins in vivo. ITCH inhibits the Wnt/β-catenin signaling pathway through ubiquitination and degradation of phosphorylated dishevelled-2 (Dvl2). A decrease in cir-ITCH expression allows increased binding of miR-7 and miR-214 to ITCH, which leads to the downregulation of ITCH expression (Fig. 1). The Wnt/β-catenin pathway is thus enhanced, promoting the development, progression, and metastasis of lung cancers. As a miR-1252 sponge, hsa_circ_0043256 binds competitively to miR-1252, thereby affecting the important negative regulator of the Wnt signaling pathway (the E3 ubiquitin ligases ITCH) [22]. Hsa_circ_0043256 upregulates ITCH expression, whereas miR-1252 partially counteracts the upregulatory effect of hsa_circ_0043256. The hsa_circ_0043256/miR-1252/ITCH axis plays an important role in cinnamaldehyde-mediated anti-tumor activity, which provides a new target for the treatment of lung cancer (Fig. 1).

CircHIPK3, a circRNA derived from the homeodomain-interacting protein kinase 3 (HIPK3) gene, and the mRNA of insulin-like growth factor 1 (IGF1) bind jointly to miR-379. CircHIPK3 regulates IGF1 expression through sponging miR-379 [23]. As a highly abundant circRNA, circHIPK3 has 18 potential miRNA binding sites [24]. In HuH-7, HCT-116, and HeLa human tumor cell lines, knockdown of circHIPK3 significantly inhibited tumor cell growth. Among six non-small cell lung cancer (NSCLC) cell lines, H1299 expressed the lowest level of circHIPK3, whereas H2170 expressed the highest level of circHIPK3. Overexpression of circHIPK3 in the NSCLC cell line NCI-H1299 significantly promoted cell proliferation, whereas interference with circHIPK3 expression in NCI-H2170 cells drastically inhibited cell proliferation [23]. circHIPK3 exerts a proliferation-promoting activity in lung cancer cell lines, indicating that it participates in the regulation of lung cancer and may become a new target for the treatment of NSCLC.

Sry, a circular transcript of the sex-determining region of Y-chromosome, has 16 conserved binding sites for miR-138. In small cell lung cancer cells, miR-138 targets H2A histone family member X (H2AX) and regulates DNA damage responses. A study found that miR-138 expression was significantly downregulated in small cell lung cancer tissues and cell lines. Overexpression of miR-138 in small cell lung cancer cell lines led to significantly decreased cell proliferation and cell cycle arrest.

Table 1 Circular RNAs in lung cancer

CircRNA	Expression level	Function	Mechanism	Diagnostic and prognostic value	Reference
circFARSA	Upregulated in tissues and plasma	To promote cell migration and invasion	Sponge miR-330-5p and miR-326; upregulate fatty acid synthase	The area under the ROC curve was 0.71	[40]
CircRNA 100876	Upregulated in tissues	Unknown	Unknown	Higher expression level associated with lower overall survival	[26]
Hsa_circ_0013958	Upregulated in tissues, cells, and plasma	To promote cell proliferation and invasion and prevent apoptosis	Sponge miR-134; upregulate cyclin D1	The area under the ROC curve was 0.815	[27]
Circular RNA-ITCH	Downregulated in tissues	To inhibit cell proliferation	Sponge miR-7 and miR-214; upregulate ITCH	Unknown	[21]
Hsa_circ_0043256	Upregulated in NSCLC cells in response to CA treatment	To inhibit cell proliferation and induce apoptosis	Sponge miR-1252; upregulate ITCH; inhibits the Wnt/β-catenin pathway	Unknown	[47]
Circ-BANP	Upregulated in tissues	To promote cell proliferation, migration, and invasion	Sponge miR-503; upregulate LARP1 expression	Higher expression level associated with lower overall survival	[36]
Circ_0067934	Upregulated in NSCLC tissues and cell lines	To promote cell proliferation, migration, and invasion	Modulate the expression levels of markers of epithelial-to-mesenchymal transition	Higher expression level associated with lower overall survival	[43]
CircRNF13	Downregulated in tissues	To inhibit cell invasion and metastasis	Sponge miR-93-5p	Unknown	[8]
CircMAN2B2	Upregulated in tissues and cell lines	To promote cell proliferation and invasion	Sponge miR-1275; upregulate FOXK1 expression	Unknown	[34]
F-circEA	Existence in plasma and H2228 cells	To promote cell migration and invasion	Unknown	F-circEA was specifically existed in EML4-AL K-positive NSCLC	[39]
Hsa_circRNA_103809	Upregulated in tissues and cell lines	To promote cell proliferation and invasion	Sponge miR-4302; upregulate the expression of ZNF121; enhance MYC protein level	Higher expression level associated with lower overall survival	[29]
CircUBAP2	Upregulated in tissues	To promote cell proliferation, invasion and prevent apoptosis	Upregulate CDK6,cyclin D1, c-IAP1, Bcl-2, Survivin, FAK, Rac1, MMP2, JNK and ERK1/2; downregulate p27 and Bax; sponge miR-339-5p, miR-96-3p and miR-135b-3p	Unknown	[28]
Hsa_circ_0000064	Upregulated in tissues and cell lines	To promote cell proliferation and cycle progression and prevent apoptosis	Upregulate caspase-3, caspase-9, bax, p21, CDK6, cyclin D1, MMP-2, and MMP-9; downregulate bcl-2	Unknown	[42]
Hsa_circ_0046264	Downregulated in tissues and cell lines	To inhibit proliferation and invasion, to promote cell apoptosis	Sponge miR-1245; upregulate BRCA2	Lower expression level associated with worse prognosis outcome	[37]
Hsa_circ_0079530	Upregulated in tissues and cell lines	To promote cell proliferation, migration, invasion and cycle progression	Unknown	The area under the ROC curve was 0.756	[41]

Table 1 Circular RNAs in lung cancer (*Continued*)

CircRNA	Expression level	Function	Mechanism	Diagnostic and prognostic value	Reference
CircRNA-FOXO3	Downregulated in tissues and cell lines	To inhibit cell proliferation, migration, and invasion	Sponge miR-155; upregulate FOXO3	The area under the ROC curve was 0.782	[33]
Hsa_circ_0012673	Upregulated in tissues	To promote cell proliferation	Sponge miR-22; upregulate ErbB3	Unknown	[32]
Hsa_circRNA_103827	Upregulated in tissues	Unknown	Unknown	Higher expression level associated with shorter overall survival	[45]
Hsa_circRNA_000122	Downregulated in tissues	Unknown	Unknown	Lower expression level associated with shorter overall survival	[45]
Hsa_circ_0014130	Upregulated in tissues	Unknown	Unknown	The area under the ROC curve was 0.878	[22]
Hsa_circ_0007385	Upregulated in tissues and cells	To promote cell proliferation, migration, and invasion	Sponge miR-181	Unknown	[35]
Circ0006916	Downregulated in 16HBE-T,A549 and H460 cell lines	To inhibit cell proliferation and cycle progression	Sponge miR-522-3p; upregulate PHLPP1	Unknown	[30]
CircPRKCI	Upregulated in tissues	To promote cell proliferation and migration	Sponge miR-545 and miR-589; upregulate E2F7 expression	Higher expression level associated with shorter overall survival	[31]
Circ_001569	Upregulated in tissues	Promote cell proliferation	Promote the Wnt/β-catenin pathway	Higher expression level associated with poorer survival outcome	[44]

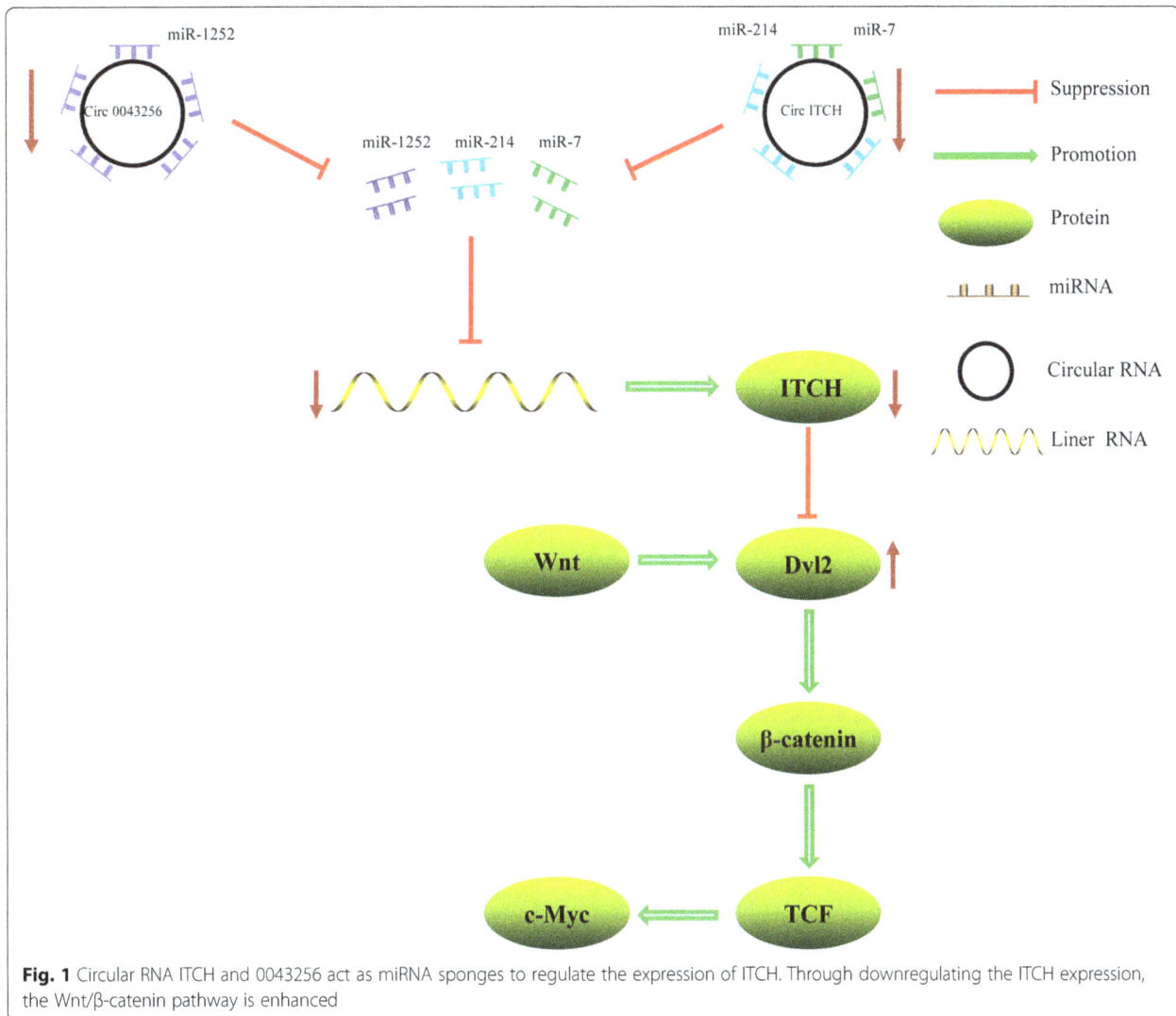

Fig. 1 Circular RNA ITCH and 0043256 act as miRNA sponges to regulate the expression of ITCH. Through downregulating the ITCH expression, the Wnt/β-catenin pathway is enhanced

H2AX knockout induced a cell inhibitory effect similar to miR-138 overexpression. It has been hypothesized that miR-138 targets H2AX and affects the proliferation and cell cycle progression of small cell lung cancer cells through inhibiting H2AX expression [25]. The Sry/miR138/H2AX axis may be involved in the regulation of small cell lung cancer, thereby possessing potential diagnostic and therapeutic intervention values.

CircRNA 100876 and the 3-UTR of matrix metalloproteinase 13 (MMP13) share common miRNA binding sites and bind jointly to miR-136 [26]. Inhibition of circRNA 100876 with small interfering RNA (siRNA) reduces the expression of MMP13, indicating that circRNA 100876 may indirectly regulate MMP13 through sponging miR-136. MMP13 is a member of the matrix metalloproteinase family that promotes lung cancer invasion and metastasis by degrading the extracellular matrix (ECM). Hsa_-circ_0013958 acts as a sponge to adsorb miR-134 and upregulates the proto-oncogene cyclin D1, thereby promoting

the proliferation and invasion of lung cancer cells [27]. It is likely that circRNA 100876 and circRNA 0013958 exert their carcinogenic effects through affecting the expression of lung cancer-related genes.

CircUBAP2 is highly expressed in lung adenocarcinoma, which is involved in tumor formation, invasion, and metastasis [28]. The results of luciferase reporter assay showed that miR-339-5p, miR-96-3p, and miR-135b-3p could act directly on circUBAP2. By analyzing the expression levels of cell proliferation and apoptosis-associated proteins (CDK6, cyclin D1, p27, c-IAP1, Bcl-2, Survivin, and Bax), it was found that CDK6, cyclin D1, and c-IAP1 expressions were downregulated, while p27 and Bax expressions were increased. CircUBAP2 silencing can inhibit the expression of Rac1 and FAK, further inhibiting the expression of MMP-2. CircUBAP2 silencing can also inhibit JNK and ERK1/2 activity. It is suggested that circUBAP2 may regulate the invasion and metastasis of tumor cells through the Rac-FAK signaling pathway and JNK signaling pathway.

Hsa_circRNA_103809 participates in the regulation of lung cancer through the miR-4302/ZNF121/MYC pathway [29]. Hsa_circRNA_103809 can promote the proliferation and invasion of lung cancer cells. Bioinformatics analysis reveals that hsa_circRNA_103809 can bind to miR-4302, while ZNF121 is the downstream target gene of miR-4302. Luciferase reporter assay showed that miR-4302 could interact with hsa_circRNA_103809 and ZNF-121. Quantitative RT-PCR further confirmed that hsa_circRNA_103809 knockdown significantly promoted miR-4302 expression, while miR-4302 overexpression inhibited ZNF121 expression. It is suggested that hsa_circRNA_103809 regulates ZNF121 expression through acting as a sponge for miR-124. The co-immunoprecipitation assay and western blot experiment further confirmed that ZNF121 can interact with MYC directly. The changes of hsa_circRNA_103809 and ZNF121 have corresponding effects on the level of MYC expression. The research of hsa_circRNA_103809 provides a new way to understand the pathogenesis of lung cancer.

Circ0006916 participates in tumor regulation through the miR-522-3P/PHLPP1 pathway [30]. Circ0006916 is downregulated in 16HBE-T, A549, and H460 cells, which inhibits cell proliferation. Luciferase reporter assay showed that circ0006916 could bind to miR-522-3P. The target gene PHLPP1 of miR-522-3P showed the same changes in the levels of mRNA and protein after the overexpression and downregulation of circ0006916. The results indicate that circ0006916 might affect the expression of PHLPP1 through miR-522-3P. The RNA pulldown experiment confirmed that RNA-binding protein TNRC6A could bind to the flanked intron region of circ0006916, and the absence of TNRC6A decreases the generation of circ0006916, indicating that TNRC6A could regulate the formation of circ0006916. This study reveals the regulatory protein in the upstream of circ0006916, and TNRC6A may participate in the growth of lung cancer cells by regulating circ0006916.

CircPRKCI participates in tumor regulation through the circPRKCI-miR-545/589-E2F7 pathway [31]. CircPRKCI is overexpressed in lung adenocarcinoma (LAC) tissues, which can promote the proliferation and migration of LAC cells. miRNA pull-down assay showed that circPRKCI could be effectively enriched by miR-589 and miR-545. RIP assay also showed that miR-545, circPRKCI, and miR-589 were effectively pulled down by anti-AGO2 antibodies. The silencing of circPRKCI did not affect the expression of miR-545 or miR-589, indicating that circPRKCI serves as a miRNA sponge, and it did not affect the expression of sponged miRNA. The results of qRT-PCR, pull-down assay, and luciferase reporter assay showed that both miR-545 and miR-589 directly bind to the 3′-UTR of E2F7 and directly downregulated the expression of E2F7, while silencing

circPRKCI also caused E2F7 downregulation, which further indicated that circPRKC could regulate E2F7 as a miR-545 and miR-589 sponge.

Hsa_circ_0012673 participates in the proliferation of lung adenocarcinoma through the miR-22/ErbB3 pathway [32]. Hsa_circ_0012673 is overexpressed in lung adenocarcinoma and has the effect of promoting cell proliferation. Luciferase reporter assay showed that miR-22 could reduce luciferase reporter activity. Knocking down hsa_circ_0012673 inhibited cell proliferation, but when miR-22 was silenced, the inhibitory effect of hsa_circ_0012673 on cells vanished. These data indicate that hsa_circ_0012673 promotes proliferation of LAC cells through miR-22. The expression of ErbB3 in tumor tissues of LAC patients was upregulated, and the expression level was positively correlated with hsa_circ_0012673, but negatively correlated with miR-22 expression. Western blot results showed that miR-22 could reduce the expression of ErbB3, while hsa_circ_0012673 increased ErbB3 protein level in LAC cells. This article describes the regulatory role of the hsa_circ_0012673/miR-22/ErbB3 pathway in proliferation and provides a new idea for the diagnosis and treatment of lung adenocarcinoma.

CircRNA-FOXO3 acts as a tumor suppressor through the miR-155/FOXO3 pathway [33]. CircRNA-FOXO3 is lowly expressed in NSCLC tissues and cell lines. Overexpression of circRNA-FOXO3 can significantly inhibit cell proliferation, metastasis, and invasion and promote apoptosis. By detecting the expression level of FOXO3 mRNA, it was found that it was downregulated in NSCLC. Spearman correlation analysis showed that the expression levels of circRNA-FOXO3 and FOXO3 mRNA were positively correlated. Bioinformatics analysis predicts that miR-155 can interact with circRNA-FOXO3 and FOXO3 mRNA. RIP assay showed that AGO2 antibody could precipitate circRNA-FOXO3 and FOXO3 mRNA. After circRNA-FOXO3 overexpression, miR-155 decreased significantly in cells. These results indicate that circRNA-FOXO3 can promote FOXO3 expression by adsorbing miR-155 and act as a tumor suppressor.

CircMAN2B2, hsa_circ_0007385, and circ-BANP were upregulated in lung cancer tissues. Hsa_circ_0046264 was downregulated in lung cancer tissues. They played regulatory roles through the adsorption of miRNAs. CircMAN2B2 can promote the expression of FOXK1 through acting as a miR-1275 sponge [34]. Knocking down circMAN2B2 can significantly inhibit the proliferation and invasion of H1299 and A549 cells, and circMAN2B2 may play a carcinogenic role in lung cancer. Hsa_circ_0007385 has the function of promoting cell proliferation, metastasis, and invasion [35]. Bioinformatics analysis and luciferase reporter assay confirmed that miR-181 can bind to hsa_circ_0007385. Circ-BANP [36] can promote cell invasion, proliferation, and metastasis. Mechanism study indicates that circ-BANP can play a regulatory role in the development of lung cancer through the miR-503/LARP1 signaling pathway. Hsa_circ_0046264 was proved to inhibit proliferation and invasion, induce apoptosis of lung cancer cells, and increase BRCA by adsorbing miR-1245 [37].

The diagnostic value of circRNAs in lung cancers

Hsa_circ_0013958 exhibits potential diagnostic value in lung cancer. Zhu et al. performed circRNA microarray to investigate the differently expressed circRNAs between lung adenocarcinoma tissues and paired adjacent non-cancerous tissues [27]. A total of 39 circRNAs were highly expressed in lung adenocarcinoma tissues, whereas 20 circRNAs were expressed at low levels in lung adenocarcinoma tissues. Quantitative polymerase chain reaction (qPCR) confirmed that hsa_circ_0013958 was highly expressed in lung adenocarcinoma tissues, plasma, and cell lines. Moreover, the expression level of hsa_circ_0013958 was related to TNM (tumor, node, and metastasis) stage and lymph node metastasis. The diagnostic accuracy of hsa_circ_0013958 was evaluated. In tissue samples, hsa_circ_0013958 yielded an AUC (the area under the receiver operating characteristic (ROC) curve) of 0.815. The sensitivity and specificity of hsa_circ_0013958 for diagnosing lung adenocarcinoma were 0.755 and 0.796, respectively. Plasma hsa_circ_0013958 had an AUC of 0.794. Moreover, hsa_circ_0013958 displayed superior diagnostic accuracy for advanced lung cancer compared with early-stage lung cancer.

Fusion-circRNA (F-circRNA) can be used as a diagnostic marker for the echinoderm microtubule-associated protein-like 4 (EML4)/anaplastic lymphoma kinase (ALK1) gene fusion mutation in lung cancer. Guarneri et al. found that aberrant chromosomal translocations and chromosomal rearrangements are involved in the occurrence of a variety of tumors [38]. Transcription of genes affected by chromosomal translocations may give rise to a new type of aberrant circRNAs, namely F-circRNAs. F-circRNAs are produced via trans-splicing during RNA editing or maturation. F-circRNAs produced via aberrant chromosomal translocation are involved in tumorigenesis and tumor regulation. As proto-oncogene-related RNAs, F-circRNAs promote cell transformation and tumor formation and play a role in treatment resistance. Lung cancer-associated EML4/ALK1 translocation also gives rise to F-circRNA, which may play an important role in the development and progression of lung cancers and serve as a novel entry point for the diagnosis of lung cancer. Tan et al. tested the EML4-ALK-positive cell line H2228 by RT-qPCR, further clarified the existence of F-circEA (fusion-circRNA from

EML4-ALK fusion gene), and found that F-circEA has the function of promoting cell proliferation and migration [39]. Further analysis of the expression of F-circEA in the tumor tissues and blood of EML4-ALK-positive patients showed that F-circEA could exist in the plasma and tumor tissues, while the mRNA of the fusion gene EML4-ALK only existed in the tumor tissue and could not be detected in the plasma. The presence of plasma F-circEA suggests that F-circEA can be used as a diagnostic marker for liquid biopsy. F-circEA has the potential value to diagnose the EML4-ALK fusion gene in NSCLC patients and guide the use of ALK inhibitor crizotinib.

CircFARSA in plasma has a diagnostic value for non-small cell lung cancer. Hang et al. have found that circFARSA is overexpressed in NSCLC tissues and plasma, and the functions of circFARSA are to promote cell migration and invasion [40]. Compared with circFARSA extracted from exosomes, the expression of circFARSA extracted from plasma is higher. It is presumed that cells can release circFARSA into the blood through other ways. By detecting plasma circFARSA from 50 patients with NSCLC and 50 healthy controls, it was found that plasma circFARSA had a diagnostic value and the AUC was 0.71. Plasma circFARSA may be used as a molecular marker for non-invasive detection of non-small cell lung cancer.

Hsa_circ_0014130 and hsa_circ_0079530 were highly expressed in NSCLC tissues. The expression of hsa_circ_0014130 was associated with TNM staging and lymph node metastasis [22]. It had a diagnostic value in differentiating lung cancer tissues and adjacent normal tissues. The area under the ROC curve was 0.878, and the sensitivity and specificity were 87% and 84.8% respectively. The expression level of hsa_circ_0075930 was correlated with tumor size and lymph node metastasis. Its AUC was 0.756, the sensitivity was 76.2%, and the specificity was 72.1% [41].

The prognostic value of circRNAs in lung cancers

CircRNA_100876 has a prognostic value in patients with lung cancer. Yao et al. examined 101 NSCLC samples, including 51 squamous cell carcinoma (SCC) samples and 50 adenocarcinoma samples [26]. The expression level of circRNA_100876 in tumor tissues was upregulated with 1.23-fold compared with normal tissues. circRNA_100876 expression level was also positively correlated with lymph node metastasis and the TNM stage of lung cancers, indicating that circRNA_100876 might be involved in the growth, proliferation, and metastasis of tumor cells. Patients expressing high levels of circRNA_100876 exhibited reduced overall survival (OS) compared with patients expressing low levels of circRNA_100876, indicating that circRNA_10087 might serve as a risk factor for predicting the prognosis of patients with NSCLC.

Hsa_circRNA_103809 and hsa_circ_0000064 were over-expressed in lung cancer tissues. Kaplan-Meier survival analysis showed that the lung cancer patients with high expression of hsa_circRNA_103809 had lower overall survival (OS), which could be used as a marker for predicting the prognosis of lung cancer [29]. The expression level of hsa_circ_0000064 is significantly correlated with metastasis and malignancy grade of lung cancer [42], and the potential value in predicting prognosis needs to be further verified by clinical research.

Circ_0067934 and circ_001569 were upregulated in NSCLC tissues. The expression of circ_0067934 is associated with TNM staging, lymph node metastasis, and distant metastasis [43]. Multivariate Cox proportional hazards analysis shows that circ_0067934 is an independent factor for poor prognosis in NSCLC patients. Circ_001569 has the function of promoting cell proliferation [44]. The expression level is related to the degree of tumor differentiation, lymph node metastasis, and TNM staging. The high expression of circ_001569 suggests that the prognosis of the patients is poor, and it may play a regulatory role through the Wnt/β-catenin pathway.

Hsa_circRNA_103827 was highly expressed in lung squamous cell carcinoma, while hsa_circRNA_000122 was lowly expressed [45]. Their expression level was correlated with the overall survival of patients. The PCR method further confirmed that Has_circRNA_404833, has_circRNA_406483, has_circRNA_006411, has_circRNA_401977, and has_circRNA_001640 have differential expression in lung cancer tissues [6], but the relationship between their expression levels and the clinicopathological features of the patients should be further studied.

The potential value of circRNAs in the treatment of lung cancers

Silencing circPRKCI can inhibit the growth of xenograft tumor in vitro and exhibit a potential therapeutic value [31]. Lin et al. injected SPC-A1 cells transfected with si-circPRKCI into subcutaneous tissue of nude mice. The tumors derived from cells transfected with si-circPRKCI had a smaller size and lower weight than the control group. Compared with xenografts derived from cell lines, patient-derived tumor xenografts (PDTX) maintain better cell differentiation ability, morphology, and architecture of the original patient tumors. The researchers injected cholesterol-conjugated si-circPRKCI and control siRNA into PDTX. Si-circPRKCI can significantly inhibit the growth of PDTX, indicating that circPRKCI is a promising therapeutic target for LAC. EGFR tyrosine kinase inhibitors (EGFR-TKIs) have been widely used in LAC patients with EGFR mutations. In order to find whether circPRKCI affects the therapeutic effects of EGFR-TKI, proliferation assays were performed.

Gefitinib combined with si-circPRKCI was more effective than gefitinib or si-circPRKCI alone, which suggested they had potential synergistic therapeutic effect, showing that circPRKCI is a potential therapeutic target.

Conclusions

Early diagnosis is an important prerequisite for effective treatment of lung cancer. Regional or distant metastasis of tumor cells is the major reason behind the poor efficacy in treatment of lung cancer patients. Computed tomography (CT) of the chest allows early detection of lung lesions. However, it is difficult to differentiate malignant from benign lesions by CT. Bronchoscopy and percutaneous pulmonary puncture allow the acquisition of pathological tissues. However, invasive procedures are often involved and are associated with certain risks. Examination of lung cancer-related protein markers in exfoliated cells and serum is a non-invasive medical procedure. Given that this procedure has limited sensitivity and specificity, new biomarkers are needed to assist in the clinical diagnosis of lung cancer. Due to their endogenous regulatory functions, closed circular structure, high stability, involvement in lung cancer development and progression, and differential expression in lung cancer tissues, circRNAs have the potential to serve as diagnostic and prognostic biomarkers for lung cancer. Given that circRNAs can be secreted to the outside of cells through exosomes and extracellular vesicles (EVs) [46] and EVs are present in a variety of body fluids (such as blood, urine, or saliva), analysis of circRNAs in body fluids is conducive to achieving non-invasive detection of tumors. Optimization of circRNA analysis methods will further improve the detection efficiency of lung cancers. With the gradual maturation of artificial circRNA construction and circRNA interference technology, regulation of circRNAs may become possible, which will provide a new approach for the treatment of lung cancers.

Acknowledgements
Not applicable.

Funding
The present study was supported by Postgraduate Research and Practice Innovation Program of Jiangsu Province, China (no. SJZZ16_0042), and the Nanjing Medical Science and Technology Development Project (no. YKK16257).

Authors' contributions
SH, YC, and SW contributed equally to this work, collected and analyzed the data, and drafted the manuscript. XW and XZ reviewed and contributed to the revision of the manuscript. All authors read and approved the final manuscript.

Competing interests
The authors declare that they have no competing interests.

References
1. Sanger HL, Klotz G, Riesner D, Gross HJ, Kleinschmidt AK. Viroids are single-stranded covalently closed circular RNA molecules existing as highly base-paired rod-like structures. Proc Natl Acad Sci U S A. 1976;73:3852–6.
2. Xu T, Wu J, Han P, Zhao Z, Song X. Circular RNA expression profiles and features in human tissues: a study using RNA-seq data. BMC Genomics. 2017;18:680.
3. Torre LA, Bray F, Siegel RL, Ferlay J, Lortet-Tieulent J, Jemal A. Global cancer statistics, 2012. CA Cancer J Clin. 2015;65:87–108.
4. Ettinger DS, Wood DE, Aisner DL, et al. Non-small cell lung cancer, version 5.2017, NCCN clinical practice guidelines in oncology. J Natl Compr Cancer Netw. 2017;15:504–35.
5. Ettinger DS, Wood DE, Akerley W, et al. NCCN guidelines insights: non-small cell lung cancer, version 4.2016. J Natl Compr Cancer Netw. 2016;14:255–64.
6. Zhao J, Li L, Wang Q, Han H, Zhan Q, Xu M. CircRNA expression profile in early-stage lung adenocarcinoma patients. Cell Physiol Biochem. 2017;44: 2138–46.
7. Memczak S, Jens M, Elefsinioti A, et al. Circular RNAs are a large class of animal RNAs with regulatory potency. Nature. 2013;495:333–8.
8. Wang L, Liu S, Mao Y, et al. CircRNF13 regulates the invasion and metastasis in lung adenocarcinoma by targeting miR-93-5p. Gene. 2018;671:170-7.
9. Guo JU, Agarwal V, Guo H, Bartel DP. Expanded identification and characterization of mammalian circular RNAs. Genome Biol. 2014;15:409.
10. Zhang Y, Zhang XO, Chen T, et al. Circular intronic long noncoding RNAs. Mol Cell. 2013;51:792–806.
11. Li Z, Huang C, Bao C, et al. Exon-intron circular RNAs regulate transcription in the nucleus. Nat Struct Mol Biol. 2015;22:256-64.
12. Du WW, Yang W, Liu E, Yang Z, Dhaliwal P, Yang BB. Foxo3 circular RNA retards cell cycle progression via forming ternary complexes with p21 and CDK2. Nucleic Acids Res. 2016;44:2846–58.
13. Du WW, Yang W, Chen Y, et al. Foxo3 circular RNA promotes cardiac senescence by modulating multiple factors associated with stress and senescence responses. Eur Heart J. 2017;38:1402–12.
14. Abe N, Hiroshima M, Maruyama H, et al. Rolling circle amplification in a prokaryotic translation system using small circular RNA. Angew Chem (Int Ed Engl). 2013;52:7004–8.
15. AbouHaidar MG, Venkataraman S, Golshani A, Liu B, Ahmad T. Novel coding, translation, and gene expression of a replicating covalently closed circular RNA of 220 nt. Proc Natl Acad Sci U S A. 2014;111:14542–7.
16. Chen X, Han P, Zhou T, Guo X, Song X, Li Y. circRNADb: a comprehensive database for human circular RNAs with protein-coding annotations. Sci Rep. 2016;6:34985.
17. Yang Y, Gao X, Zhang M, et al. Novel role of FBXW7 circular RNA in repressing glioma tumorigenesis. J Natl Cancer Inst. 2018;110(3):304–15.
18. Hansen TB, Kjems J, Damgaard CK. Circular RNA and miR-7 in cancer. Cancer Res. 2013;73:5609–12.
19. Webster RJ, Giles KM, Price KJ, Zhang PM, Mattick JS, Leedman PJ. Regulation of epidermal growth factor receptor signaling in human cancer cells by microRNA-7. J Biol Chem. 2009;284:5731–41.
20. Chou YT, Lin HH, Lien YC, et al. EGFR promotes lung tumorigenesis by activating miR-7 through a Ras/ERK/Myc pathway that targets the Ets2 transcriptional repressor ERF. Cancer Res. 2010;70:8822–31.
21. Wan L, Zhang L, Fan K, Cheng ZX, Sun QC, Wang JJ. Circular RNA-ITCH suppresses lung cancer proliferation via inhibiting the Wnt/beta-catenin pathway. Biomed Res Int. 2016;2016:1579490.
22. Zhang S, Zeng X, Ding T, et al. Microarray profile of circular RNAs identifies hsa_circ_0014130 as a new circular RNA biomarker in non-small cell lung cancer. Sci Rep. 2018;8:2878.
23. Tian F, Wang Y, Xiao Z, Zhu X. Circular RNA CircHIPK3 promotes NCI-H1299 and NCI-H2170 cell proliferation through miR-379 and its target IGF1. Zhongguo Fei Ai Za Zhi. 2017;20:459–67.
24. Zheng Q, Bao C, Guo W, et al. Circular RNA profiling reveals an abundant circHIPK3 that regulates cell growth by sponging multiple miRNAs. Nat Commun. 2016;7:11215.
25. Yang H, Luo J, Liu Z, Zhou R, Luo H. MicroRNA-138 regulates DNA damage response in small cell lung cancer cells by directly targeting H2AX. Cancer Investig. 2015;33:126–36.
26. Yao JT, Zhao SH, Liu QP, et al. Over-expression of CircRNA_100876 in non-small cell lung cancer and its prognostic value. Pathol Res Pract. 2017;213:453–6.
27. Zhu X, Wang X, Wei S, et al. hsa_circ_0013958: a circular RNA and potential novel biomarker for lung adenocarcinoma. FEBS J. 2017;284:2170–82.
28. Yin Y, Gao H, Guo J, Gao Y. Effect of circular RNA UBAP2 silencing on proliferation and invasion of human lung cancer A549 cells and its mechanism. Zhongguo Fei Ai Za Zhi. 2017;20:800–7.
29. Liu W, Ma W, Yuan Y, Zhang Y, Sun S. Circular RNA hsa_circRNA_103809 promotes lung cancer progression via facilitating ZNF121-dependent MYC expression by sequestering miR-4302. Biochem Biophys Res Commun. 2018; 500:846–51.
30. Dai X, Zhang N, Cheng Y, et al. RNA-binding protein trinucleotide repeat-containing 6A regulates the formation of circular RNA 0006916, with important functions in lung cancer cells. Carcinogenesis. 2018;39:981–92.
31. Qiu M, Xia W, Chen R, et al. The circular RNA circPRKCI promotes tumor growth in lung adenocarcinoma. Cancer Res. 2018;78:2839–51.
32. Wang X, Zhu X, Zhang H, et al. Increased circular RNA hsa_circ_0012673 acts as a sponge of miR-22 to promote lung adenocarcinoma proliferation. Biochem Biophys Res Commun. 2018;496:1069–75.
33. Zhang Y, Zhao H, Zhang L. Identification of the tumorsuppressive function of circular RNA FOXO3 in nonsmall cell lung cancer through sponging miR155. Mol Med Rep. 2018;17:7692–700.
34. Ma X, Yang X, Bao W, et al. Circular RNA circMAN2B2 facilitates lung cancer cell proliferation and invasion via miR-1275/FOXK1 axis. Biochem Biophys Res Commun. 2018;498:1009–15.
35. Jiang MM, Mai ZT, Wan SZ, et al. Microarray profiles reveal that circular RNA hsa_circ_0007385 functions as an oncogene in non-small cell lung cancer tumorigenesis. J Cancer Res Clin Oncol. 2018;144:667–74.
36. Han J, Zhao G, Ma X, et al. CircRNA circ-BANP-mediated miR-503/LARP1 signaling contributes to lung cancer progression. Biochem Biophys Res Commun. 2018;503:2429-35.
37. Yang L, Wang J, Fan Y, Yu K, Jiao B, Su X. Hsa_circ_0046264 up-regulated BRCA2 to suppress lung cancer through targeting hsa-miR-1245. Respir Res. 2018;19:115.
38. Guarnerio J, Bezzi M, Jeong JC, et al. Oncogenic role of fusion-circRNAs derived from cancer-associated chromosomal translocations. Cell. 2016;165:289–302.
39. Tan S, Gou Q, Pu W, et al. Circular RNA F-circEA produced from EML4-ALK fusion gene as a novel liquid biopsy biomarker for non-small cell lung cancer. Cell Res. 2018;28:693–5.
40. Hang D, Zhou J, Qin N, et al. A novel plasma circular RNA circFARSA is a potential biomarker for non-small cell lung cancer. Cancer Med. 2018;7:2783–91.
41. Li J, Wang J, Chen Z, Chen Y, Jin M. Hsa_circ_0079530 promotes cell proliferation and invasion in non-small cell lung cancer. Gene. 2018;665:1–5.
42. Luo YH, Zhu XZ, Huang KW, et al. Emerging roles of circular RNA hsa_circ_0000064 in the proliferation and metastasis of lung cancer. Biomed Pharmacother. 2017;96:892–8.
43. Wang J, Li H. CircRNA circ_0067934 silencing inhibits the proliferation, migration and invasion of NSCLC cells and correlates with unfavorable prognosis in NSCLC. Eur Rev Med Pharmacol Sci. 2018;22:3053–60.
44. Ding L, Yao W, Lu J, Gong J, Zhang X. Upregulation of circ_001569 predicts poor prognosis and promotes cell proliferation in non-small cell lung cancer by regulating the Wnt/beta-catenin pathway. Oncol Lett. 2018;16:453–8.
45. Xu J, Shu J, Xu T, et al. Microarray expression profiling and bioinformatics analysis of circular RNA expression in lung squamous cell carcinoma. Am J Transl Res. 2018;10:771–83.
46. Lasda E, Parker R. Circular RNAs co-precipitate with extracellular vesicles: a possible mechanism for circRNA clearance. PLoS One. 2016;11:e0148407.
47. Tian F, Yu CT, Ye WD and Wang Q: Cinnamaldehyde induces cell apoptosis mediated by a novel circular RNA hsa_circ_0043256 in non-small cell lung cancer. Biochem Biophys Res Commun. 2017;493:1260-6.

22

Prognostic significance of metastatic lymph node ratio: the lymph node ratio could be a prognostic indicator for patients with gastric cancer

Yi Hou, Xudong Wang and Jing Chen*⑩

Abstract

Background: To demonstrate the prognostic significance and value of lymph node ratio (LNR) and evaluate the possibility of becoming a new indicator to enhance the current Union for International Cancer Control (UICC)/ American Joint Committee on Cancer (AJCC) tumor, lymph node, metastasis (TNM) staging system.

Methods: Our retrospective study included 221 patients who got gastric cancer and underwent curative gastrectomy between 2005 and 2012 at the Fourth Hospital Affiliated of China Medical University. The log-rank test was used to compare the clinicopathological variables. The Kaplan-Meier method and Cox proportional hazard regression model was used to perform the univariate analysis and multivariate statistical survival analysis.

Results: The patients with a better differentiated pathological type; an earlier stage of T staging, N staging, and TNM staging; and a lesser LNR would have a longer survival time according to the univariate analysis. As for the multivariate analysis, the Grade, T stage, N stage, and LNR had the statistical significance. Both in group 1 (the number of lymph nodes examined $\geq$ 15, namely LN $\geq$ 15) and group 2 (LN < 15), the LNR had statistical significance and the median survival time would decrease with the increase of the LNR. It was still statistically significant between group LNR1 and group LNR2 which were regrouped by the new cut-off value.

Conclusion: The LNR could estimate the prognosis of patients with curative gastrectomy regardless of the number of lymph nodes examined. Thus LNR could become a new indicator to enhance the current TNM stage system.

Keywords: Gastric cancer, Lymph node ratio, Survival analysis, Multivariate analysis, Prognosis

Background

The study aimed to demonstrate the prognostic significance and value of lymph node ratio (LNR) and evaluate the possibility of becoming a new indicator to enhance the current Union for International Cancer Control (UICC)/American Joint Committee on Cancer (AJCC) tumor, lymph node, metastasis (TNM) staging system.

* Correspondence: chenjing55@126.com
Department of Gastrointestinal Surgery, The Fourth Affiliated Hospital of China Medical University, Chongshan road 4th, Huanggu district, Shenyang 110032, Liaoning, China

Main text

Introduction

Gastric cancer is one of the most common malignancies and was one of the five most commonly diagnosed cancers in China in 2015. The estimated incidence in 2015 was 679,100, including 477,700 men and 201,400 women. It was also the second leading cause of cancer death in China, with an estimated total mortality of 498,000, including 339,300 men and 158,700 women. Worldwide, gastric cancer was also the fourth most common cancer. [1, 2]. Thereby, adequate and timely treatment is necessary for patients with gastric cancer. Curative resection remains the most essential treatment for patients with gastric cancer. However, postoperative clinical pathological staging is equally crucial for guiding postoperative therapy. The most commonly and extensively used staging system for gastric cancer is the Union for International Cancer Control (UICC)/American Joint Committee on Cancer (AJCC) tumor, lymph node, and metastases (TNM) staging system. The TNM staging system classifies patients with gastric cancer into various stages based on the depth of primary tumor invasion (T stage), regional lymph node metastases (N stage), and distant metastases (M stage) [3–5]. However, "stage migration" is frequent and occurs in 10–25% of cases [6]. The 7th edition TNM staging system requires that at least 15 lymph nodes be examined to obtain an accurate lymph node metastatic category. However, the surgeon's technical expertise, the pathologist's experience, and other unavoidable conditions may result in less than 15 lymph nodes examined, which has been deemed inadequate [7].

The phenomenon of stage migration is caused by an insufficient number of lymph nodes examined [4, 5, 8]. This phenomenon can lead to inaccurate classification and may affect guidance for postoperative therapy. In order to reduce stage migration, some investigators have proposed using the LNR, namely the ratio between positive lymph nodes compared with the total number of lymph nodes examined, as a new prognostic indicator for gastric cancer. LNR has been confirmed to be a simple and reproducible prognostic tool, even in the case of limited lymph node dissection [6]. There have been a series of reports that show that LNR may effectively reduce the phenomenon of stage migration. Additionally, some studies have reported LNR to be an independent prognostic factor [8–13].

In the present study, we retrospectively evaluated the prognostic significance of LNR in 221 gastric cancer patients. We aimed to evaluate the prognostic significance and clinical value of the metastatic LNR in patients who underwent curative gastrectomy, with a potential goal of enhancing and the 7th edition TNM staging system.

Methods

Patients

This retrospective study included 221 patients who underwent curative gastrectomy for a definite histological diagnosis of gastric cancer between 2005 and 2012 at the Fourth Hospital Affiliated of China Medical University. All 221 candidates had undergone chest radiography, abdominal computed tomography (CT), and gastroscopy. Patient eligibility criteria included the following: [1] R0 curative gastrectomy, [2] accurate histopathological examination, [3] no less than a D2 lymph node dissection, [4] no identifiable distant metastasis in the liver, peritoneum, and so on, [5] no recurrent gastric carcinoma or gastric stump carcinoma, [7] survived the perioperative period, [8] no neoadjuvant chemotherapy

or other preoperative chemotherapy, and [9] complete medical record and follow-up data.

R0 curative gastrectomy was defined as no macroscopic and microscopic remaining tumor tissue in the margin of the resected specimens. D2 lymphadenectomy involved the removal of the N1 nodes, defined as the perigastric lymph node stations 1, 3, and 5 along the lesser curvature of the stomach and perigastric lymph node stations 2, 4, and 6 along the greater curvature of the stomach. N2 was defined as perigastric lymph node stations 7 (along the left gastric artery), 8 (along the common hepatic artery), 9 (along the celiac artery), and 10 (along the splenic artery) [14].

Study patients were divided to two groups. Group 1 included 178 patients who had 15 or more lymph nodes examined (sufficient group). Group 2 included 43 patients who had less than 15 lymph nodes examined (insufficient group).

Our study was performed in accordance with the ethical standards of the World Medical Association Declaration of Helsinki. All 221 patients provided their written informed consent to participate in this study. Our study was approved by the independent ethics committees at the Fourth Hospital Affiliated of China Medical University.

Statistical analysis

SPSS (Statistical Product and Service Solutions) software version 19.0 for Windows (SPSS Inc. Chicago, IL, USA) was used for all statistical analyses. The differences between clinicopathological variables were compared by the Kaplan-Meier method. The statistical significance of the differences between different survival curves was examined by the log-rank test. The Cox proportional hazard regression model was used to perform multivariate statistical survival analysis. The cut-off values of subgroups of T stage, N stage, and TNM stage were based on the 7th AJCC/UICC TNM staging system. The cut-off values of LNR were 0, 0.13 (2/15), and 0.4 (6/15). The subgroups of LNR were defined as R0 (LNR = 0), R1 ($0 <$ LNR ≤ 0.13), R2 ($0.13 <$ LNR ≤ 0.4), and R3 (LNR $>$ 0.4). The independent variables analyzed were as follows: [1] sex (male versus female), [2] age (< 65 versus ≥ 65), [3] tumor location (lower third versus middle third versus upper third), [4] grade (poorly differentiated versus well differentiated and moderately differentiated), [5] T stage (T1 versus T2 versus T3 versus T4), [7] N stage (N0 versus N1 versus N2 versus N3), [8] TNM stage (I versus II versus III), [9] total number of examined lymph nodes (< 15 versus ≥ 15), and [10] the ratio between metastatic lymph nodes and examined lymph nodes (R0 versus R1 versus R2 versus R3). A p value of less than 0.05 was defined as statistically significant for all analyses in this study.

Results

Clinical and histopathology data

Of 221 patients, 160 (72.4%) patients were male and 61 (27.4%) were female. The median age was 64 (range 37 to 85) years. The median survival time was 42 months with a 5-year survival rate of 29.0%. There was a total of 6606 lymph nodes resected with an average of 29.9 ± 1.1 (mean ± standard error) and a median of 30 (range 1 to 105). The number of patients who had greater than or equal to 15 lymph nodes resected was 178 (80.5%); 43 patients (19.5%) had fewer than 15 lymph nodes resected. There were 1503 positive lymph nodes in the entire cohort, with an average of 6.8 ± 0.7 (mean ± standard error) and a median of 2 (range 0 to 50). Regarding tumor grade, 51 (23.1%) patients had tumors that were well differentiated or moderately differentiated histologically; 170 (76.9%) had poorly differentiated tumors. Regarding tumor location, there were 180 (81.4%), 13 (5.9%), and 28 (12.7%) tumors in the lower, middle, and upper groups, respectively. Patients were divided to four groups based on T stage (T1, T2, T3, and T4); there were 23 (10.4%), 39 (17.6%), 98 (44.3%), and 61 (27.6%) patients in each group respectively. Concerning N stage, there were 67 (30.3%), 46 (20.8%), 34 (15.4%), and 74 (33.5%) patients in the N0, N1, N2, and N3 groups, respectively. With regard to TNM stage, all patients were divided into three groups according to stage I, II, and III; there were 43 (19.5%), 63 (28.5%), and 115 (52.0%) patients in each staging group, respectively. All clinical and histopathology data is presented in Table 1.

Univariate and multivariate analysis

In the univariate analysis, there were nine clinicopathological variables tested to verify statistical significance in comparing overall survival (OS) among all 221 patients. The clinicopathological variables included sex, age at surgery, tumor grade, tumor location, T stage, N stage, TNM stage, LN (the number of lymph nodes resected), and LNR (the ratio between metastatic lymph nodes and examined lymph nodes). Ultimately, tumor grade ($p < 0.001$), T stage ($p < 0.001$), N stage ($p < 0.001$), TNM stage ($p < 0.001$), and LNR ($p < 0.001$) were statistically significant (Fig. 1). The results of the univariate analysis, which included median survival time and p value, are presented in Table 2. All nine clinicopathological variables were included in the multivariate analysis by the Cox proportional-hazards model (forward stepwise procedure). The multivariate analysis showed that tumor grade, T stage, N stage, and LNR still had statistical significance. The result of the multivariate analysis is presented in Table 3.

In this study, we focused on LNR (the ratio between metastatic lymph nodes and examined lymph nodes) in the sufficient group (group 1, LN ≥ 15) and

Table 1 Clinical and histopathology data of all 221 patients

Variables	Number of patients	Percent (%)
Sex		
Male	160	72.4
Female	61	27.6
Age (years)		
≥ 65	100	45.2
< 65	121	54.8
Grade		
Well or moderately differentiated	51	23.1
Poorly differentiated	170	76.9
Location		
Lower	180	81.4
Middle	13	5.9
Upper	28	12.7
T stage		
T1	23	10.4
T2	39	17.6
T3	98	44.3
T4	61	27.6
N stage		
N0	67	30.3
N1	46	20.8
N2	34	15.4
N3	74	33.5
TNM stage		
I	43	19.5
II	63	28.5
III	115	52.0
LN		
< 15	43	19.5
≥ 15	178	80.5
LNR		
0	68	30.8
0–0.13	47	21.3
0.13–0.4	54	24.4
> 0.4	52	23.5

The depth of primary tumor invasion (T stage), classification of regional metastasis lymph nodes (N stage), and TNM stage were based on the 7th edition TNM staging system; LN: number of lymph nodes examined; LNR: ratio between the positive lymph nodes and the total number of lymph nodes examined

the insufficient group (group 2, LN < 15). In group 1, the total number of patients who had greater than or equal to 15 lymph nodes resected was 178; there were 57 (32.0%), 38 (21.3%), 45 (25.3%), and 38 (21.3%) patients in the r0 (LNR = 0), r1 (0 < LNR ≤ 0.13), r2 (0.13 < LNR ≤ 0.4), and r3 (LNR > 0.4) groups, respectively.

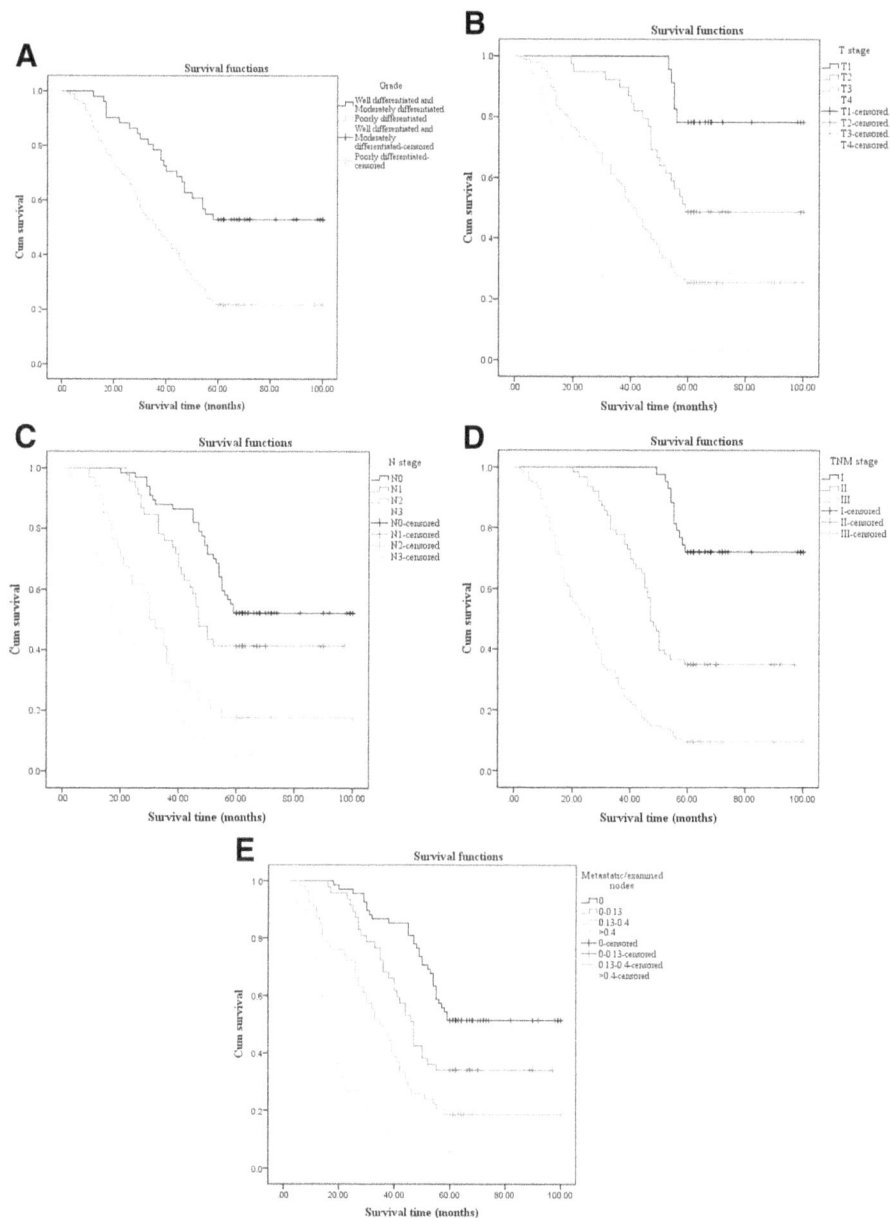

Fig. 1 The factors with statistical significance of univariate analysis and panels **a** to **e** reveal the survival curves of grade, T stage, N stage, TNM stage, and LNR, respectively

The univariate analysis showed a statistically significant result ($p < 0.001$) in comparing LNR (Fig. 2a). On the other hand, there were 43 patients who had fewer than 15 lymph nodes in group 2. This group had the following resection rates: r0 (LNR = 0), r1 ($0 < LNR \leq 0.13$), r2 ($0.13 < LNR \leq 0.4$), and r3 (LNR > 0.4) had 11 (25.6%), 9 (20.9%), 9 (20.9%), and 14 (32.6%) patients, respectively. We still obtained a statistically significant result ($p < 0.001$) in the univariate analysis (Fig. 2b). The results of the univariate analysis of LNR in groups 1 and 2 are presented in Table 4.

Although the univariate analysis showed a statistically significant result in group 2, we abandoned the method that divided patients in group 2 into four subgroups. We found another way to evaluate prognostic significance of LNR in group 2, to make the result more accurate. We compared all 221 patients who had R0 resections with those who had R1, R2, and R3 resections, respectively. Then, we found that R3 had the maximum chi-square value. These results are shown in Table 5. Finally, we chose 0.4 as a new cut-off value in group 2 and divided patients into two groups, LNr1 (LN $\leq$ 0.4) and LNr2 (LN

Table 2 Univariate Analysis of 221 Patients with curative gastrectomy

Variables	Median survival (month)	p value
Sex		0.824
Male	44.0	
Female	41.0	
Age (years)		0.482
≥ 65	41.0	
< 65	42.0	
Grade		< 0.001
Well or moderately differentiated	61.0	
Poorly differentiated	36.0	
Location		0.405
Lower	40.5	
Middle	45.0	
Upper	50.0	
T stage		< 0.001
T1	64.0	
T2	59.0	
T3	41.5	
T4	25.0	
N stage		< 0.001
N0	60.0	
N1	47.0	
N2	31.0	
N3	18.5	
TNM stage		< 0.001
I	62.0	
II	47.0	
III	26.0	
LN		0.895
< 15	44.0	
≥ 15	41.5	
LNR		< 0.001
0	60.0	
0–0.13	47.0	
0.13–0.4	35.5	
> 0.4	17.0	

The depth of primary tumor invasion (T stage), classification of regional metastasis lymph nodes (N stage) and TNM stage were based on the 7th edition TNM staging system; LN: number of lymph nodes examined; LNR: ratio between the positive lymph nodes and the total number of lymph nodes examined

Table 3 Multivariable analysis of all Variables using Cox proportional hazard regression model

Variables	HR	p value	95.0% CI	
			Lower	Upper
Grade				
Well or moderately differentiated	1			
Poorly differentiated	0.442	< 0.001	0.284	0.689
T stage				
T1	1			
T2	0.086	< 0.001	0.033	0.228
T3	0.225	< 0.001	0.128	0.395
T4	0.277	< 0.001	0.189	0.407
N stage				
N0	1			
N1	0.066	0.009	0.009	0.507
N2	0.341	0.002	0.172	0.674
N3	0.580	0.036	0.348	0.965
LNR				
0	1			
0–0.13	2.358	0.402	0.317	17.519
0.13–0.4	0.721	0.342	0.368	1.414
> 0.4	0.427	< 0.001	0.277	0.659

CI: confidence interval

Discussion

Gastric cancer, one of the most common malignant neoplasms in the world, results in the death of thousands every year, especially in China [1, 5, 15]. After curative resection of gastric cancer was implemented, the possibility to extend survival has been a topic of exploration for investigators globally, as extending life is always a consistent goal. Thus, the factors that influence prognosis after curative resection in gastric cancer have been extensively studied. Indisputably, lymph node stage (N stage) is one of the foremost prognostic factors [16–18]. Many studies have shown that the 5-year survival rate of gastric cancer patients with positive lymph nodes is significantly lower than in those without lymph node metastasis. Moreover, as the number of lymph node metastases increases, prognosis gradually decreases. Not only metastasis lymph node stage but also the total number of lymph nodes examined is an important factor that influences prognosis. It has been demonstrated that the number of lymph nodes is an independent prognostic factor and a larger number of lymph nodes can lead to a higher 5-year overall survival rate [19–24]. The TNM staging system, a tool to evaluate prognosis of patients who had curative resection of gastric cancer, is current and accepted comprehensively by surgeons. In the 7th Union for International Cancer Control (UICC)/American Joint Committee on Cancer (AJCC) tumor, lymph node, metastasis (TNM) staging system

> 0.4). We were then able to obtain a statistically significant result (p value < 0.001) by comparing these two subgroups (Fig. 3). The LNr1 and LNr2 groups had 29 (67.4%) and 14 (32.6%) patients, respectively.

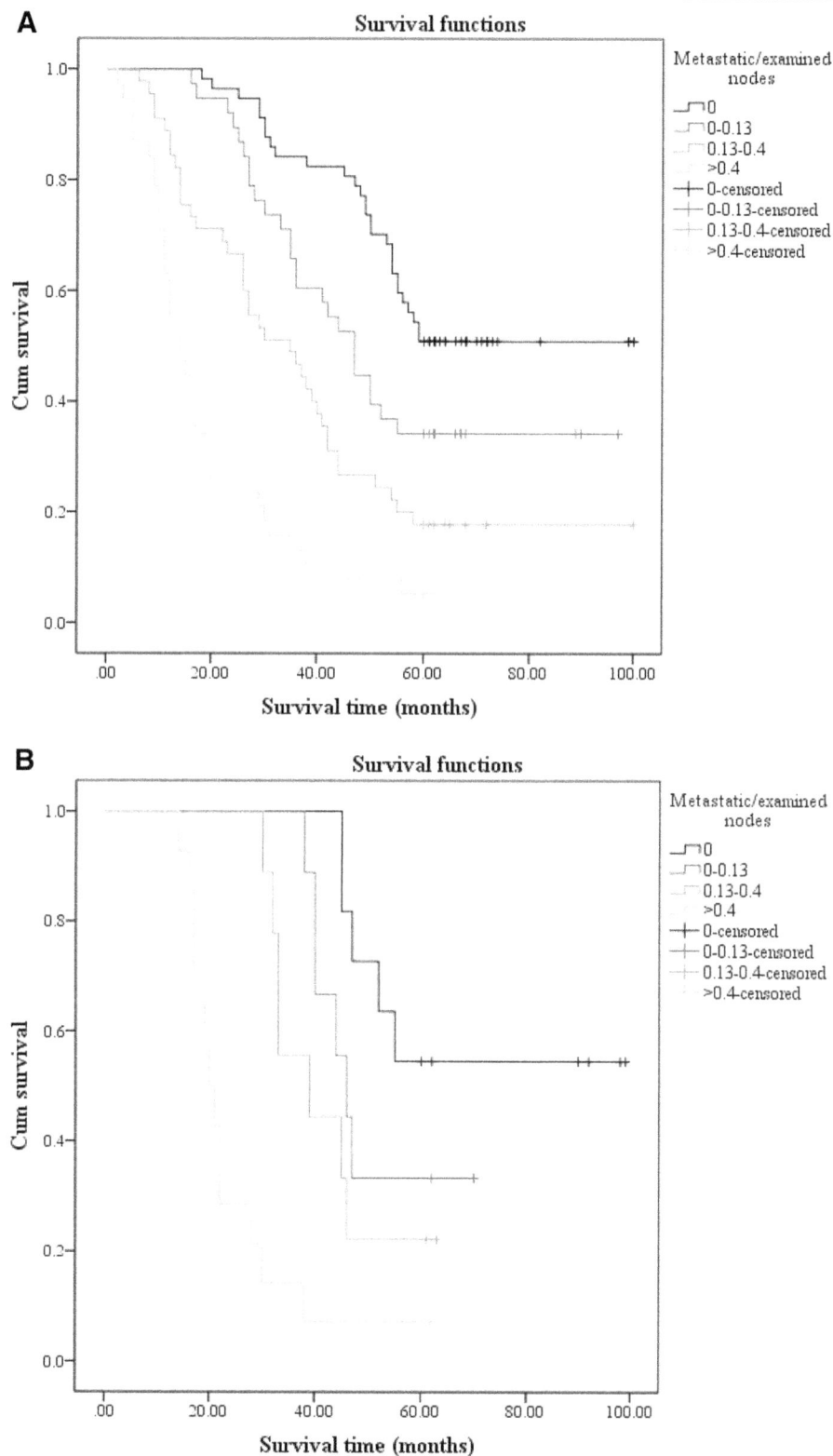

Fig. 2 The survival curves of LNR in group 1 (LN ≥ 15) and group 2 (LN < 15), respectively. Panels **a** and **b** reveal the survival curves of LNR in group 1 (LN ≥ 15) and LNR in group 2 (LN < 15), respectively

Table 4 Univariate analysis of LNR in groups with ≥ 15 and <
15 lymph nodes examined

	Number of patients	Percent (%)	Median survival (month)	p value
Group 1				
LNR				< 0.001
0	57	32.0	60.0	
0–0.13	38	21.3	47.0	
0.13–0.4	45	25.3	35.0	
> 0.4	38	21.3	14.0	
Group 2				
LNR				< 0.001
0	11	25.6	60.0	
0–0.13	9	20.9	46.0	
0.13–0.4	9	20.9	39.0	
> 0.4	14	32.6	20.5	

published in 2010, metastatic lymph nodes are essential in prognostication. However, properly classifying lymph node metastasis is limited by the number of lymph nodes. This system requires that at least 15 lymph nodes be examined postoperatively to obtain precise N staging, in order to avoid inaccurate staging. When the number of lymph nodes is > 15, the number of lymph node metastases is more accurate in assessing prognosis. However, if the number of lymph nodes is insufficient, the phenomenon of stage migration occurs [4, 5, 8, 10]. In addition, increasing the number of lymph nodes examined can lead to a higher 5-year survival rate. Hence, obtaining more lymph nodes from the postoperative specimen was deemed to be necessary and useful. Most surgeons follow the UICC/AJCC guide and remove a sufficient number of lymph nodes. Nevertheless, there are still some reasons that lead to fewer than 15 lymph nodes being obtained at surgery. Insufficiency of the technique itself, surgeon experience, or the lymph nodes in the specimen being too small may be reasons leading to a lesser number of lymph nodes being examined [7, 25]. Thus, many investigators have investigated finding a method to reduce that phenomenon. In recent years, LNR has been provided superior prognostic information over the N category according to the TNM classification in breast, colon, and rectal cancer [26]. Some investigators have proposed that LNR could be a new prognostic indicator and have demonstrated LNR to be an

Table 5 Comparisons of overall survival between R0 and R1, R2, or R3

	Median survival (month)	Chi-square	p value
R1	47.0	6.999	0.008
R2	35.5	28.101	< 0.001
R3	17.0	82.490	< 0.001

independent prognostic factor in gastric cancer. It has also been attested that the LNR may reduce the phenomenon of stage migration [10, 13, 27–29].

We aimed to determine the prognostic significance of the metastatic LNR as a new tool to evaluate prognosis of patients with curative gastrectomy. In our study, we found that tumor grade, T stage, N stage, TNM stage, and LNR were the factors that influenced prognosis of patients according to the univariate analysis. Patients with a better differentiated pathological type, an earlier stage of T staging, N staging, and TNM staging, and a lower LNR have improved survival rates. However, when all nine factors are entered into the Cox proportional-hazards model, the multivariable analysis showed that only grade, T stage, N stage, and LNR showed statistical significance. LNR still had statistical significance in both the univariate and multivariable analysis. Thus, our study again demonstrated that LNR was an independent prognostic factor. With increased LNR, OS decreases. Thus, LNR may have value for evaluating prognosis. LNR could become a new tool to estimate prognosis in patients who undergo curative gastrectomy.

Although LNR is an independent prognostic factor, further research is required. We have evaluated the influence of LNR on prognosis in group 1 (LN ≥ 15) and group 2 (LN < 15). In our study, we set cut-off values (0, 0.13, and 0.4) based on N stage of the TNM staging system. The advantages of and reasons for choosing this cut-off value were convenience and ease, which should be important characteristics for any prognostic system used by physicians. Ultimately, we divided all patients in each group into four subgroups (R0, R1, R2, and R3) according to LNR, respectively.

In group 1, there were 178 patients, who were divided into the following four subgroups: r0 (LNR = 0), r1 (0 < LNR ≤ 0.13), r2 (0.13 < LNR ≤ 0.4), and r3 (LNR > 0.4). We compared the four subgroups with regard to survival time, and the univariate analysis showed statistical significance between the four subgroups. Patients in the r0 group had a maximal median survival time of 60.0 months, and the median survival time of patients in the r3 group was minimal (14.0 months). Thus, we considered that when LN ≥ 15, the LNR had value in evaluating prognosis of patients with curative gastrectomy and the median survival time decreased with increasing LNR. In group 2, we still obtained a statistically significant result between r0 (LNR = 0), r1 (0 < LNR ≤ 0.13), r2 (0.13 < LNR ≤ 0.4), and r3 (LNR > 0.4). The univariate analysis showed that different LNRs can lead to different prognoses.

It appeared that LNR may be a prognostic indicator for patients, regardless of number of lymph nodes examined, according to our study results. However, we did not think that the method of grouping that divided all patients into four groups was suitable for group 2. On the one hand, we had a small sample size and the number of patients with

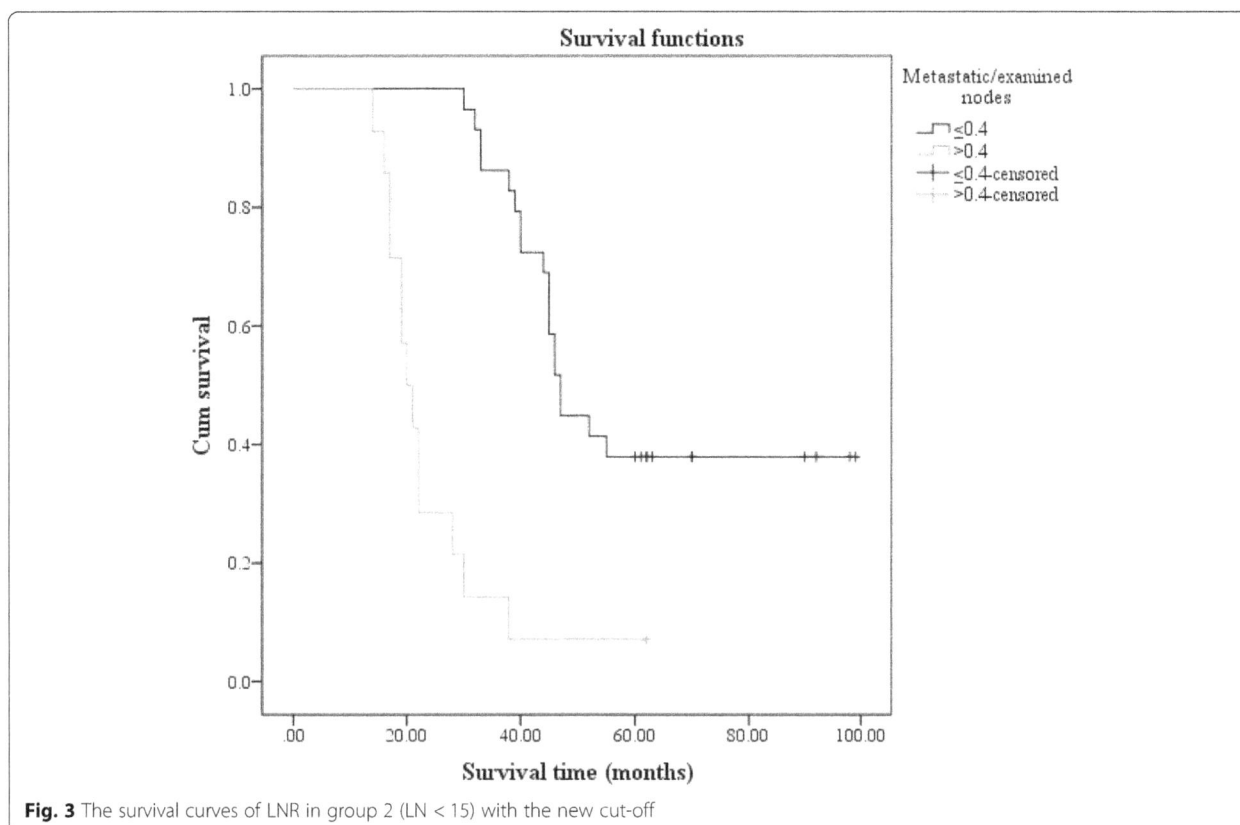

Fig. 3 The survival curves of LNR in group 2 (LN < 15) with the new cut-off

LN < 15 examined was only 43. On the other hand, when the number of lymph nodes examined was less than 15, increasing or decreasing the number by one lymph node would lead to a larger variation of LNR. For example, when the number of metastatic lymph nodes increased by one for patients with five lymph nodes examined, the LNR would increase by 0.2. But the LNR would increase by only 0.07 when the total number of lymph nodes examined was 15. Thus, it would be imprecise for prognostication if we divided the patients with fewer than 15 lymph nodes into too many subgroups.

Finally, we decided to divide our patients into two subgroups: LNr1 and LNr2. The cut-off value was chosen in this way: we compared all four subgroups of LNR, regardless of the number of lymph nodes examined. We compared R0 with R1, R2, and R3 and found that R3 had the largest significant statistical difference compared with R0. Ultimately, we chose 0.4 as the cut-off value and divided patients with LN < 15 examined into two subgroups. The univariate analysis showed a statistically significant result (Fig. 3). And the median survival time of patients with LNR that greater than 0.4 was 20.5 months. The other patients who had an LNR less than or equal to 0.4 had a higher median survival time (47.0 months). That result meant that LNR had value in evaluating prognosis of patients with fewer than 15

lymph nodes examined and the median survival time decreased with increasing LNR.

The TNM staging system has some disadvantages that could be improved. LNR, as a new research direction, has been shown to have value in estimating prognosis. Our study demonstrated that LNR was an independent prognostic factor. Either in patients with greater than or equal to 15 LN examined, or fewer than 15 LN, LNR could estimate prognosis and OS was shown to decrease with increasing LNR. We found that there was no correlation between LNR and the total number of harvested LNs. In other words, patients with identical LNR, even with differing numbers of detected metastatic nodes, will have a similar outcome. Conversely, among patients with the same number of metastatic nodes, those with a higher LNR will have an unfavorable outcome [30]. Thus, the LNR could be a new prognostic indicator to enhance the TNM staging system.

Conclusions

In conclusion, LNR can estimate prognosis in patients who undergo curative gastrectomy, regardless of the number of LNs examined. Thus, LNR may become a new indicator to evaluate prognosis after curative gastrectomy and enhance the current TNM staging system.

Abbreviations
AJCC: American Joint Committee on Cancer; CT: Computed tomography; LNR: Lymph node ratio; OS: Overall survival; SPSS: Statistical Product and Service Solutions; TNM: Tumor, lymph node, metastasis; UICC: Union for International Cancer Control

Acknowledgements
We thank International Science Editing (http://www.internationalscienceediting.com) for editing this manuscript.

Authors' contributions
XW collected data of the patients who got gastric cancer and underwent curative gastrectomy. YH and JC analyzed and interpreted the patient data. YH wrote the paper and was a major contributor in writing the manuscript. All authors read and approved the final manuscript.

Competing interests
The authors declare that they have no competing interests.

References
1. MD WCPD, Zheng R, Baade PD, et al. Cancer statistics in China, 2015 [J]. Ca A Cancer J Clinicians. 2016;66(2):115–32.
2. Kamangar F, Dores GM, Anderson WF. Patterns of cancer incidence, mortality, and prevalence across five continents: defining priorities to reduce cancer disparities in different geographic regions of the world [J]. J Clin Oncol. 2006;24(14):2137–50.
3. Coburn NG, Swallow CJ, Kiss A, et al. Significant regional variation in adequacy of lymph node assessment and survival in gastric cancer. [J]. Cancer. 2006;107(9):2143–51.
4. Sobin LHGM, Wittekind CH. International Union Against Cancer (UICC) TNM classification of malignant tumors. 7th ed. New York: Wiley-Lwass; 2010.
5. Edge SB, Byrd DR, Compton CC, Fritz AG, Greene FL, Trotti A, editors. AJCC Cancer staging manual. 7th ed. New York: Springer; 2010.
6. Pedrazzani C, Sivins A, et al. Ratio between metastatic and examined lymph nodes (N ratio) may have low clinical utility in gastric cancer patients treated by limited lymphadenectomy: results from a single-center experience of 526 patients [J]. World J Surg. 2010;34(1):85–91.
7. Chen S, Zhao BW, Li YF, et al. The prognostic value of harvested lymph nodes and the metastatic lymph node ratio for gastric cancer patients: results of a study of 1,101 patients [J]. PLoS One. 2011;7(11):e49424.
8. Manzoni GD, Verlato G, Roviello F, et al. The new TNM classification of lymph node metastasis minimizes stage migration problems in gastric cancer patients [J]. Br J Cancer. 2002;87(2):171–4.
9. Okusa T, Nakane Y, Boku T, et al. Quantitative analysis of nodal involvement with respect to survival rate after curative gastrectomy for carcinoma. [J]. Surg Gynecol Obstet. 1990;170(6):488–94.
10. Inoue K, Nakane Y, Iiyama H, et al. The superiority of ratio-based lymph node staging in gastric carcinoma [J]. Ann Surg Oncol. 2002;9(1):27–34.
11. Nitti D, Marchet A, Olivieri M, et al. Ratio between metastatic and examined lymph nodes was an independent prognostic factor after D2 resection for gastric cancer: analysis of a large European Monoinstitutional experience [J]. Ann Surg Oncol. 2003;10(9):1077–85.
12. Celen O, Yildirim E, Berberoglu U. Prognostic impact of positive lymph node ratio in gastric carcinoma [J]. J Surg Oncol. 2007;96(2):95–101.
13. Marchet A, Mocellin S, Ambrosi A, et al. The ratio between metastatic and examined lymph nodes (N ratio) is an independent prognostic factor in gastric cancer regardless of the type of lymphadenectomy: results from an Italian multicentric study in 1853 patients.[J]. Ann Surg. 2007;245(4):543–52.
14. Association J G C. Japanese classification of gastric carcinoma: 3rd English edition [J]. Gastric Cancer. 2011;14(2):101–12.
15. Jemal A, Siegel R, Ward E, et al. Cancer statistics, 2009[J]. Ca A Cancer J Clinicians. 2009;59(4):225–49.
16. Siewert JR, Böttcher K, Stein HJ, et al. Relevant prognostic factors in gastric cancer: ten-year results of the German gastric cancer study. [J]. Ann Surg. 1998;228(4):449–61.
17. Wu CW, Hsieh MC, Lo SS, et al. Relation of number of positive lymph nodes to the prognosis of patients with primary gastric adenocarcinoma[J]. Gut. 1996;38(4):525–7.
18. Yokota T, Kunii Y, Teshima S, et al. Significant prognostic factors in patients with early gastric cancer. [J]. Int Surg. 2000;85(4):286–90.
19. Chu X, Yang ZF. Impact on survival of the number of lymph nodes resected in patients with lymph node-negative gastric cancer [J]. World J Surg Oncol. 2015;13(1):1–8.
20. Hsu JT, Lin CJ, Sung CM, et al. Prognostic significance of the number of examined lymph nodes in node-negative gastric adenocarcinoma [J]. Eur J Surg Oncol. 2013;39(11):1287–93.
21. Jiao XG, Deng JY, Zhang RP, et al. Prognostic value of number of examined lymph nodes in patients with node-negative gastric cancer. [J]. World J Gastroenterol. 2014;20(13):3640.
22. Smith DD, Schwarz RR, Schwarz RE. Impact of total lymph node count on staging and survival after gastrectomy for gastric cancer: data from a large US-population database. [J]. J Clin Oncol. 2005;23(23):7114–24.
23. Schwarz RE, Smith DD. Clinical impact of lymphadenectomy extent in resectable gastric cancer of advanced stage [J]. Ann Surg Oncol. 2007; 14(2):317–28.
24. Song W, Yuan Y, Wang L, et al. The prognostic value of lymph nodes dissection number on survival of patients with lymph node-negative gastric cancer. [J]. Gastroenterol Res Pract. 2014;2014(1):603194.
25. Wong SL, Hong J, Hollenbeck BK, et al. Hospital lymph node examination rates and survival after resection for colon cancer [J]. JAMA. 2007;298(18):2149–54.
26. Lemmens VEPP, Dassen AE, et al. Lymph node examination among patients with gastric cancer: variation between departments of pathology and prognostic impact of lymph node ratio [J]. Eur J Surg Oncol. 2011;37(6):488–96.
27. Alatengbaolide LD, Li Y, et al. Lymph node ratio is an independent prognostic factor in gastric cancer after curative resection (R0) regardless of the examined number of lymph nodes[J]. Am J Clin Oncol. 2013;36(4):325.
28. Maduekwe UN, Lauwers GY, Fernandezdelcastillo C, et al. A new metastatic lymph node ratio system reduces stage migration in patients undergoing D1 lymphadenectomy for gastric adenocarcinoma [J]. Ann Surg Oncol. 2010;17(5):1267–77.
29. Ibrahim S, Dogu et al. does N ratio affect survival in D1 and D2 lymph node dissection for gastric cancer? World J Gastroenterol. 2011;17(35):4007–12.
30. Persiani R, Rausei S, et al. Ratio of metastatic lymph nodes: impact on staging and survival of gastric cancer [J]. Eur J Surg Oncol. 2008;34(5):519–24.

23

Application of red light phototherapy in the treatment of radioactive dermatitis in patients with head and neck cancer

Xudong Zhang[†], Hongfei Li[†], Qian Li, Ying Li, Chao Li, Minmin Zhu, Bing Zhao and Guowen Li[*]

Abstract

Background: To observe the effect of red light phototherapy (RLPT) on radioactive dermatitis (RD) caused by radiotherapy in patients with head and neck cancer (HNC).

Methods: Sixty patients with HNC admitted to our hospital were randomly divided into experimental group and control group, 30 patients in each group. The control group received routine daily care during radiotherapy treatment. In the experimental group, in addition to routine daily care during radiotherapy treatment, photon therapy apparatus RLPT was added, 10 min/time, 2 times/day, and lasted until the end of radiotherapy. The pain and conditions of the patients' skin were assessed daily, and the skin pain and dermatitis grades of the two groups were compared.

Results: In terms of the reaction degree of RD, experimental group was mainly grade 0–2, and control group was mainly grade 2–3, with a significant difference ($P < 0.05$). In terms of skin pain, according to the pain records at week 2, 3, and 4, the pain degree increased with time. However, the score of wound pain in experimental group was significantly lower than that in control group, and there was a significant difference between the two groups ($P < 0.05$).

Conclusions: The application of RLPT in the treatment of RD can help accelerate wound healing and significantly shorten healing time. It can not only reduce wounds pain of patients, promote inflammation and ulcer healing, but also ensure the smooth progress of patients' radiotherapy and improve their quality of lives, which is worth popularization and application in the clinical practice.

Keywords: Radioactive dermatitis, Red light phototherapy, Nasopharyngeal carcinoma, Head and neck cancer

Background

Head and neck cancer (HNC), represented by nasopharyngeal carcinoma (NPC), is one of the most frequent cancers in China and Southeast Asia countries, and its incidence is increasing gradually. Due to its anatomical and pathological characteristics, radiotherapy is still the main method to treat NPC [1]. However, radiation-induced skin reaction is the most common complication of tumor radiotherapy, and its incidence is high. About 87% of patients with radiotherapy will have erythema and more serious radioactive skin reactions [2, 3]. Radioactive dermatitis (RD) is mainly caused by skin exposure to high energy physical radiation, resulting in skin mucosal inflammatory damage. It manifests as erythema, epithelial shedding, skin ulcers, and pain. Severe cases can cause local or systemic infection. As the red light of visible light (the wavelength is 600–700 nm), photochemical effect has a physiotherapy effect on the body [4]. The application of red light phototherapy (RLPT) to systemic burn wounds has achieved good results in relieving pain and preventing cross infection [5, 6]. Based on the clinical practice of our hospital, we have done some summative research to confirm the positive therapeutic effect of RLPT on RD.

Methods
Patients
Sixty patients with HNC admitted to our hospital from January 2017 to July 2017 were selected in this research. Among them, 52 cases were NPC, 4 cases were laryngeal

* Correspondence: guowenli12@sohu.com
†Xudong Zhang and Hongfei Li contributed equally to this work.
Radiotherapy inpatient Ward II, The First Affiliated Hospital of Zhengzhou University, No.1 Eastern Jianshe Road, Zhengzhou 450000, Henan, China

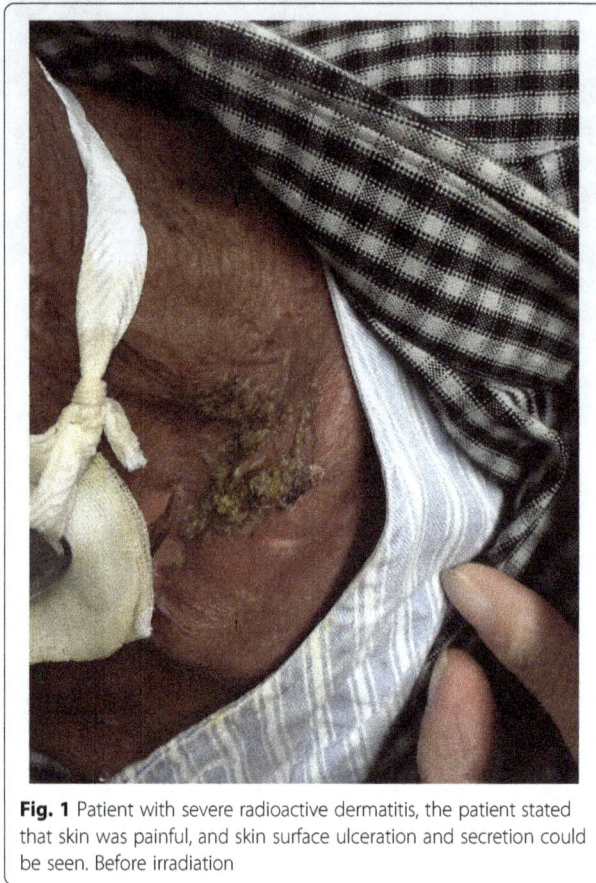

Fig. 1 Patient with severe radioactive dermatitis, the patient stated that skin was painful, and skin surface ulceration and secretion could be seen. Before irradiation

cancer, 2 cases were tonsillar carcinoma, and 2 cases were tongue cancer. And males were 42 cases, accounting for 70%; females were 18 cases, accounting for 30%; aged 24–75 years. In addition, education background below junior high school was 14 cases, accounting for

Table 1 Comparison of general data between two groups

Item	Experimental group ($n = 30$)	Control group ($n = 30$)	x^2/t	P
Gender [n (%)]				
Male	22 (73.3)	20 (66.7)	0.317	0.574
Female	8 (26.7)	10 (33.3)		
Education background [n (%)]				
Below junior high school	6 (20)	8 (26.7)	0.373	0.523
Above junior high school	24 (80)	22 (73.3)		
Payment method [n (%)]				
Medical insurance	29 (96.7)	28 (93.3)		0.500[a]
Self-supporting	1 (3.3)	2 (6.7)		
Age	46.4 ± 11.91	45.23 ± 12.70	0.453	0.667

[a]Fisher's exact test result, no chi-square value

Table 2 Comparison of the degree of radioactive dermatitis reaction between the two groups (n)

Group	Number	Grade 0–1	Grade 2	Grade 3	U	P
Experimental group	30	18	12	0	4.79	0.000
Control group	30	2	19	9		

23%; education background above junior high school was 46 cases, accounting for 77%. All patients received three-dimensional intensity-modulated radiation therapy with 30 to 32 irradiations for 6 weeks. The study not only received informed consent from all patients, but also received the support of the ethics committee of the First Affiliated Hospital of Zhengzhou University (Fig. 1).

Inclusion criteria were ① pathologically diagnosed; ② received chemotherapy and radiotherapy for the first time; and ③ signed the informed consent and willing to involve in this research.

Exclusion criteria were ① patients with communication disorders; and ② patients who were unwilling to take part in this treatment.

Table 3 Comparison of occurrence of skin pain at different times between the two groups

	Group E ($n = 30$)	Group C ($n = 30$)	x^2	P
End of second week				
Mild	2	16	15.56	0.000
Moderate	0	0		
Severe	0	0		
End of third week				
Mild	7	26	24.31	0.000
Moderate	0	0		
Severe	0	0		
End of fourth week				
Mild	16	26	7.94	0.005
Moderate	0	0		
Severe	0	0		
End of fifth week				
Mild	27	30	3.61	0.076
Moderate	0	0		
Severe	0	0		
End of sixth week				
Mild	27	27	1.65	0.098
Moderate	0	3		
Severe	0	0		
x^2	65.083	27.091		
P	0.000	0.000		

Note: Group E is experimental group, and group C is control group

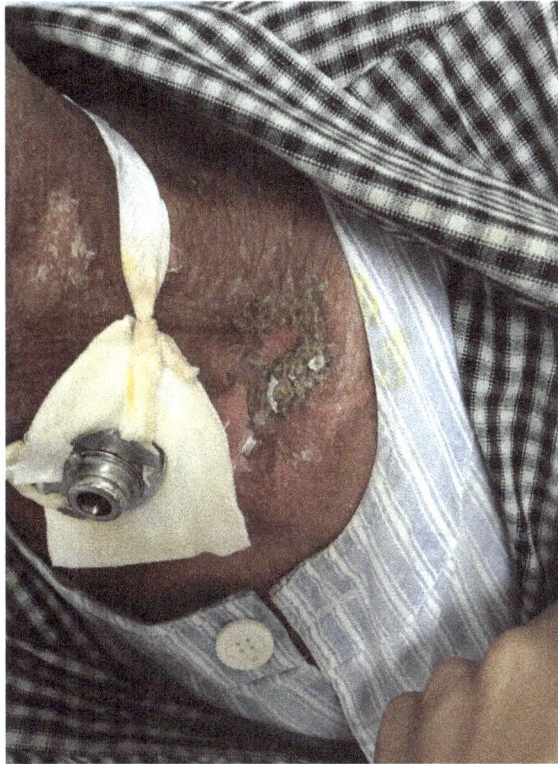

Fig. 2 Patient with severe radioactive dermatitis, the patient stated that skin was painful, and skin surface ulceration and secretion could be seen. The second irradiation, the wound was basically dry and the pain was less than before

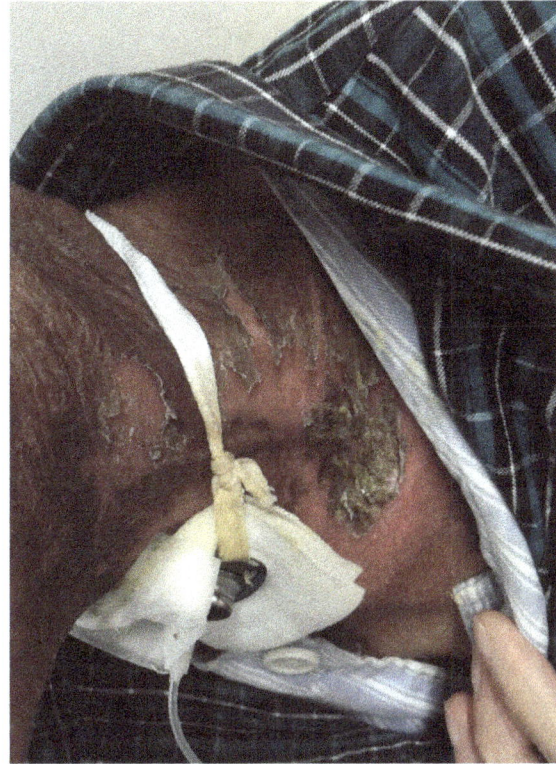

Fig. 3 Patient with severe radioactive dermatitis, the patient stated that skin was painful, and skin surface ulceration and secretion could be seen. The fifth irradiation, the scabs came off, and pain was almost gone

All patients were randomly divided into two groups, control group (*n* = 30) and experimental group (*n* = 30). There was no significant difference in the general data between the two groups, gender distribution ($P > 0.05$), educational background distribution ($P > 0.05$), and payment methods ($P > 0.05$). In terms of age distribution, the experimental group was 46.4 ± 11.91 years old, and the control group was 45.23 ± 12.70 years old; there was no significant difference between the two groups ($P > 0.05$) (Table 1).

Methods

Control group: routine methods of nursing were given during radiotherapy, including health education, skin self-care, and skin protective agent. 0.9% normal saline cotton balls were used to gently clean the wound and remove necrotic tissue, and the wound were dried with sterile gauze.

Experimental group: in addition to gently cleaning the wound with 0.9% normal saline cotton ball to remove the necrotic tissue, the RLPT treatment was also used. The patient was in a supine position, and the radiation field skin was fully exposed. The irradiation time was 10 min, 2 times/day, the lampshade was 15–20 cm from the wound surface, and the wound temperature was 30 °C. In the process of irradiation, doctors and patients should wear sunglasses to avoid eye injuries caused by strong light and the doctors should ask the patients if they are uncomfortable in time. If there is any abnormality, they should timely handle it and record it.

Observation index and curative effect evaluation

The degree of skin reaction and pain in the neck were observed daily during the treatment. Radioactive skin lesions were graded according to the acute radiation response scoring criterion of American Radiation Therapy Oncology Group [7]. Grade 0: no change; grade 1: follicular dark red spots, dry desquamation, depilation, hair loss, and sweat reduction; grade 2: tender or bright red spots, patchy erosion, and moderate edema; grade 3: external position erosion of skin wrinkles and pitting edema; grade 4: ulcer, bleeding, and necrosis. The degree of pain was assessed by the numerical rating scale (NRS), and the degree of pain was expressed as a

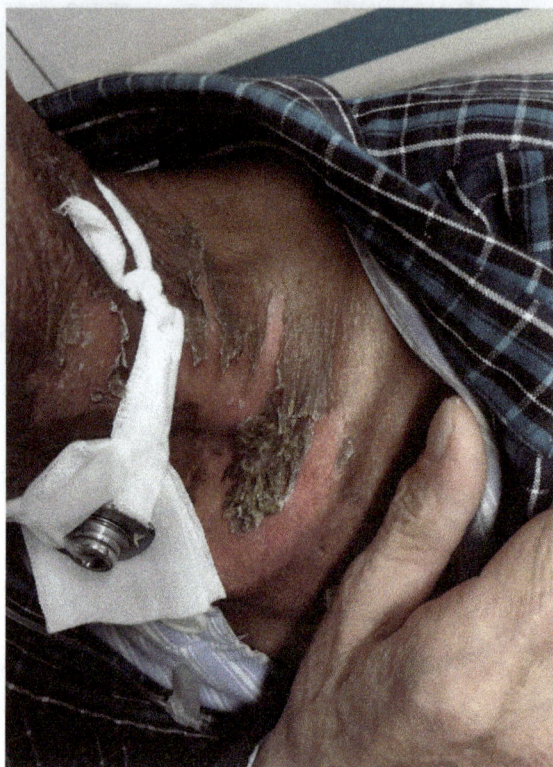

Fig. 4 Patient with severe radioactive dermatitis, the patient stated that skin was painful, and skin surface ulceration and secretion could be seen. The sixth irradiation

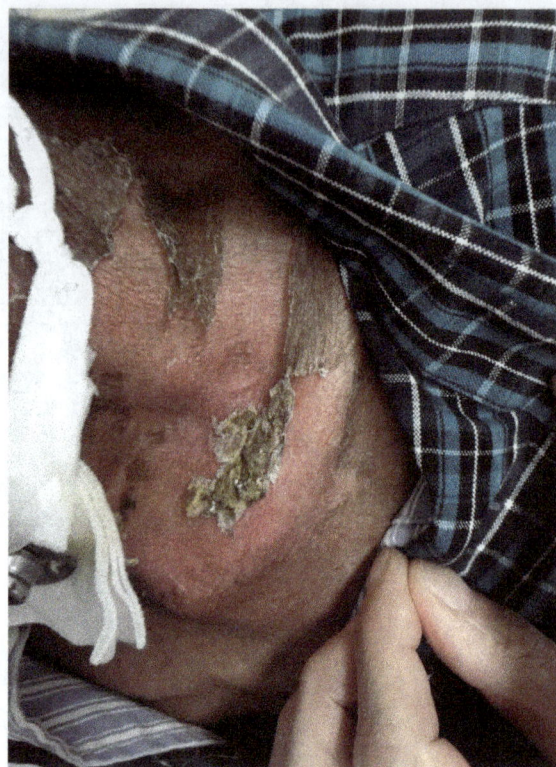

Fig. 5 Patient with severe radioactive dermatitis, the patient stated that skin was painful, and skin surface ulceration and secretion could be seen. The seventh irradiation

number from 0 to 10. 0 was painless; 1–3 was mild pain, which can be tolerated; 4–6 was moderate pain, which is severely disturbed, accompanied by irritability or passive position [8]. The participants chose one of the numbers according to their personal pain feelings. NRS had good reliability and validity, and was easy to record.

Statistical analysis

SPSS17.0 software was used for statistical analysis, and descriptive statistical analysis was performed on general data. Measurement data were expressed as mean ± standard deviation, and the difference between groups was tested by independent sample t test. Chi-square test was used to compare the difference between groups of enumeration data, and non-parametric rank sum test was used to compare the rank data. There was a significant difference at $P < 0.05$.

Results

Comparison of the degree of RD reaction between the two groups

In the experimental group and control group, there was a significant difference in the degree of RD reaction

between the two groups. The experimental group was mainly composed of grade 0–2 RD, including 18 cases (60.00%) of grade 0–1 and 12 cases (40.00%) of grade 2. The control group was mainly composed of grade 2–3 RD, including 19 cases of grade 2 (63.33%), 9 cases of grade 3 (30.00%) and only 2 cases of grade 0–1 (6.67%). It showed that the degree of inflammatory response of the experimental group was lighter than that of the control group. There was a significant difference between the two groups (Table 2).

Comparison of occurrence of skin pain at different times between the two groups

In Table 3, the results showed that there was a significant difference in the occurrence of skin pain at the end of second, third, and fourth week between the two groups ($P < 0.05$), but there was no significant difference at the end of fifth and sixth week between the two groups ($P > 0.05$). Comparison within groups, the chi-square test results of occurrence of skin pain at different time points in the experimental group and the control group were $\chi^2 = 65.083$ and $\chi^2 =$

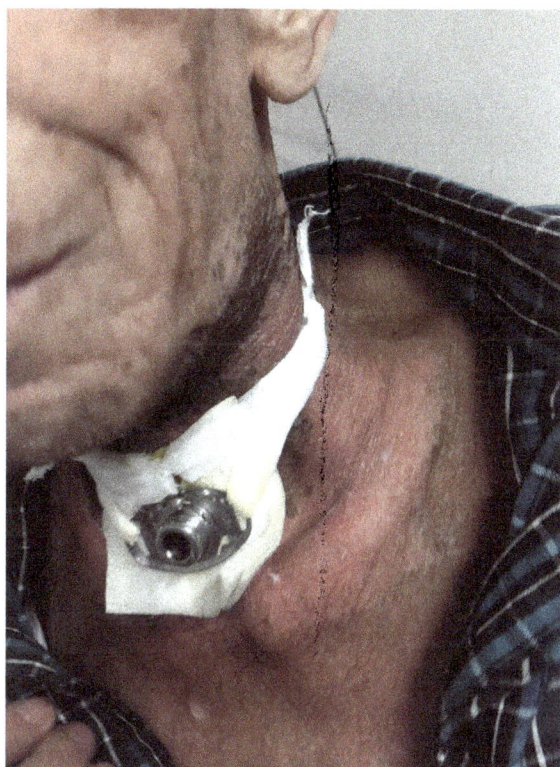

Fig. 6 Patient with severe radioactive dermatitis, the patient stated that skin was painful, and skin surface ulceration and secretion could be seen. The eighth irradiation, and the new skin was basically formed

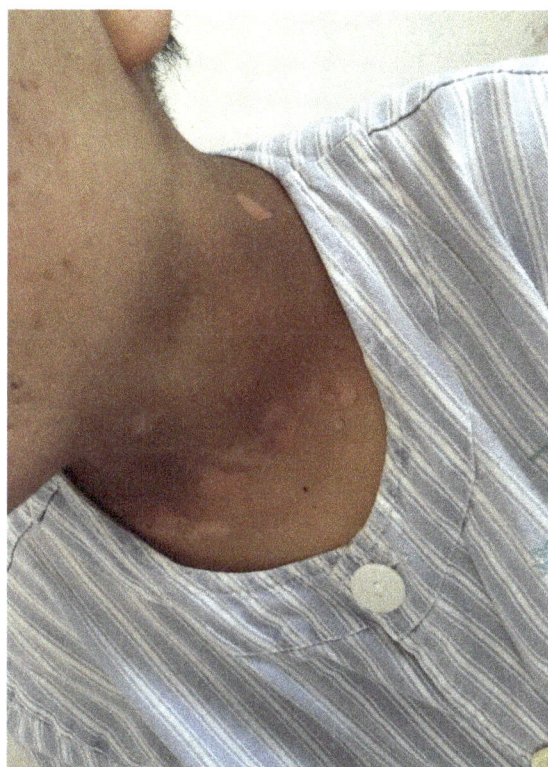

Fig. 7 Patient with severe radioactive dermatitis, the patient stated tingling in the irradiation area, the skin was gray, with multiple small ulcerations and a small amount of seepage

27.091, respectively, with significant differences ($P <$ 0.05). It showed that there was a linear trend in each group, and the occurrence of skin pain increased with time (Figs. 2, 3, and 4).

Discussion

The incidence of HNC ranks sixth in all tumor types and mortality ranks eighth. Radiation therapy is still the main method for treating such cancers [9–11]. The skin reaction caused by radiation is the most common complication of tumor radiotherapy, and its incidence is high. About 87% of patients with radiotherapy will have erythema and more serious radiation skin reactions. For early lesions, 10-year disease-related survival rate, recurrence-free survival rate, and distant metastasis-free survival rate were 98%, 94%, and 98%, respectively. However, due to the high dose of radiotherapy, radiation would cause certain damage to the skin of the irradiated field to form RD [12–15].

RD is mainly due to the skin receives high energy physical radiation, which directly damage the human epidermal cell DNA molecules. It is an inflammatory damage of the skin mucosa caused by radiation (mainly β, γ, and x rays). It is characterized by erythema, epithelial shedding, skin ulcers, and pain. Severe cases can cause local or systemic infection. Acute radioactive skin reactions often cause itching and pain, and delays in treatment can affect appearance and lower quality of life [15–18].

Infrared therapy apparatus adopts high-energy semiconductor chip to integrate cold light source. Its specific wavelength red light photons and high efficient biochemical enzymatic reaction mechanism significantly stimulate fibroblast and endothelial cell growth, promote granulation formation, relieve pain, and accelerate wound healing. Specifically, long-wave infrared light can reach the shallow layer of the skin, while short-wave infrared light may reach deep skin or even subcutaneous tissue, and the red light band (620–760 am) can cause deep tissue vasodilation and circulation improvement [19]. After the application of close-range RLPT in RD, red light is strongly absorbed by the mitochondria of human cells. Through photochemical action, it promotes material metabolism, strengthens the cell activity, promotes the proliferation of epithelial tissue in the wound of the patient, improves the local blood circulation, and speeds up the formation of granulation tissue. On the basis of ensuring skin integrity, it promotes the healing

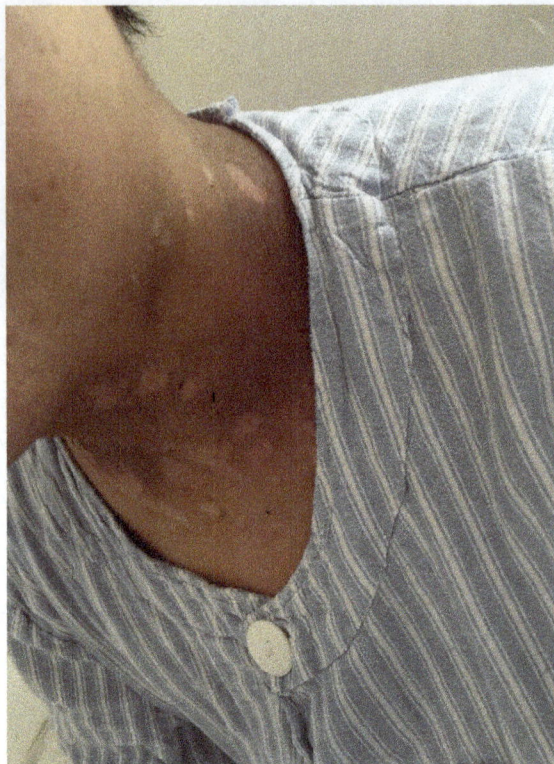

Fig. 8 The second irradiation

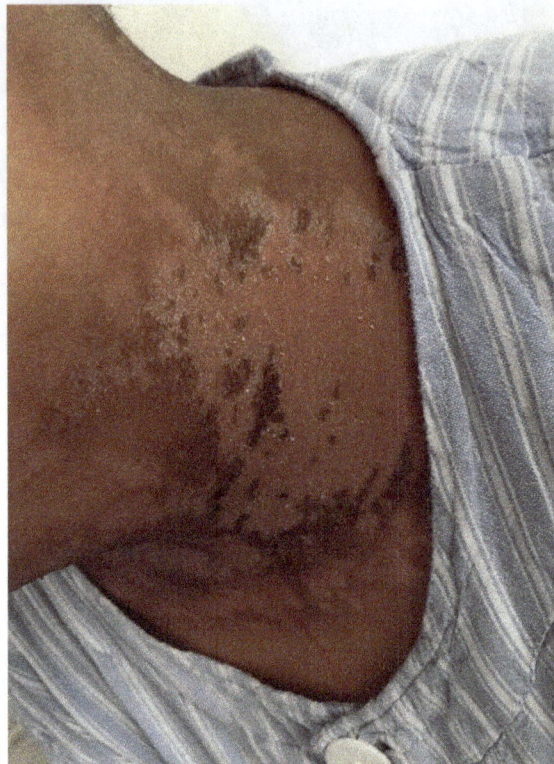

Fig. 10 The fifth irradiation

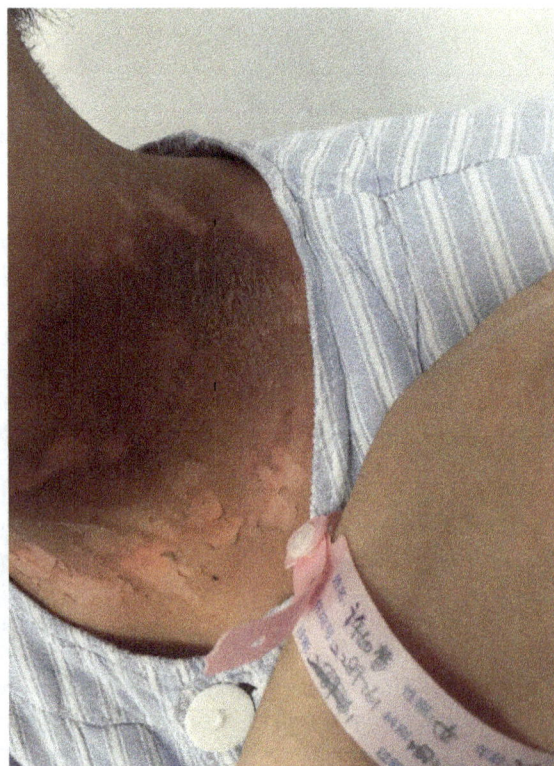

Fig. 9 The forth irradiation, the skin was dry and part of started to peel off

of tissues, shortens the time of treatment, and relieves the pain of patients [20, 21]. In terms of safety, studies have shown that RLPT has little adverse reaction and even no adverse reactions occur [22].

The results of this study indicated that close-range RLPT had a good therapeutic effect on RD. After the application of RLPT, the degree of RD reaction in the experimental group was lighter than that in the control group ($P < 0.05$, Table 2). This indicated that RLPT promoted the healing of inflammation and shortened the healing time, which could not only reduce the complications such as infection caused by mucosal damage, but also further improve the control rate of tumor. The results of pain score in the patients who participated in the experiment showed (Table 3) that the wound pain score of the experimental group was significantly lower than that of the control group, with a significant difference ($P < 0.05$). It is suggested that RLPT can effectively relieve or alleviate wound pain and reduce the pain caused by skin reaction (Figs. 5, 6, 7, 8, 9, 10, 11, 12, 13, 14, and 15).

Conclusions

In conclusion, RLPT can accelerate the healing ability of wound and significantly shorten the healing time. It can not only relieve the pain of patients' wounds and promote the healing of inflammation and ulcer,

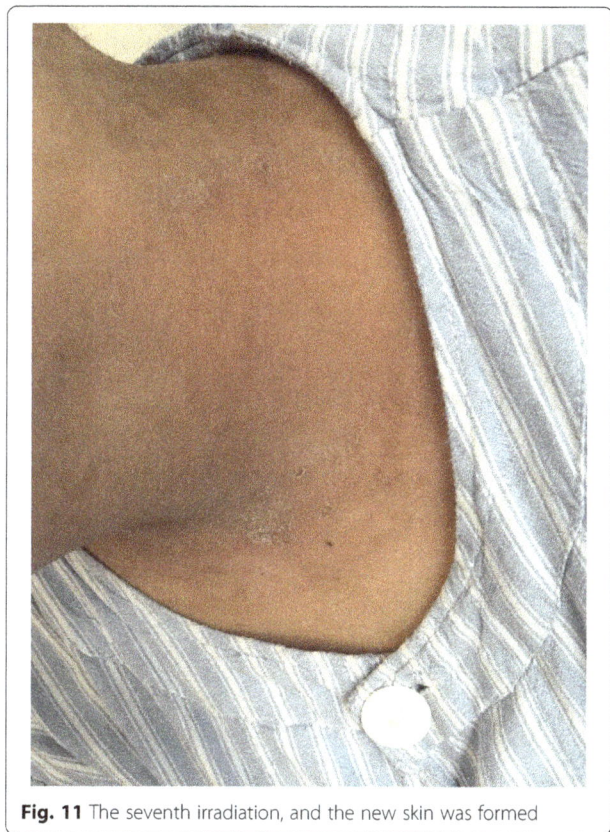

Fig. 11 The seventh irradiation, and the new skin was formed

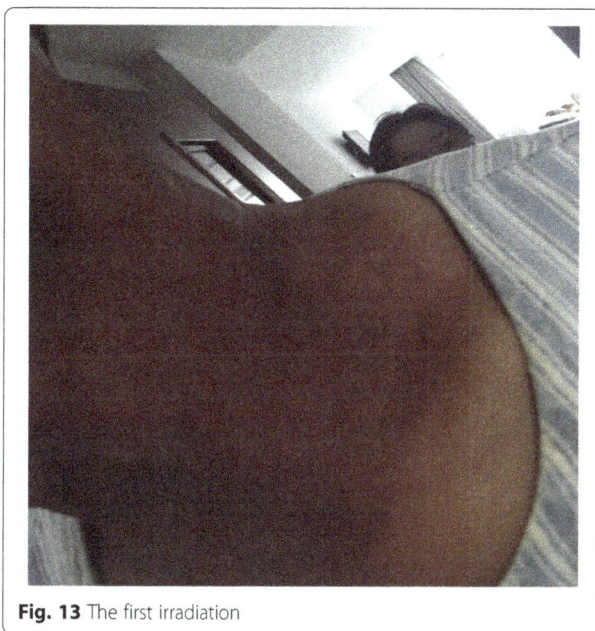

Fig. 13 The first irradiation

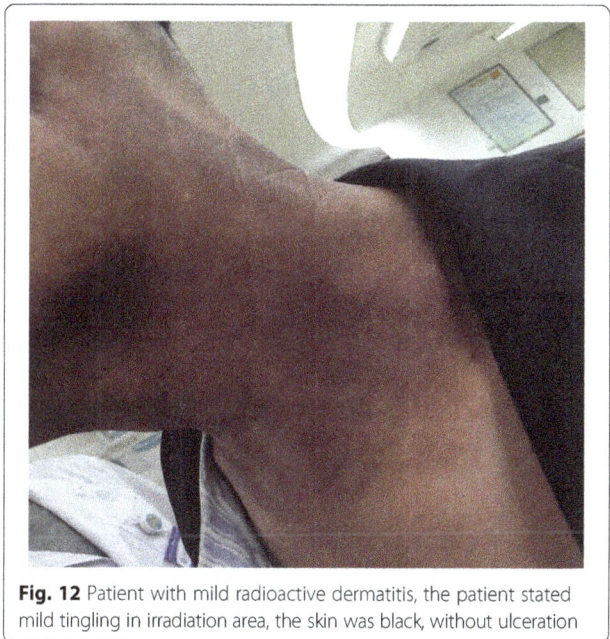

Fig. 12 Patient with mild radioactive dermatitis, the patient stated mild tingling in irradiation area, the skin was black, without ulceration

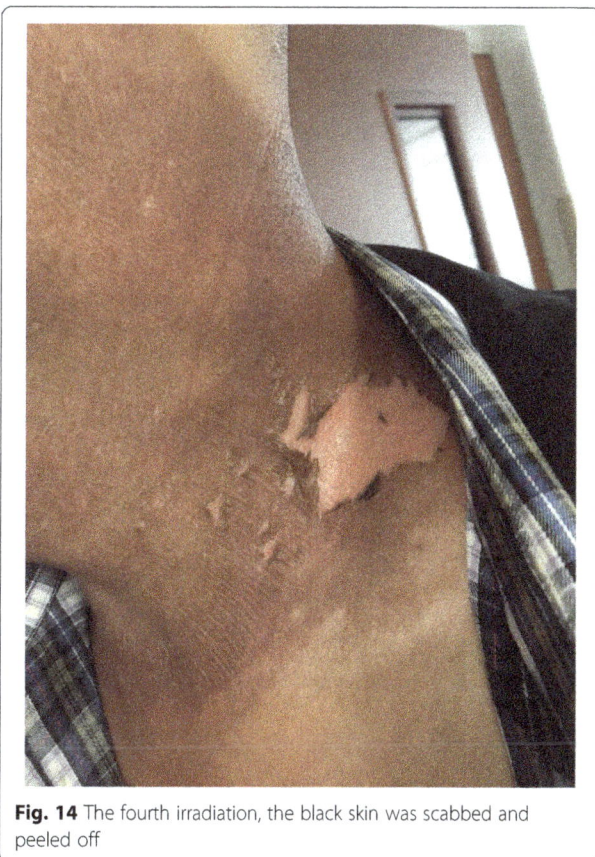

Fig. 14 The fourth irradiation, the black skin was scabbed and peeled off

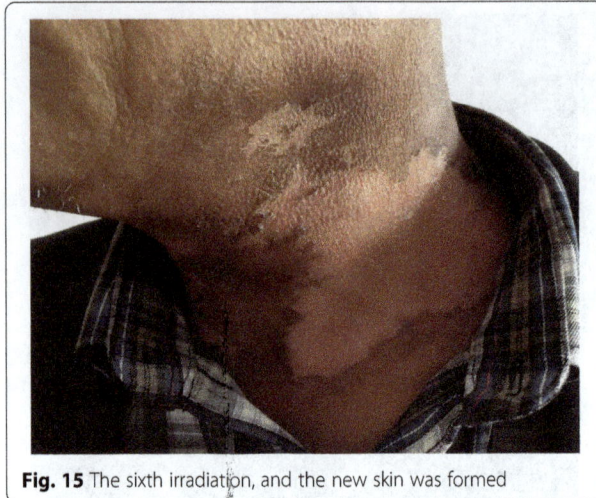

Fig. 15 The sixth irradiation, and the new skin was formed

but also guarantee the smooth progress of the patients' radiotherapy and improve their quality of lives, which is worth the popularization and application in the clinical practice.

Abbreviations
HNC: Head and neck cancer; NPC: Nasopharyngeal carcinoma; NRS: Numerical rating scale; RD: Radioactive dermatitis; RLPT: Red light phototherapy

Acknowledgements
Not applicable.

Funding
None.

Authors' contributions
All authors had full access to all the data in the study and take responsibility for the integrity of the data and the accuracy of the data analysis. XZ and HL contributed to the study concept and design. QL, YL, and CL helped in the acquisition of data. MZ and BZ contributed to the analysis and interpretation of data. XZ and ZL helped in writing of the article. All authors contributed to the critical revision of the article for important intellectual content. HL carried out the statistical analysis. All authors helped in the administrative, technical, and material support. GL supervised the study. All authors read and approved the final manuscript.

Competing interests
The authors declare that they have no competing interests.

References
1. Zhang W, Chen Y, Zhou G, Liu X, Chen L, Tang L, et al. Pretreatment serum lactate dehydrogenase and N classification predict long-term survival and distant metastasis in patients with nasopharyngeal carcinoma who have a positive family history of cancer. Medicine. 2015;94:e1505.
2. Silander E, Nyman J, Bove M, Johansson L, Larsson S, Hammerlid E. Impact of prophylacticpercutaneous endoscopic gastrostomy on malnutrition and quality of life in patients with head and neck cancer: a randomized study. Head Neck. 2012;34:1–9.
3. Lam TC, Wong FC, Leung TW, Ng SH, Tung SY. Clinical outcomes of 174 nasopharyngeal carcinoma patients with radiation-induced temporal lobe necrosis. Int J Radiat Oncol Biol Phys. 2012;82:e57–65.
4. Zhou Q, Han F, Tai A, Deng X. Prognostic factors of local control after re-irradiation with intensity modulated radiation therapy of locally recurred nasopharyngeal carcinoma. Int J Radiat Oncol Biol Phys. 2014;90:S525.
5. Mertens R, Granzen B, Lassay L, Bucsky P, Hundgen M, Stetter G, Heimann G, Weiss C, Hess CF, Gademann G. Treatment of nasopharyngeal carcinoma in children and adolescents: definitive results of a multicenter study (NPC-91-GPOH). Cancer. 2005;104:1083–9.
6. Korreman SS. Motion in radiotherapy: photon therapy. Phys Med Biol. 2012; 57:R161–91.
7. Harms W, Krempien R, Grehn C, Berns C, Hensley FW, Debus J. Daytime pulsed dose rate brachytherapy as a new treatment option for previously irradiated patients with recurrent oesophageal cancer. Br J Radiol. 2005;78: 236–41.
8. Skiveren J, Kjaerby E, Nordahl Larsen H. Cooling by frozen gel pack as pain relief during treatment of axillary hyperhidrosis with botulinum toxin a injections. Acta Derm Venereol. 2008;88:366–9.
9. Francis D. Trends in incidence of head and neck cancers in India. Eur J Cancer. 2018;92:S23.
10. Carvalho AL, Nishimoto IN, Califano JA, Kowalski LP. Trends in incidence and prognosis for head and neck cancer in the United States: a site-specific analysis of the SEER database. Int J Cancer. 2005;114:806–16.
11. McCarthy CE, Field JK, Rajlawat BP, Field AE, Marcus MW. Trends and regional variation in the incidence of head and neck cancers in England: 2002 to 2011. Int J Oncol. 2015;47:204–10.
12. Kong M, Hong SE, Choi J, Kim Y. Comparison of survival rates between patients treated with conventional radiotherapy and helical tomotherapy for head and neck cancer. Radiat Oncol J. 2013;31:1–11.
13. Zheng M, Li L, Tang Y, Liang XH. How to improve the survival rate of implants after radiotherapy for head and neck cancer? J Periodontal Implant Sci. 2014;44:2–7.
14. Pugliano FA, Piccirillo JF, Zequeira MR, Fredrickson JM, Perez CA, Simpson JR. Clinical-severity staging system for oropharyngeal cancer: five-year survival rates. Otolaryngol Head Neck Surg. 1999;120:38–45.
15. Zhang H, Feng L. The clinical effect of Kang Fuxin combined vitamin B_(12) solution in treating fourth-degree radioactive dermatitis. J Am Geriatr Soc. 1990;38:659–62.
16. Chen X, Wang Q, Deng C, Wang G, Liu H, Li G. Clinical observation of Kangfuxin fluid combined with medical anti-radiation spray on injury dermatitis induced by radiation in head and neck tumor patients. Laboratory Medicine & Clinic; 2017.
17. Koppes SA, Engebretsen KA, Agner T, Angelova-Fischer I, Berents T, Brandner J, et al. Current knowledge on biomarkers for contact sensitization and allergic contact dermatitis. Contact Dermatitis. 2017;77:1–16.
18. Vieira Crespo PA, Jorge RDFP, Micaela DSC, Ferreira Pinto MA. Photon radiation therapy monitoring apparatus. FreePatentsOnline; 2012.
19. Toya R, Murakami R, Saito T, Murakami D, Matsuyama T, Baba Y, et al. Radiation therapy for nasopharyngeal carcinoma: the predictive value of interim survival assessment. J Radiat Res. 2016;57:541–7.
20. Hong JS, Jung JY, Yoon JY, Suh DH. Acne treatment by methyl aminolevulinate photodynamic therapy with red light vs. intense pulsed light. Int J Dermatol. 2013;52:614–9.
21. Liu J, Fang Q, Zheng J, Dou Y, Zhang Q, Liao Z, et al. Efficacy and safety evaluation of systemic red light therapy for burn wound repair. Zhongguo Yi Liao Qi Xie Za Zhi. 2010;34:293–6.
22. Na JI, Suh DH. Red light phototherapy alone is effective for acne vulgaris: randomized, single-blinded clinical trial. Dermatol Surg. 2007;33:1228–33.

24

Postoperative morbidity of complete mesocolic excision and central vascular ligation in right colectomy: a retrospective comparative cohort study

Gian Andrea Prevost[1,2]* (iD), Manfred Odermatt[1], Markus Furrer[1,2] and Peter Villiger[1]

Abstract

Background: To investigate morbidity and mortality following complete mesocolic excision (CME) and central vascular ligation (CVL) in patients undergoing right colectomy.

Methods: Data from consecutive patients undergoing elective right colectomy at a university-affiliated referral centre were retrospectively analysed. Patients who underwent conventional right-sided colonic cancer surgery (January 2001–April 2009, $n = 84$) were compared to patients who underwent CME/CVL (May 2009–January 2015, $n = 71$). The primary end point was anastomotic leak. Secondary end points were delayed gastric emptying, severe respiratory failure, mortality and length of hospital stay.

Results: No significant difference was found in the rate of anastomotic leak (1.2% in the conventional versus 5.6% in the CME/CVL group, $p = 0.108$). Patients in the CME/CVL group had a higher 90-day mortality rate (7.0% versus 0.0%, $p = 0.019$). Four out of five deceased patients suffered from aspiration with consecutive respiratory failure. There was a tendency towards delayed gastric emptying in the CME/CVL group (12.7% versus 7.1%, $p = 0.246$). Clavien-Dindo complication grades ≥ 2 were similar in both groups with 16 (19%) in the conventional and 15 (21.1%) in the CME/CVL group ($p = 0.747$). CME/CVL patients had a shorter mean length of stay with 11 versus 14 days ($p < 0.001$).

Conclusions: Complete mesocolic excision with central vascular ligation in right colectomy seems to have a higher aspiration rate leading to severe respiratory failure and to higher mortality compared to conventional resection methods. Patient selection for this procedure may therefore be crucial.

Keywords: Right colectomy, Complete mesocolic excision, Central vascular ligation, Morbidity, Mortality

Background

Total mesorectal excision (TME) is a well-established technique for the management of rectal cancer which has significantly reduced local recurrence rate [1]. In recent years, the concept of complete mesocolic excision (CME) with dissection adhering to embryological planes and central vascular ligation (CVL) has also been adopted to colonic resection [2–6]. While data exist describing an increased disease-free survival in patients who have undergone right colectomy using CME [7], little is known about the perioperative morbidity and mortality associated with CME/CVL in the specific anatomical proximity of pancreas and duodenum [8–11]. Although the CME/CVL procedure has proven to be feasible and may even prolong disease-free survival, in our experience, a specific array of postoperative problems seems to occur more commonly in CME/CVL than in conventional right colectomy. In particular, delayed gastric emptying with consecutive pulmonary aspiration and anastomotic leaks seem to have increased since the introduction of CME/CVL. Due to the lack of randomised controlled trials confirming an increased overall survival of CME/CVL for right colectomy, it is questionable whether the potentially increased

* Correspondence: gianandreapre@hotmail.com
[1]Department of Surgery, Kantonsspital Graubünden, Loëstrasse 170, CH-7000 Chur, Switzerland
[2]Private University of the Principality of Liechtenstein, Triesen, Principality of Liechtenstein

complication rate outweighs the probable oncological benefits of this method.

We therefore conducted a single-centre retrospective cohort study to determine whether there is an increase in morbidity associated with CME/CVL compared to conventional right colectomy.

Material and methods
Patients and methods

From January 2001 to December 2014, a total of 266 patients underwent right colectomy in our university-affiliated referral hospital. Only adult patients (> 18 years) who underwent elective right colectomy for confirmed or suspected primary malignant tumours were included as shown in Fig. 1. Exclusion criteria were multi-visceral resections, concomitant inflammatory bowel disease and patients denying consent for analysis of their personal data. A total of 155 patients met the inclusion criteria whose characteristics are shown in Table 1. Patients with suspected malignant tumours were operated in the same technique as patients with confirmed malignancies. Therefore, short-term outcome should not differ significantly between those groups allowing for inclusion of both groups for final analysis.

The CME/CVL method was implemented in May 2009 after observerships in institutions already using this method, video tutorials and practical workshops. In the later period of conventionally performed resections, laparoscopy has increasingly been adopted and became the primary approach. Patients being in the conventional control group had surgery from January 2001 to May 2009 whilst the CME/CVL group underwent surgery from May 2009 to January 2015.

The tested alternative hypothesis was that CME/CVL has higher perioperative morbidity than conventional resection. The primary end point was anastomotic leak. Secondary end points were delayed gastric emptying,

severe respiratory failure, mortality and length of hospital stay.

Ninety-day institutional mortality was reported because Byrne et al. [12] showed that extending mortality reporting to 90 days identifies a greater number of operation and hospitalisation-associated deaths when compared to the 30-day period. Delayed gastric emptying was defined as nasogastric tube removal after postoperative day 3. Severe respiratory failure was defined as required intubation or non-invasive treatment with continuous positive airway pressure. Chronic kidney disease was defined as a glomerular filtration rate of < 45 ml/min/1.73 m^2 at admission, estimating the glomerular filtration rate with the CKD-EPI (Chronic Kidney Disease Epidemiology Collaboration) equation [13].

Procedures
Conventional resection

After lateral to medial mobilisation of the right colon, division of the transverse colon and the terminal ileum by electrocautery followed. The mesocolon was dissected in a V-shape manner towards the origin of the ileocolic and right colic vessels which were ligated. The anastomoses were mainly fashioned in a hand-sewn end-to-end technique. In the few cases of conventional procedures performed laparoscopically, the same technique as in the corresponding open operation was used. Resection of the exteriorised bowel as well as the anastomosis was performed via a transverse supraumbilical incision where a wound protector was applied.

Complete mesocolic excision and central vascular ligation

CMEs with CVL were usually performed laparoscopically with open procedures limited to selected patients with bulky tumours. In contrast to the technique of CME/CVL described by Hohenberger et al. [14],

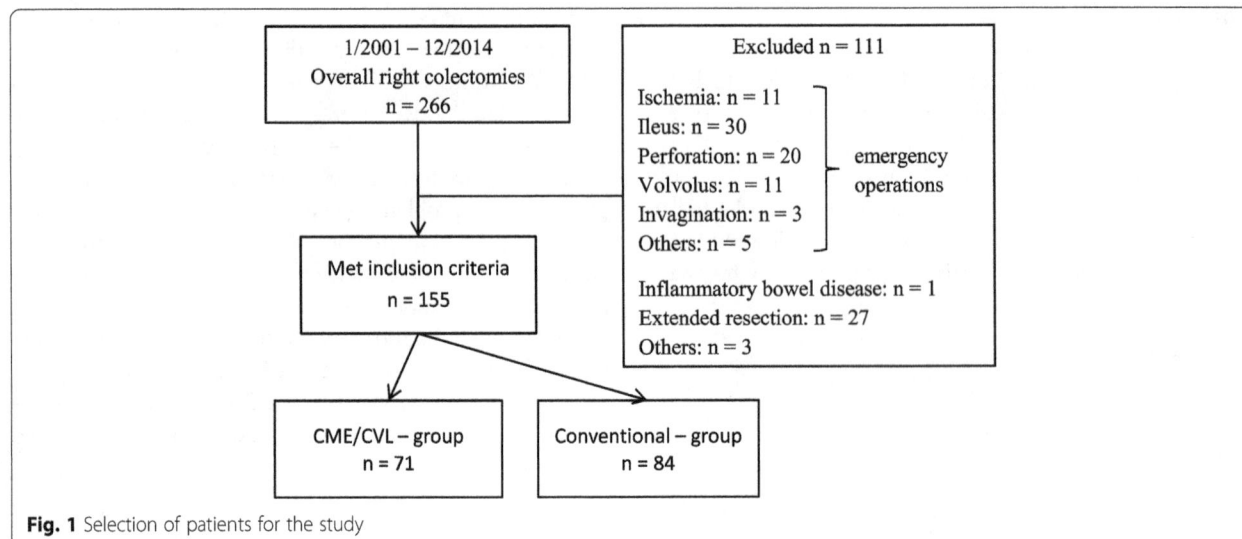

Fig. 1 Selection of patients for the study

Table 1 Baseline parameters

	Conventional group	CME/CVL group	p value
	n = 84	n = 71	
Patient characteristics			
Female gender	42 (50.0)	32 (45.1)	0.540
Age (years)*	73.8 (21.0–88.9)	73.6 (33.0–88.9)	0.843
Arterial hypertension	34 (38.6)	38 (52.1)	0.088
Coronary artery disease	10 (11.9)	12 (16.9)	0.374
Cerebrovascular insult	0 (0.0)	5 (7.0)	0.019
Diabetes mellitus	5 (6.1)	13 (18.3)	0.019
Chronic kidney disease	4 (4.8)	7 (9.9)	0.218
Dialysis	0 (0.0)	2 (2.8)	0.208
Chronic obstructive pulmonary disease	5 (6.0)	4 (5.6)	1.000
Body mass index**	24.9 (4.3) (16.6–34.9)	25.5 (3.7) (18.1–35.6)	0.361
Smoker	16 (19.0)	9 (12.7)	0.283
Alcohol abuse	9 (10.7)	3 (4.2)	0.132
Steroids	2 (2.4)	2 (2.8)	1.000
Previous abdominal surgery	46 (54.8)	41 (57.7)	0.709
ASA 1	3 (3.6)	2 (2.8)	
ASA 2	56 (66.7)	48 (67.6)	
ASA 3	25 (29.8)	21 (29.6)	0.964
Perioperative parameters			
Operation time (minutes)**	155 (52) (62–315)	174 (48) (105–374)	0.020
Anaesthesia time (minutes)**	279 (67) (140–510)	292 (52) (204–465)	0.179
First surgeon: consultant	35 (41.7)	47 (66.2)	0.002
Laparoscopic operation	0 (0.0)	22 (31.0)	< 0.001
Laparoscopy-assisted operation	10 (11.9)	28 (39.4)	< 0.001
Extended right colectomy	6 (7.1)	5 (7.0)	0.981
Stapler anastomosis	57 (67.9)	70 (98.6)	< 0.001
Side-to-side anastomosis	57 (67.9)	69 (97.2)	< 0.001
Insertion of drains intraoperatively	45 (53.6)	49 (69.0)	0.050
Intraoperative fluid balance (ml)**	2642 (1021) (500–5800)	1558 (803) (180–4890)	< 0.001
Continuous epidural analgesia	65 (77.4)	62 (87.3)	0.109
Preoperative bowel preparation	26 (31.0)	2 (2.8)	< 0.001

With percentages in parentheses unless indicated otherwise

ASA American Society of Anesthesiologists classification

*Values are median (range)

**Values are mean (standard deviation) (range)

Kocherisation of the duodenum to harvest the retro-pancreatic central lymph nodes was not performed routinely.

In open CME/CVL, mobilisation of the right colon started laterally and continued centrally between the mesocolic surface layer and Gerota's fascia. The ileocolic, the right colic, and the right branch of the middle colic vessels were divided at their origin. In extended right colectomies, the middle colic vessels were divided centrally at the level of the superior mesenteric artery and vein preserving the ileocolic trunk if present. Lymph node clearance around the central vessels and the superior mesenteric vein was performed. The greater omentum was divided at the resection level of the transverse colon and detached from the stomach. An isoperistaltic side-to-side stapler anastomosis was performed in most cases.

In contrast to the open resection, a medial to lateral mobilisation was performed in laparoscopic CME/CVL. The dissection started medial of the ileocolic vessels with creating a window in the mesentery. Following the ileocolic pedicle, the superior mesenteric vein was identified and cleared from lymphatic tissue up to and including the ileocolic trunk. The ileocolic as well as the right branch of the middle colic vessels were ligated and divided centrally. The medial to lateral mobilisation exposed the duodenum and head of the pancreas. Lateral division completed the mobilisation of the right colon. In complete laparoscopic procedures, the bowel was divided with endoscopic linear staplers and the specimen retrieved over a small suprapubic transverse laparotomy using a wound retractor. Finally, a laparoscopic side-to-side stapler anastomosis was performed. For laparoscopy-assisted procedures, a transverse supraumbilical incision was made wide enough to exteriorise and resect the mobilised bowel and to fashion the anastomosis by stapler.

Assessment of the specimen

From May 2009 onwards, specimens were examined adhering to the grading system used for the MRC CLASSIC trial complemented with the subsequently introduced fourth category [15]. In this grading system, specimens were classified as follows:

- Grade 1/"poor": moderate bulk of mesocolon and disruptions extending down onto the muscularis propria
- Grade 2/"moderate": moderate bulk of mesocolon, disruptions not reaching down onto the muscularis propria
- Grade 3/"good": intact mesocolon and smooth peritoneal-lined surface
- Grade 4: pathologist's classification as grade 3 and surgeon reports central dissection

Perioperative management

The patient was admitted the day before surgery. Bowel preparation was a routine procedure in the conventional group only. Single-shot antibiotic prophylaxis with Cefazolin and Metronidazole was administered in both groups. Abdominal drains and nasogastric tubes were inserted routinely. Nasogastric tubes were removed either immediately after the operation or on the following day in cases with low tube output. The time of drain removal was decided by the primary surgeon. Liquids and solid food were administered as soon as tolerated. There was no change in postoperative nutrition policy over the study period. In particular, there was no enhanced recovery program established for both groups.

Data analysis

Data were collected from clinical records and pooled in an electronic database. Statistical analysis was performed using SPSS version 18 (SPSS Inc., an IBM Company

Chicago, Illinois, USA). Discrete variables were compared with the chi-square test or Fisher exact test, as appropriate. Means of continuous data were compared using the Student's t test for normally distributed data and the Mann-Whitney U test for not normally distributed data. Normality was determined graphically using histograms. P values ≤ 0.05 were considered to be significant.

Results

Included for analysis were 155 patients with 84 patients in the conventional group and 71 patients in the CME/CVL group. Baseline parameters of the two groups are shown in Table 1. Characteristics of the malignant tumours are listed in Table 2.

The primary end point, namely anastomotic leak, was reached in only one case (1.2%) in the conventional group versus four cases (5.6%) in the CME/CVL group, the difference not being statistically significant ($p = 0.180$). However, a significant difference was found in the postoperative 90 day institutional mortality rate with zero cases in the conventional group and five cases (7.0%) in the CME/CVL group ($p = 0.019$). The first patient, a 78-year-old man with an adenocarcinoma of the ascending colon, died on postoperative day 5 most likely from aspiration caused by repeated vomiting. The second patient, an 89-year-old man with a cecal adenocarcinoma died on postoperative

Table 2 Malignant tumour characteristics

	Conventional group	CME/CVL group	p value
	n = 71 (84.5)	59 (83.1)	0.810
Tumour locations			
Ileocoecal (ileum, appendix, coecum)	29 (40.8)	34 (57.6)	
Ascending colon	29 (40.8)	16 (27.1)	
Right flexure and transverse colon	13 (18.3)	9 (15.3)	0.149
T-stage			
Tumour in situ (Tis)	1 (1.4)	1 (1.7)	
T1	5 (7.0)	5 (8.5)	
T2	7 (9.9)	9 (15.3)	
T3	51 (71.8)	36 (61.0)	
T4	7 (9.9)	8 (13.6)	0.771
N-stage			
N0	38 (53.5)	41 (69.5)	
N1	18 (25.4)	8 (13.6)	
N2	15 (21.1)	10 (16.9)	0.143
M-stage			
M0	60 (84.5)	55 (93.2)	
M1	9 (12.7)	4 (6.8)	
Mx	2 (2.8)	0 (0.0)	0.217

With percentages in parentheses

day 8 in the intensive care unit from respiratory insufficiency after aspiration and consecutive pneumonia. The third patient, an 82-year-old female patient with a metastasised adenocarcinoma of the caecum, died on the 53rd postoperative day due to prolonged gastroparesis and consecutive aspiration. The fourth patient, a 74-year-old man with a large adenoma of the ascending colon, died on the 7th postoperative day from a cardiovascular arrest after fulminant aspiration. A septic shock caused by an anastomotic insufficiency led to a consecutive abdominal compartment syndrome requiring emergency laparotomy and an ileostomy on postoperative day 7 where the patient died the same day because of cardiac organ failure. The fifth patient, a 77-year-old man with an adenocarcinoma of the transverse colon, died on postoperative day 19 from a pulmonary embolism after an operative revision of an anastomotic leak on postoperative day 12. All four patients with aspiration had a nasogastric tube reinserted because of nausea and vomiting. Overall however, the frequency of complications Clavien-Dindo ≥ 2 was not significantly different in the two groups with 16 (19%) in the conventional and 15 (21.1%) in the CME/CVL group ($p = 0.747$).

Intra- and postoperative complications are listed in Table 3.

The mean harvested lymph node count was 23.3 (SD 12.5) in the conventional and 32.2 (SD 17.4) in the CME/CVL group ($p = 0.001$). For the resection quality analysis, there were 12 cases missing. The median of the specimen resection quality in the CME/CVL group was 3. Twenty-nine (49.2% of the analysed specimen) had a resection quality of 4, 15 (25.4%) had a resection quality of 3, 14 (23.7%) of 2 and 1 (1.7%) of 1.

Details about the postoperative course are summed up in Table 4.

Discussion

Our study shows a higher mortality in the CME/CVL group with aspiration and consecutive respiratory failure as the leading cause. Previous studies comparing CME/CVL to conventional right colectomies regarding perioperative morbidity are limited. Bertelsen et al. [8] revealed a higher postoperative morbidity in CME/CVL patients with a higher rate of intraoperative injury including splenic and superior mesenteric vein injuries and a higher rate of postoperative sepsis. Consistent to our data, Bertelsen et al. also found a higher respiratory failure rate in this collective compared to the conventionally operated group (8.1% versus 3.4%, $p < 0.001$). In contrast, a case series by Prochazka et al. [11] of 63 patients in a conventional group versus 20 patients in a CME/CVL group showed no difference in morbidity. Although in our study, the mortality rate of 7% seems to be unacceptably high, similar mortality rates for CME/CVL of the right colon have been reported in the past

Table 3 Complications

	Conventional group	CME/CVL group	p value
	n = 84	n = 71	
Intraoperative apparent complications	12 (14.3)	14 (19.7)	0.367
Vascular injuries	4 (4.8)	7 (9.9)	0.218
Blood loss (ml)*	300 (50–4000)	100 (40–800)	< 0.001
Post-operative complications			
Clavien-Dindo ≥ 2	16 (19)	15 (21.1)	0.747
Surgical site infections			
Superficial and deep incisional	13 (15.5)	8 (11.3)	0.446
Organ/space	3 (3.6)	4 (5.6)	0.703
Anastomotic leak	1 (1.2)	4 (5.6)	0.180
Iatrogenic small bowel perforation	1 (1.2)	1 (1.4)	1.000
Bleeding	4 (4.8)	2 (2.8)	0.688
Sepsis	0 (0.0)	2 (2.8)	0.208
Pneumonia	3 (3.6)	4 (5.6)	0.703
Severe respiratory failure	0 (0.0)	5 (7.0)	0.019
Pulmonary embolism	1 (1.2)	2 (2.8)	0.593
Cardiac decompensation or atrial fibrillation	1 (1.2)	3 (4.2)	0.333
Acute renal insufficiency	0 (0.0)	3 (4.2)	0.094
Urinary tract infection	4 (4.8)	1 (1.4)	0.376
Urinary retention	4 (4.8)	0 (0.0)	0.125
90-day institutional mortality rate	0 (0.0)	5 (7.0)	0.019

With percentages in parentheses unless indicated otherwise
*Values are median (range)

[16]. Our seemingly high mortality rate may be explained by the extended time period of 90 days defining institutional mortality. Furthermore, all of the deceased patients were of advanced age (median 78, range 74–89) and had substantial comorbidities (80% ASA 3).

Aspiration with respiratory failure proved to be the main cause of death (4 out of 5 patients) in CME/CVL patients. There was also a tendency towards longer nasogastric tube drainage in this group indicating prolonged postoperative gastroparesis as a risk factor for aspiration. This may be explained by the extensive mobilisation of the mesenteric root at the duodenal knee and pancreas head specific to CME/CVL right colectomy.

Two out of the five deceased patients suffered from anastomotic leakage, and one of them had a fulminant aspiration. Anastomotic leakage in colorectal surgery is a leading factor for postoperative morbidity. Bowel paralysis and gastroparesis are well-known disorders secondary

Table 4 Postoperative course

	Conventional group	CME/CVL group	p value
	n = 84	n = 71	
Duration of hospital stay (d)*	14 (8–43)	11 (6–35)	< 0.001
ICU postoperative	3 (3.6)	4 (5.6)	0.703
Reintervention	3 (3.6)	8 (11.3)	0.063
Needed antibiotic therapy	14 (16.7)	11 (15.5)	0.843
Time to first mobilisation (pod)**	1.10 (0.51) (0–4)	1.13 (0.58) (0–3)	0.722
Time to first flatus (pod)**	2.62 (1.13) (1–6)	2.04 (1.06) (1–6)	0.005
Time to first bowel movement (pod)**	4.17 (1.86) (1–11)	3.37 (1.61) (1–8)	0.005
Time to normal diet (pod)*	7 (4–26)	5 (1–18)	< 0.001
Delayed gastric emptying	6 (7.1)	9 (12.7)	0.246
Total length of stay of NGT (d)*	2 (1–12)	4.5 (1–14)	0.207
Urine catheter removal (pod)**	4.64 (3.02) (1–21)	3.27 (1.71) (0–9)	0.001
Drain removal (pod)*	5 (1–20)	3 (1–15)	0.002
Maximal weight gain (kg)**	4.47 (2.92) (−2–11)	3.78 (2.85) (−2–11)	0.138
Total days with CEA*	5 (0–12)	4 (0–9)	0.029

With percentages in parentheses unless indicated otherwise
ICU intensive care unit, *pod* postoperative day, *d* days, *CEA* continuous epidural analgesia, *NGT* nasogastric tube
*Values are median (range)
**Values are mean (standard deviation) (range)

to anastomotic leakage, but compared to other resection areas, right colectomy seems to have a negative impact on gastric emptying even in otherwise uneventful courses.

Increased rates of vascular injury, though not statistically significant, occurred in the CME/CVL group which may be caused by the more extensive dissection along the superior mesenteric vein. On the other hand, median intraoperative blood loss was significantly higher in the conventional group most likely because of the higher rate of open procedures in this group. Increased blood loss has been proven to adversely impact the operative outcome especially regarding anastomotic leakage [17]. Although lymphatic leaks are to be expected due to the more extensive lymphadenectomy, we did not experience isolated lymphatic leaks being clinically obvious and needing any specific treatment. However, we did not systematically screen for asymptomatic lymphoceles and some complications as abscesses or prolonged ileus might have been caused by lymphatic leaks in the first place.

Compared to the conventional group, a significant higher amount of procedures have been performed by a consultant in the CME/CVL group (66.2% versus 41.7%, p = 0.002). This was primarily due to the new and more demanding operation technique.

The main limitation of our study is its retrospective nature, the long observation period associated with changes in perioperative and adjuvant management and the lack of power because of small sample size. Though some of the differences in short-term outcomes seem to be clinically relevant, they did not reach statistical significance which may solely be due to small sample sizes.

The differences of operative and postoperative management in the two groups due to changing methods and modified managements in the last two decades may explain some of the differing results. Additionally, the whole learning curve of CME/CVL right colectomy, in particular laparoscopic CME/CVL, is included in the consecutive cases potentially increasing the complication rate in the CME/CVL group. Multiple previous studies have shown significant advantages of laparoscopic compared to open procedures including perioperative morbidity [18–22] which is in contrast to our results where more complications in the CME/CVL group occurred where most procedures were performed laparoscopically. Likewise did other factors like less intraoperative blood loss, better intraoperative fluid balance and less postoperative weight gain in the CME/CVL group not translate in a better short-term outcome. On the other hand, the prolonged gastroparesis in this group may support our hypothesis, namely that CME/CVL for right colectomy adversely affects gastrointestinal function postoperatively. Though ASA did not differ between the two groups, some risk factors may have increased the risk for complications in the CME/CVL group. In particular, diabetes mellitus and cerebrovascular disease rates were more frequently reported in the CME/CVL group and may partially explain the worse short-term outcome in this group. Diabetes mellitus as a known risk factor for delayed gastric emptying may have increased this effect in the CME/CVL group [23]. On the other hand, the abovementioned differences in baseline morbidities might be due to underreporting in the historic control group. At that time, Switzerland had a reimbursement system mainly focusing on the principal diagnosis so that comorbidity reporting in health records was not as rigorous as it became in later periods. This explanation may be supported by the fact that for example chronic kidney disease was reported significantly more commonly in the CME/VLE group although the average glomerular filtration rate at admission was similar in both group. Though not decreasing overall morbidity, the higher rate of laparoscopic procedures may explain the shorter hospital stay in the CME/CVL group. Also the aforementioned implementation of a new reimbursement system in Switzerland with Diagnoses Related Groups (SwissDRG) in January 2012 and its economic impact on health care might be a reason for shorter hospital stays [24].

Conclusions

Taking into account the lack of randomised controlled trials and that current data [7] only strongly suggest a survival benefit for patients operated with the CME/CVL standard, careful patient selection to avoid the increased morbidity of the clearly more extensive procedure may be crucial especially in elderly patients. While mesocolic excision undisputedly has to be considered the standard of tumour surgery, the benefit of central vascular ligation and extensive lymph node clearing beyond the level of vessel ligation as a rigid oncologic principle to be applied in all patients remains unclear. As recent data [7] has been unable to show clear superiority of CME/CVL in regard to disease-free survival, an adequately powered randomised controlled trial is in our opinion ethically justifiable to determine the real long-term impact of CVL with extensive lymphatic tissue clearance as an independent factor besides newer chemotherapeutic regimens.

Abbreviations

ASA: American Society of Anesthesiologists classification; CEA: Continuous epidural analgesia; CME: Complete mesocolic excision; CVL: Central vascular ligation; ICU: Intensive care unit; NGT: Nasogastric tube; Pod: Postoperative day; TME: Total mesorectal excision

Acknowledgements

We would like to thank Mrs. Jaime Duffield for the proofreading of this study.

Funding

None

Authors' contributions

All authors made substantial contributions to the conception and design of the study and read and approved the final manuscript. GAP collected and analysed the data and was a major contributor in writing the manuscript. MO was a major contributor in interpreting data.

Competing interests

The authors declare that they have no competing interests.

References

1. Birgisson H, Talback M, Gunnarsson U, et al. Improved survival in cancer of the colon and rectum in Sweden. Eur J Surg Oncol. 2005; 31:845–53.
2. Sondenaa K, Quirke P, Hohenberger W, et al. The rationale behind complete mesocolic excision (CME) and a central vascular ligation for colon cancer in open and laparoscopic surgery: proceedings of a consensus conference. Int J Color Dis. 2014;29:419–28.
3. Tagliacozzo S, Tocchi A. Extended mesenteric excision in right hemicolectomy for carcinoma of the colon. Int J Color Dis. 1997;12:272–5.
4. Eiholm S, Ovesen H. Total mesocolic excision versus traditional resection in right-sided colon cancer - method and increased lymph node harvest. Dan Med Bull. 2010;57:A4224.
5. West NP, Hohenberger W, Weber K, et al. Complete mesocolic excision with central vascular ligation produces an oncologically superior specimen compared with standard surgery for carcinoma of the colon. J Clin Oncol. 2010;28:272–8.
6. West NP, Kobayashi H, Takahashi K, et al. Understanding optimal colonic cancer surgery: comparison of Japanese D3 resection and European complete mesocolic excision with central vascular ligation. J Clin Oncol. 2012;30:1763–9.
7. Gouvas N, Agalianos C, Papaparaskeva K, et al. Surgery along the embryological planes for colon cancer: a systematic review of complete mesocolic excision. Int J Color Dis. 2016;31:1577–94.
8. Bertelsen CA, Neuenschwander AU, Jansen JE, et al. Short-term outcomes after complete mesocolic excision compared with 'conventional' colonic cancer surgery. Br J Surg. 2016;103:581–9.
9. Rasulov AO, Malikhov AG, Rakhimov OA, et al. Short-term outcomes of complete mesocolic excision for right colon cancer. Khirurgiia (Mosk). 2017; 8:79–86.
10. Kim IY, Kim BR, Choi EH, et al. Short-term and oncologic outcomes of laparoscopic and open complete mesocolic excision and central ligation. Int J Surg. 2016;27:151–7.
11. Prochazka V, Zetelova A, Grolich T, et al. Complete mesocolic excision during right hemicolectomy. Rozhl Chir. 2016;95:359–64.
12. Byrne BE, Mamidanna R, Vincent CA, et al. Population-based cohort study comparing 30- and 90-day institutional mortality rates after colorectal surgery. Br J Surg. 2013;100:1810–7.
13. Stevens PE, Levin A. Evaluation and management of chronic kidney disease: synopsis of the kidney disease: improving global outcomes 2012 clinical practice guideline. Ann Intern Med. 2013;158:825–30.
14. Hohenberger W, Weber K, Matzel K, et al. Standardized surgery for colonic cancer: complete mesocolic excision and central ligation--technical notes and outcome. Color Dis. 2009;11:354–64 discussion 64-5.
15. West NP, Morris EJ, Rotimi O, et al. Pathology grading of colon cancer surgical resection and its association with survival: a retrospective observational study. Lancet Oncol. 2008;9:857–65.
16. Bertelsen CA. Complete mesocolic excision an assessment of feasibility and outcome. Dan Med J. 2017;64(2).
17. McDermott FD, Heeney A, Kelly ME, et al. Systematic review of preoperative, intraoperative and postoperative risk factors for colorectal anastomotic leaks. Br J Surg. 2015;102:462–79.
18. Sun J, Jiang T, Qiu Z, et al. Short-term and medium-term clinical outcomes of laparoscopic-assisted and open surgery for colorectal cancer: a single center retrospective case-control study. BMC Gastroenterol. 2011;11:85.
19. Li JC, Leung KL, Ng SS, et al. Laparoscopic-assisted versus open resection of right-sided colonic cancer--a prospective randomized controlled trial. Int J Color Dis. 2012;27:95–102.
20. Storli KE, Sondenaa K, Furnes B, et al. Outcome after introduction of complete mesocolic excision for colon cancer is similar for open and laparoscopic surgical treatments. Dig Surg. 2013;30:317–27.
21. Guillou PJ, Quirke P, Thorpe H, et al. Short-term endpoints of conventional versus laparoscopic-assisted surgery in patients with colorectal cancer (MRC CLASICC trial): multicentre, randomised controlled trial. Lancet. 2005;365:1718–26.
22. Hewett PJ, Allardyce RA, Bagshaw PF, et al. Short-term outcomes of the Australasian randomized clinical study comparing laparoscopic and conventional open surgical treatments for colon cancer: the ALCCaS trial. Ann Surg. 2008;248:728–38.
23. Halland M, Bharucha AE. Relationship between control of glycemia and gastric emptying disturbances in diabetes mellitus. Clin Gastroenterol Hepatol. 2016;14:929–36.
24. Busato A, von Below G. The implementation of DRG-based hospital reimbursement in Switzerland: a population-based perspective. Health Res Policy Syst. 2010;8:31.

25

Appropriate preoperative membranous urethral length predicts recovery of urinary continence after robot-assisted laparoscopic prostatectomy

Daiki Ikarashi* (ID), Yoichiro Kato, Mitsugu Kanehira, Ryo Takata, Akito Ito, Mitsutaka Onoda, Renpei Kato, Tomohiko Matsuura, Kazuhiro Iwasaki and Wataru Obara

Abstract

Purpose: We investigated that preoperative membranous urethral length (MUL) would be associated with the recovery of urinary continence after robot-assisted laparoscopic prostatectomy (RALP).

Patients and methods: We studied 204 patients who underwent RALP between May 2013 and March 2016. All patients underwent pelvic magnetic resonance imaging (MRI) preoperatively to measure MUL. Urinary continence was defined as the use of one pad or less (safety pad). The 204 patients were divided into two groups: continence group, those who achieved recovery of continence at 3, 6, and 12 months after RALP, and incontinence group, those who did not. We retrospectively analyzed the patients in terms of preoperative clinical factors including age, body mass index (BMI), estimated prostate volume, neurovascular bundle salvage, history of preoperative hormonal therapy, and MUL.

Results: The safety pad use rate was 69.6%, 86.9%, and 91.1% at 3, 6, and 12 months, respectively. On univariate and multivariate analyses, MUL were significant factors in every term of recovery of urinary continence in both groups. According to the receiver operating characteristic (ROC) curve analysis, the preoperative MUL that could best predict early recovery of urinary continence at 3 months after RALP was 12 mm.

Conclusions: We suggest that preoperative MUL > 12 mm would be a predictor of early recovery of urinary continence after RALP.

Keywords: Membranous urethral length, Urinary continence, Robot-assisted laparoscopic prostatectomy

Introduction

Urinary incontinence is one of the most unfavorable complications influencing the quality of life for patients after radical prostatectomy (RP). In early 2000, the initial robot-assisted laparoscopic prostatectomy (RALP) was performed with the da Vinci surgical system [1]. Currently, RALP has become a more popular surgical procedure for RP in Japan. RALP is expected to achieve better outcomes regarding recovery of urinary continence than did the conventional procedure. Its advanced technology provides a three-dimensional operative view and laparoscopic instruments that mimic the movement of the human wrist. For the robotic approach, a meta-analysis of 51 studies showed statistically significant improvement in urinary continence recovery at 12 months with RALP compared to retropubic and laparoscopic RP [2].

Predictive factors for recovery of urinary continence after RP, such as patient age, body mass index (BMI), and prostate volume, have been reported [2, 3]. Membranous urethral length (MUL) as measured by magnetic resonance imaging (MRI) also was reported to be a strong predictive factor for recovery of urinary continence in a systematic review and meta-analysis [4]. These reports demonstrated that preoperative MUL is associated significantly and positively with a return to continence following RP. However, few reports exist on the

* Correspondence: heart-of-albirex1@hotmail.co.jp
Department of Urology, Iwate Medical University School of Medicine, 19-1, Uchimaru, Morioka-shi, Iwate 020-8505, Japan

association of MUL and recovery of urinary continence after RALP in the Japanese population.

We evaluated the association of preoperative MUL with the recovery of urinary incontinence after RALP in Japanese patients.

Patients and methods

We performed RALP using the da Vinci Si surgical system in 204 consecutive patients from whom we could collect the Expanded Prostate Cancer Index Composite (EPIC) questionnaire [5] at least preoperatively and 3 months after RALP between May 2013 and March 2016. All patients underwent pelvic MRI preoperatively. Most patients had no urinary incontinence before surgery; only ten patients had incontinence more than once a week. All surgical procedures were performed by four surgeons (YK, MK, RT, and WO). All surgeons are over 10 years as urologists, and each surgeon experienced RALP in more than 40 cases. RALP was performed via the conventional transperitoneal approach using the four-armed da Vinci surgical robot system [6]. In all cases, we performed the Rocco technique for posterior reconstruction of Denonvillier's facia [7], anterior preservation [8], and bladder neck preservation [9] for preventing incontinence. Hemi–nerve sparing was performed depending on the cancer status [10]. Pelvic lymph node dissection also was performed in patients with a high risk of cancer according to the D'Amico criteria. We also offered all patients pelvic floor exercise education during the operative period.

The MUL was measured by T2-weighted coronal and sagittal sections as a distance from the prostatic apex to the level of the urethra at the penile bulb on preoperative pelvic MRI (Fig 1) [11]. In terms of measuring the MUL, a number of urologists evaluated MUL of each case at the preoperative conference. Thereafter, the data of MUL was remeasured by a researcher.

Urinary continence was evaluated at 3, 6, and 12 months after RALP using question 5 of the EPIC questionnaire [5]. Continence was defined as the use of one pad or less as a safety pad. We also examined the quality of life (QOL) score regarding urinary continence pre- and postoperatively using question 12 of the EPIC questionnaire [5].

The patients were divided into two groups: continence group, those who achieved recovery of urinary continence within 3, 6, 12 months, and incontinence group, those who did not.

Univariate analysis was performed with the t test, analysis of variance, chi-square, and Fisher's exact test between continence and incontinence group regarding preoperative clinical factors including patient age, BMI, estimated prostate volume, clinical stage, neurovascular bundle salvage, history of preoperative hormonal therapy, positive surgical margin, leakage at vesicourethral anastomosis, and MUL. Multivariate analysis was performed using a logistic regression model, and significances were tested using a likelihood ratio test. Statistical analyses were performed using JMP software (SAS Institute, Inc., Cary, NC, USA). For all statistical comparisons, differences with $P < 0.05$ were considered statistically significant.

Result

Mean patient age was 65 years, BMI was 23.7 kg/m^2, prostate-specific antigen (PSA) was 6.5 ng/ml, and MUL was 13.1 mm. Preoperative hormonal therapy was given in 34 (16.7%) patients, and hemi–nerve sparing was performed in 70 (34.6%; Table 1). The safety pad rate was 69.6%, 86.9%, and 91.1% at 3, 6, and 12 months, respectively, and the pad-free rate was 33.8%, 49.7%, and 64.3%, respectively. The QOL regarding the urinary condition

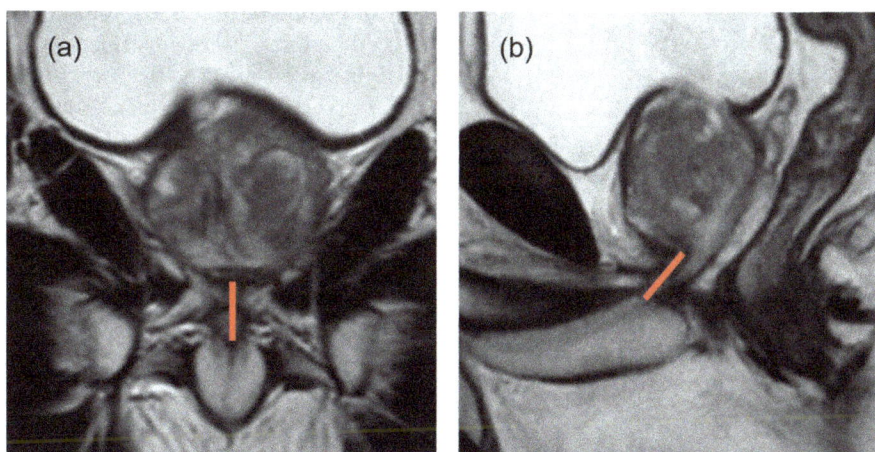

Fig. 1 The preoperative membranous urethral length as the distance from the prostatic apex to the level of the urethra at the penile bulb is measured in the T2-weighted MRI **a** coronal and **b** sagittal planes

Table 1 Patient characteristics

Characteristic	Total ($n = 204$)
Median (range)	
Observation period, days	350 (82–545)
Age, years	65 (41–76)
BMI, kg/m^2	23.7 (17.2–37.6)
PSA level, ng/ml	6.5 (3.5–46.4)
Preoperative MUL, mm	13.1 (4.5–22.9)
Estimated prostate volume, g	38 (7–94)
Console time, min	143 (87–351)
Operation time without console, min	52 (18–93)
Intraoperative bleeding, ml*	70 (10–1243)
N (%)	
Clinical stage	
^T2a	159 (77.9%)
T2b	24 (11.8%)
^T2c	21 (10.3%)
Preoperative hormonal therapy history	34 (16.7%)
Lymph node dissection	58 (28.4%)
Neurovascular bundle saving	70 (34.6%)
Positive surgical margin	59 (28.9%)
Leakage at the vesicourethral anastomosis	17 (8.3%)

*Including urine

after RALP was worst at 3 months. It improved gradually, and at 1 year postoperatively, it had improved to the preoperative status (Fig. 2).

In the univariate analysis for recovery of urinary continence 3 months after RALP, patient age ($P = 0.034$), and MUL ($P < 0.001$) were statistically significantly associated

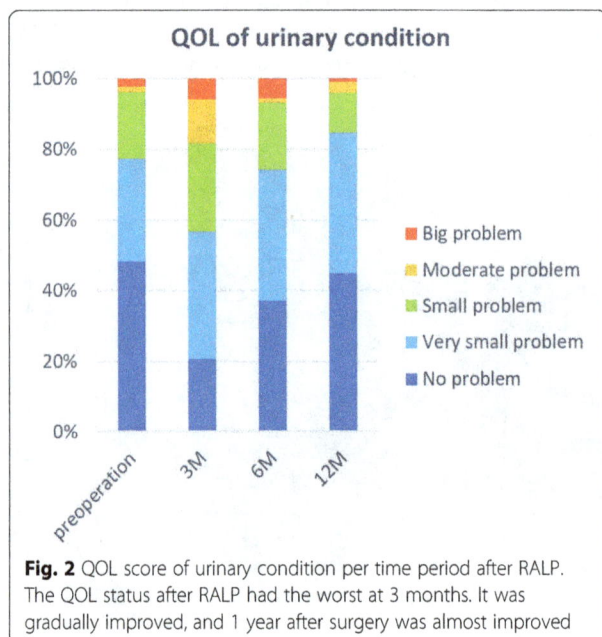

Fig. 2 QOL score of urinary condition per time period after RALP. The QOL status after RALP had the worst at 3 months. It was gradually improved, and 1 year after surgery was almost improved

with safety pad use. At 6 months after RALP, MUL ($P = 0.004$), console time, and leakage at vesicourethral anastomosis were statistically significant. At 12 months after RALP, MUL ($P = 0.023$) was statistically significant (Table 2). On multivariate analysis, patient age, leakage at vesicourethral anastomosis, and MUL achieved statistical significance with safety pad use. Among them, MUL was the most statistically significant with safety pad at 3 months after RALP (Table 3). Moreover, we estimated the optimal length of the MUL that could best classify between the continence and incontinence group. The cutoff point of MUL for recovery of urinary continence at 3 months after RALP was determined using the receiver operating characteristic (ROC) analysis. We identified a reasonable cutoff point of MUL to be 12 mm (Fig. 3). MUL > 12 mm was a favorable predictor of recovery of urinary continence at 3 months after RALP. Furthermore, using the cutoff point of MUL 12 mm, our cases were classified into continence and incontinence groups with a sensitivity of 80% and specificity of 70% (Fig. 3).

Discussion

RALP is expected to affect not only cancer control but also functional outcomes, such as continence and potency [12]. Especially, many reviews reported that patients who underwent RALP would tend to recover urinary continence within 1 year postoperatively earlier than patients who underwent retropubic RP (RRP) [12–14]. Early recovery of urinary continence is one of the strongest points of RALP. However, some patients suffer severe urinary incontinence after RALP. Therefore, we conducted this study to investigate factors that influence recovery of urinary continence in patients undergoing RALP.

Several preoperative predictive factors for recovery of urinary continence after RALP, such as age, body mass index, prostate size, medical comorbidities, history of transurethral resection of the prostate (TURP), and history of preoperative urinary continence or lower urinary tract symptoms, were identified as studied previously. MUL based on preoperative imaging also is a predictive factor associated with urinary continence [15]. Coakley et al. [16] reported the first study using endorectal MRI to measure preoperative MUL and showed a correlation of MUL with urinary continence after RRP [13]. They demonstrated that a longer preoperative MUL was associated with a faster recovery of continence; at 1 year postoperatively, 120 of 134 patients (89%) with preoperative MUL > 12 mm were completely continent, compared to only 35 of 46 (76%) whose preoperative MUL was ≤ 12 mm. Despite the preoperative median length of MUL seems to be a minor difference among continence and incontinence groups in our study, in prior studies, an increase in MUL as low as 1 mm can increase the odds of return to continence up to 200%

Table 2 Univariate analysis

Parameters	Continence at 3 months (n = 204)			Continence at 6 months (n = 175)			Continence at 12 months (n = 112)		
	Continence (n = 142)	Incontinence (n = 62)	P	Continence (n = 152)	Incontinence (n = 23)	P	Continence (n = 102)	Incontinence (n = 10)	P
Median (range)									
Age, years	65 (41–74)	67 (51–76)	0.034	66 (58–76)	64 (41–75)	0.989	66 (50–76)	64 (58–73)	0.689
BMI, kg/m²	23.6 (17.2–37.6)	23.9 (18.9–33.1)	0.213	23.8 (17.2–37.6)	23.6 (18.9–33.1)	0.507	23.7 (17.2–32.7)	24.5 (18.9–33.1)	0.391
PSA level, ng/ml	6.7 (3.5–46.4)	5.6 (4.2–24.1)	0.178	6.4 (3.5–46.4)	6.6 (4.2–14.5)	0.833	6.2 (3.8–32.1)	6.8 (4.2–16.7)	0.669
Preoperative MUL, mm	13.6 (8.3–22.9)	11.1 (4.5–17.9)	<.001	13.5 (6.5–22.9)	11.1 (4.5–17.3)	0.004	13.4 (6.5–22.9)	10.8 (4.5–17.3)	0.023
Estimated prostate volume, g	38 (7–94)	38 (17–92)	0.481	38 (7–94)	41 (20–92)	0.119	39 (14–94)	49 (30–92)	0.758
Console time, min	140 (87–351)	150 (99–339)	0.062	139 (89–253)	157 (99–280)	0.028	135 (89–253)	177 (99–280)	0.059
Operation time without console, min	51 (18–93)	54 (23–86)	0.792	49 (18–93)	54 (23–86)	0.477	51 (24–93)	56 (23–86)	0.506
Intraoperative bleeding, ml	68 (10–1243)	83 (16–535)	0.759	66 (14–1243)	85 (20–397)	0.696	70 (14–1243)	78 (26–320)	0.967
N (%)									
Clinical stage			0.218			0.763			0.532
^T2a	109 (76.8%)	50 (80.6%)		119 (78.3%)	18 (78.2%)		83 (81.4%)	9 (90%)	
T2b	20 (14.1%)	4 (6.5%)		19 (12.5%)	2 (8.7%)		13 (12.7%)	1 (10%)	
^T2c	13 (9.1%)	8 (12.9%)		14 (9.2%)	3 (13.1%)		6 (5.9%)	0	
Preoperative hormonal therapy history	21 (14.8%)	13 (20.9%)	0.276	20 (13.2%)	5 (21.7%)	0.298	11 (10.8%)	3 (30%)	0.122
Lymph node dissection	40 (28.2%)	18 (29%)	0.901	43 (28.3%)	6 (26.1%)	0.825	25 (24.5%)	2 (20%)	0.746
Neurovascular bundle saving	52 (36.6%)	18 (29%)	0.312	57 (37.5%)	8 (34.8%)	0.901	39 (38.2%)	4 (40%)	0.951
Positive surgical margin	43 (30.3%)	17 (27.4%)	0.678	45 (29.6%)	4 (17.4%)	0.224	29 (28.4%)	1 (10%)	0.209
Leakage at vesicourethral anastomosis	9 (6.3%)	9 (14.5%)	0.068	8 (5.3%)	7 (30.4%)	0.007	5 (4.9%)	2 (20%)	0.059

BMI body mass index, *PSA* prostate-specific antigen, *MUL* membranous urethral length

[17]. Our study demonstrated that preoperative MUL > 12 mm was the strongest factor indicating recovery of urinary continence 3 months after RALP. We identified 3 months after RALP as the early period for recovery of urinary continence because the result of QOL testing at 3 months after RALP was by no means satisfactory, and there still was room for improvement.

A previous study reported that MUL has anatomical variation [14]. Our study showed similar data as those reported in Korean patients [18, 19]. The average MUL in Asian patients may be approximately 12 mm. On the other hand, MUL in reports from the USA and Europe is slightly longer than that of Asians, but the racial difference is not clear because the number of reports is too small [15, 20].

MUL also has been associated with urinary continence recovery after RP [4, 15, 17–19]. Papaerl et al. [11] reported that a loss ratio of MUL between pre- and postoperatively

Table 3 Multivariate analysis

Parameters	Continence at 3 months (n = 204)			Continence at 6 months (n= 175)			Continence at 12 months (n = 112)		
	OR	95%CI	P	OR	95%CI	P	OR	95%CI	P
Age, years	1.074	1.01–1.15	0.028	–			–		
Preoperative MUL, mm	0.635	0.53–0.74	<.0001	0.699	0.56–0.85	0.0002	0.743	0.56–0.96	0.026
Console time, min	–			1.007	0.99–1.02	0.167	0.997	0.95–1.05	0.09
Leakage at vesicourethral anastomosis	–			0.123	0.03–0.43	0.0014	–		

OR odds ratio, *CI* confidence interval

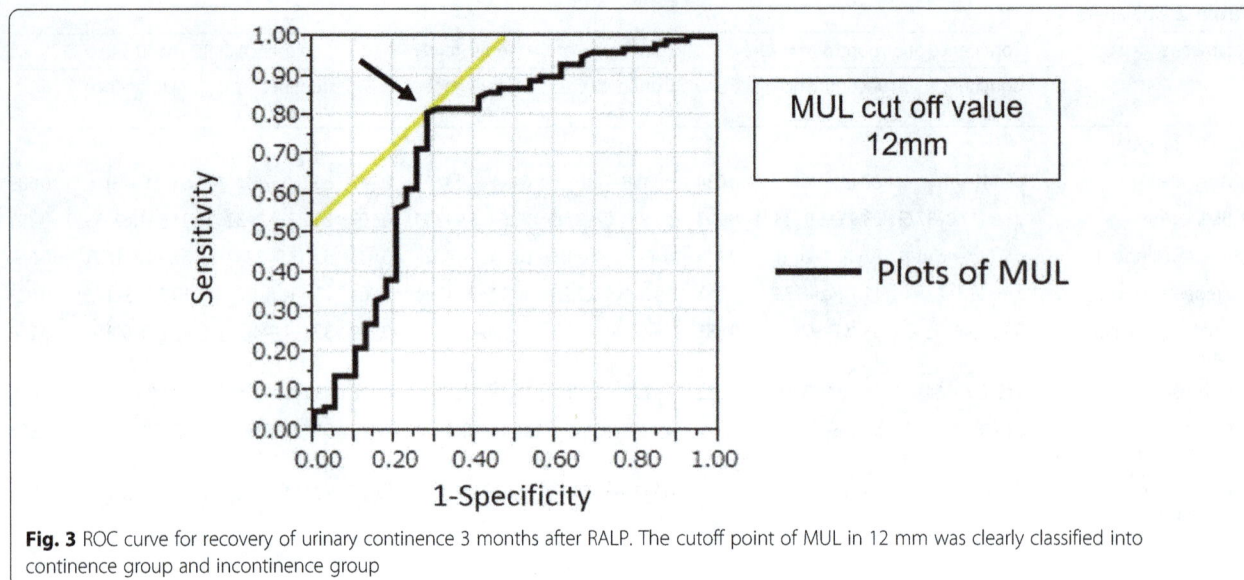

Fig. 3 ROC curve for recovery of urinary continence 3 months after RALP. The cutoff point of MUL in 12 mm was clearly classified into continence group and incontinence group

was associated with postoperative incontinence. They suggested that preserving MUL is important for time-to-recovery and degree of recovery. The membranous urethra contains smooth muscle fibers along its entire length and is surrounded by the rhabdosphincter [21–23]. Decreasing intraoperative trauma when preserving the MUL, which includes a greater amount of smooth muscle fibers and rhabdosphincter, has an important role in continence after RP because it contributes to maintaining and increasing urethral closure pressure [24].

Our result suggested that a longer preoperative MUL has advantages for early urinary continence recovery after RALP. In the open era, MUL might not have been taken into account as an operator's factor, but in the RALP era, the anatomical difference is evident more clearly and objectively. Therefore, not only the different operator technique, but also the MUL would relate directly to the early recovery of urinary continence.

In multivariate analysis, increasing patient age also was a risk factor for incontinence after RALP. Several studies showed a greater impact on urinary continence recovery with increasing age [25, 26]. Meanwhile, Basto et al. [27] reported urinary continence recovery rates after RALP in older men that were comparable to their younger counterparts, and thus, this should not be a reason to deny older men with a reasonable life-expectancy curative treatment for localized prostate cancer. In addition, leakage at vesicourethral anastomosis was one of the risk factors for incontinence after RALP in multivariate analysis. Leakage at vesicourethral anastomosis causes inflammatory change followed by fibrotic tissue development around the anastomotic site and sometimes causes a refractory fistula. Stavros et al. [28] reported leakage at vesicourethral anastomosis causes

complications including incontinence after prostatectomy. When the MUL is < 12 mm, the patient is older or complication of leakage at vesicourethral anastomosis, early recovery of urination would not be easy. Therefore, we suggested that MUL is an important factor for preoperative informed consent regarding continence.

Our study has several limitations. First, there are some inherent limitations of pad use as an outcome measure. We defined continence as the use of one pad or less per day and did not measure pad weight. What is important in actual clinical situations is whether the number of pads is related to QOL improvement. Therefore, we investigated a QOL questionnaire for the use of a security pad. Second, MRI was performed before RALP, while MUL was measured retrospectively. In terms of measuring MUL, we evaluated MUL by a number of urologists at the preoperative conference. Therefore, the data of MUL which were summarized by a urologist who was blinded to clinical data would be more reproducible and for less selective bias in this study. Third, there was a negative impact between urinary continence and nerve sparing in our study. The aim of nerve preservation was not only for urinary continence but also for the prevention of erectile dysfunction. We also considered that cancer control was more important. Therefore, we have performed nerve preservation on one side where cancer was not detected. There was no case of bilateral nerve preservation. Although 70 cases were performed on nerve preservation, no significant difference in urinary incontinence rate between preservation group and no preservation group was shown ($p = 0.312$). Steineck et al. [10] reported that there is a relation between nerve preservation and urinary incontinence, but their study examined nerve preservation on both sides. In contrast, Pick et al. [29] reported no significant difference was found in continence rates after RALP between hemi–nerve sparing and no nerve sparing. We consider that a more detailed examination about an association between nerve sparing and urinary incontinence is necessary. Finally, the retrospective design also might be a limitation. We currently are performing a prospective examination of a modified procedure on the prostatic apex according to the MUL during RALP.

Conclusion

In conclusion, preoperative MUL > 12 mm would be a predictive factor for the recovery of urinary continence at 3 months after RALP. Evaluation of preoperative MUL would be useful in clinical settings because it is easy to measure and to acquire beneficial informed consent. This result should be validated by well-conducted prospective randomized controlled trials in the future.

Abbreviations

BMI: Body mass index; EPIC: Expanded Prostate Cancer Index Composite; MRI: Magnetic resonance imaging; MUL: Membranous urethral length; PSA: Prostate-specific antigen; QOL: Quality of life; RALP: Robot-assisted laparoscopic prostatectomy; ROC: Receiver operating characteristic; RP: Radical prostatectomy; TURP: Transurethral resection of the prostate

Acknowledgements
Not applicable

Funding
None

Authors' contributions
DI contributed to the project development, data collection and management, data analysis, and manuscript drafting. YK contributed to the project development and manuscript editing. MK and RT contributed to the data analysis. AI, MO, RK, and TM contributed to the data collection. KI and WO contributed to the project development and manuscript editing. All authors read and approved the final manuscript.

Competing interests
The authors declare that they have no competing interests.

References
1. Binder J, Kramer W. Robotically-assisted laparoscopic prostatectomy. BJU Int. 2001;87:408.
2. Bauer RM, Gozzi C, Hubner W, et al. Contemporary management of postprostatectomy incontinence. Eur Urol. 2011;59:985.
3. Sandhu JS, Eastham JA. Factors predicting early return of continence after radical prostatectomy. Curr Urol Rep. 2010;11:191.
4. Mungovan SF, Sandhu JS, Akin O, et al. Preoperative membranous urethral length measurement and continence recovery following radical prostatectomy: a systematic review and meta-analysis. Eur Urol. 2017;71(3):368.
5. Wei JT, Dunn RL, Litwin MS, Sandier HM, Sanda MG. Development and validation of the expanded prostate cancer index composite (EPIC) for comprehensive assessment of health-related quality of life in men with prostate cancer. Urology. 2000;56(6):899.
6. Yasui T, Tozawa K, Kurokawa S, et al. Impact of prostate weight on perioperative outcomes of robot-assisted laparoscopic prostatectomy with a posterior approach to the seminal vesicle. BMC Urol. 2014;14:6.
7. Rocco F, Carmignani L, Acquati P, et al. Restoration of posterior aspect of rhabdosphincter shorten continence time after retropubic prostatectomy. J Urol. 2006;175:2201–6.
8. Hurtes X, Roupret M, Vaessen C, et al. Anterior suspension combined with posterior reconstruction during robotic assisted radical prostatectomy: results from a phase II randomized clinical trial. J Urol. 2011;185:1262–7.
9. Freire MP, Weinberg AC, Lei Y, et al. Anatomic bladder neck preservation during robotic-assisted laparoscopic radical prostatectomy: description of technique and outcomes. Eur Urol. 2009;56:972–80.
10. Steineck G, Bjartell A, Hugosson J, et al. Degree of preservation of the neurovascular bundles during radical prostatectomy and urinary continence 1 year after surgery. Eur Urol. 2015;67:559.
11. Paparel P, Akin O, Sandhu JS, et al. Recovery of urinary continence after radical prostatectomy: association with urethral length and urethral fibrosis measured by preoperative and postoperative endorectal magnetic resonance imaging. Eur Urol. 2009;55:629.
12. Di Pierro GB, Baumeister P, Stucki P, et al. A prospective trial comparing consecutive series of open retropubic and robot-assisted laparoscopic prostatectomy in a centre with a limited caseload. Eur Urol. 2011;59(1):1.
13. Ficarra V, Novara G, Rosen RC, et al. Systematic review and meta-analysis of studies reporting urinary continence after robot-assisted radical prostatectomy. Eur Urol. 2012;62:405.
14. Krambeck AE, DiMarco DS, Rangel LJ, et al. Radical prostatectomy for prostatic adenocarcinoma: a matched comparison of open retropubic and robot-assisted techniques. BJU Int. 2009;103(4):448.
15. Matsushita K, Kent MT, Vickers AJ, et al. Preoperative predictive model of recovery of urinary continence after radical prostatectomy. BJU Int. 2015;116:577.
16. Coakley FV, Eberhardt S, Kattan MW, et al. Urinary continence after radical retropubic prostatectomy: relationship with membranous urethral length on preoperative endorectal magnetic resonance imaging. J Urol. 2002;168:1032.
17. Lee H, Kim K, Hwang SI, et al. Impact of prostatic apical shape and protrusion on early recovery of continence after robot-assisted radical prostatectomy. Urology. 2014;84:844.
18. Jeong SJ, Yeon JS, Lee JK, et al. Development and validation of nomograms to predict the recovery of urinary continence after radical prostatectomy: comparisons between immediate, early, and late continence. World J Urol. 2014;32:437.
19. Son SJ, Lee SC, Jeong CW, et al. Comparison of continence recovery between robot-assisted laparoscopic prostatectomy and open radical retropubic prostatectomy: a single surgeon experience. Korean J Urol. 2013;54(9):598.
20. Tienza A, Hevia M, Benito A, Pascual JI, Zudaire JJ, Robles JE. MRI factors to predict urinary incontinence after retropubic/laparoscopic radical prostatectomy. Int Urol Nephrol. 2015;47:1343.
21. Strasser H, Ninkovic M, Hess M, Bartsch G, Stenzl A. Anatomic and functional studies of the male and female urethral sphincter. World J Urol. 2000;18:324.
22. Strasser H, Pinggera GM, Gozzi C, et al. Three-dimensional trans-rectal ultrasound of the male urethral rhabdosphincter. World J Urol. 2004;22:335.
23. Dalpiaz O, Mitterberger M, Kerschbaumer A, et al. Anatomical approach for surgery of the male posterior urethra. BJU Int. 2008;102:1448.
24. Bentzon DN, Graugaard-Jensen C, Borre M. Urethral pressure profile 6 months after radical prostatectomy may be diagnostic of sphincteric incontinence: preliminary data after 12 months' follow-up. Scand J Urol Nephrol. 2009;43:114.
25. Sacco E, Preyer-Galetti T, Pinto F, et al. Urinary incontinence after radical prostatectomy: influence by definition, risk factors and temporal trend in a large series with a long-term follow-up. BJU Int. 2006;97:1234.
26. Eastham JA, Kattan MW, Rogers E, et al. Risk factors for urinary incontinence after radical prostatectomy. J Urol. 1996;156:1707.
27. Basto MY, Vidyasagar C, Marvelde L, et al. Early urinary continence recovery after robot-assisted radical prostatectomy in older Australian men. BJU Int. 2014;114:29.
28. Tyritzis SI, Katafigiotis I, Constantinides CA, et al. All you need to know about urethrovesical anastomotic urinary leakage following radical prostatectomy. J Urol. 2012;188:369–76.
29. Pick DL, Osann K, Skarecky D, et al. The impact of cavernosal nerve preservation on continence after robotic radical prostatectomy. BJU Int. 2011;108:1492–6.

26

Assessment of expression of *interferon γ* (*IFN-G*) gene and its antisense (*IFNG-AS1*) in breast cancer

Hajar Yaghoobi[1,2], Hakim Azizi[3], Vahid Kholghi Oskooei[4], Mohammad Taheri[5,6]* 🆔 and Soudeh Ghafouri-Fard[4]*

Abstract

Background: The role of long non-coding RNAs has been extensively appreciated in the contexts of cancer. *Interferon γ-antisense RNA1* (*IFNG-AS1*) is an lncRNA located near to IFN-γ-encoding (*IFNG*) gene and regulates expression of *IFNG* in Th1 cells.

Methods: In the present study, we evaluated expression of *IFNG* and *IFNG-AS1* in 108 breast samples including tumoral tissues and their adjacent non-cancerous tissues (ANCTs) using real-time PCR. *IFNG-AS1* was significantly upregulated in tumoral tissues compared with ANCTs (expression ratio = 2.23, $P = 0.03$).

Results: Although the expression of *IFNG* was higher in tumoral tissues compared with ANCTs (relative expression = 1.89), it did not reach the level of significance ($P = 0.07$). *IFNG* expression was significantly higher in HER2-negative tumoral tissues compared with HER2-positive ones ($P = 0.01$) and in grade 1 samples compared with grade 2 ones ($P = 0.03$). No other significant difference was found in expressions of genes between other groups.

Conclusion: Significant strong correlations were detected between expression of *IFNG* and *IFNG-AS1* in both tumoral tissues and ANCTs. The present study provides evidences for participation of *IFNG* and *IFNG-AS1* in the pathogenesis of breast cancer and warrants future studies to elaborate the underlying mechanism.

Keywords: IFNG, IFNG-AS1, Breast cancer

Background

Long non-coding RNAs (lncRNAs) are increasingly acknowledged as principal regulators of gene expression in the contexts of both cancer [1] and immunological disorders [2]. Considering the prominent role of immune system in control of carcinogenesis process, lncRNAs with regulatory roles on both immune cells and cancer cells are of particular value as tumor biomarkers or therapeutic targets. *Interferon γ-antisense RNA1* (*IFN-G-AS1*) is located near to IFN-γ-encoding (*IFNG*) gene. This lncRNA is regarded as a fundamental checkpoint that participates in IFNG expression in Th1 cells [3]. Targeting immune checkpoint molecules has been suggested as a new approach in cancer treatment. The specific pattern of expression of non-coding RNAs in tumoral

tissues and their participation in initial phases of modulation of immune responses have potentiate them as novel candidates for changing the tumor microenvironment [4]. As IFN-based strategies along with immune checkpoint inhibitors are putative therapeutic options for malignancies [4], therapeutic modulation of *IFNG-AS1* expression would exert beneficial effects in cancer patients from diverse aspects. Elevated expression of *IFNG-AS1* lncRNA has been reported in Hashimoto's thyroiditis (HT) patients in correlation with the proportion of circulating Th1 cells and *IFNG* gene expression [5]. The role of IFN-γ has been documented in both breast cancer pathogenesis and patients' response to treatments. IFN-γ has been initially recognized for its role in antitumor host immunity which is exerted through induction of Th1 polarization and activation of both cytotoxic T cells (CTLs) and dendritic cells. Nevertheless, in certain conditions, IFN-γ function is in

* Correspondence: Mohammad_823@yahoo.com; s.ghafourifard@sbmu.ac.ir
[5]Student Research Committee, Shahid Beheshti University of Medical Sciences, Tehran, Iran
[4]Department of Medical Genetics, Shahid Beheshti University of Medical Sciences, Tehran, Iran
Full list of author information is available at the end of the article

Table 1 The nucleotide sequences of primers used for expression analysis

Gene name	Primer sequence	Primer length	Product length
B2M	F: AGATGAGTATGCCTGCCGTG	20	104
	R: CGGCATCTTCAAACCTCCA	19	
IFNG	F: GGCAAGGCTATGTGATTACAAGG	23	96
	R:CATCAAGTGAAATAAACACACAACCC	26	
IFNG-AS1	F: AGGAAGCTGGGTAATTGAATGC	22	94
	R: CTTAGGAGGAGAATTTTGGGAGAG	24	

favor of tumor progression which has been documented by the observed negative effect of IFN-γ treatment on patient survival in some clinical trials. The underlying mechanism for such negative effect might be irresponsiveness to IFN-γ, downregulation of the MHC complex, or overexpression of other genes such as programmed cell death 1 ligand 1 (PD-L1) [6]. On the other hand, overexpression of IFN/STAT1-related genes has been suggested as prognostic markers of response to chemotherapy in estrogen receptor (ER) negative breast cancers [7]. More importantly, IFN-γ treatment in conjunction with anti-erbB2/neu mAb has significantly suppressed tumor growth in animal models [8]. In spite of several efforts to evaluate the efficiency of IFN-γ treatment in breast cancer, data regarding expression of IFNG gene in breast cancer tissues is scarce. In the present study, we assessed expression of IFNG gene and its natural occurring antisense RNA in 108 breast samples including tumoral tissues and their adjacent non-cancerous tissues (ANCTs) using real-time

PCR in association with patients clinicopathological characteristics.

Methods

Patients

The current study enrolled 54 breast cancer patients. All patients had invasive ductal carcinoma of breast based on the histological examination. All of them have been recently diagnosed as having breast cancer and had no previous chemo/radiotherapy. The patients were admitted to Sina and Farmanieh hospitals over the years 2016–2017. The research protocol was approved by the ethical committee of Shahid Beheshti University of Medical Sciences (IR.SBMU.RETECH.REC.1397.403). All methods were performed in accordance with the relevant guidelines and regulations. Informed written consent was obtained from all patients. Tumoral tissues and ANCTs (0.5 cm × 0.5 cm) were excised from all patients during surgery, transferred in liquid nitrogen to the genetic laboratory of Shahid Beheshti University of Medical Sciences. Tissue samples were assessed by pathologists to endorse the diagnosis.

Expression analysis

Relative expressions of IFNG and IFNG-AS1 genes were assessed in tumoral tissues and paired ANCTs in the rotor gene 6000 Corbett Real-Time PCR System. Total RNA was extracted from tissue samples using TRIzol™ Reagent (Invitrogen, Carlsbad, CA, USA), and cDNA was synthesized by using RevertAid First Strand cDNA Synthesis Kit (TaKaRa, Japan). Al samples were treated with DNAse I to remove DNA contamination. SYBR

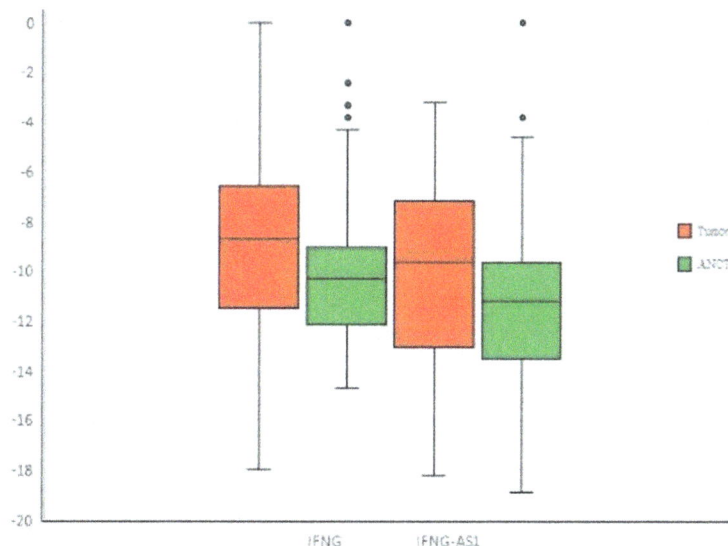

Fig. 1 The relative expression of IFNG and IFNG-AS1 in tumoral tissues (n = 54) and ANCTs (n = 54) as presented by –delta CT values (CT housekeeping - CT target gene) in each set of samples

Green RT-PCR Master Mix (TaKaRa, Japan) was used for expression analysis of genes. Expressions of genes were normalized to expression of *Beta 2 microglobulin* (*B2M*). The nucleotide sequences of primers are shown in Table 1. All experiments were performed in duplicate.

Statistical analysis

Student's paired *t* test was used for analysis of differences in gene expression between paired samples. The association between clinicopathological data and transcript levels of each gene was assessed using chi-square test. Tukey's honest significance test was used to assess the difference between mean values of transcript levels between different groups. The efficiency-corrected calculation model was used for assessment of fold changes of expression levels in tumoral tissues vs. ANCTs. The pairwise correlation between relative transcripts levels of *IFNG* and *IFNG-AS1* genes was calculated using the regression model. For all statistical tests, the level of significance was set at $P < 0.05$. The receiver operating characteristic (ROC) curve was designed to assess the properness of gene expression levels for differentiating tumoral vs. ANCTs. The Youden index (j) was used to escalate the difference between sensitivity (true-positive rate) and 1 − specificity (false-positive rate).

Results

Elevated levels of *IFNG* and *IFNG-AS1* can be used to identify breast cancer

IFNG-AS1 was significantly upregulated in tumoral tissues compared with ANCTs (expression ratio = 2.23, $P = 0.03$). Although the expression of *IFNG* was higher in

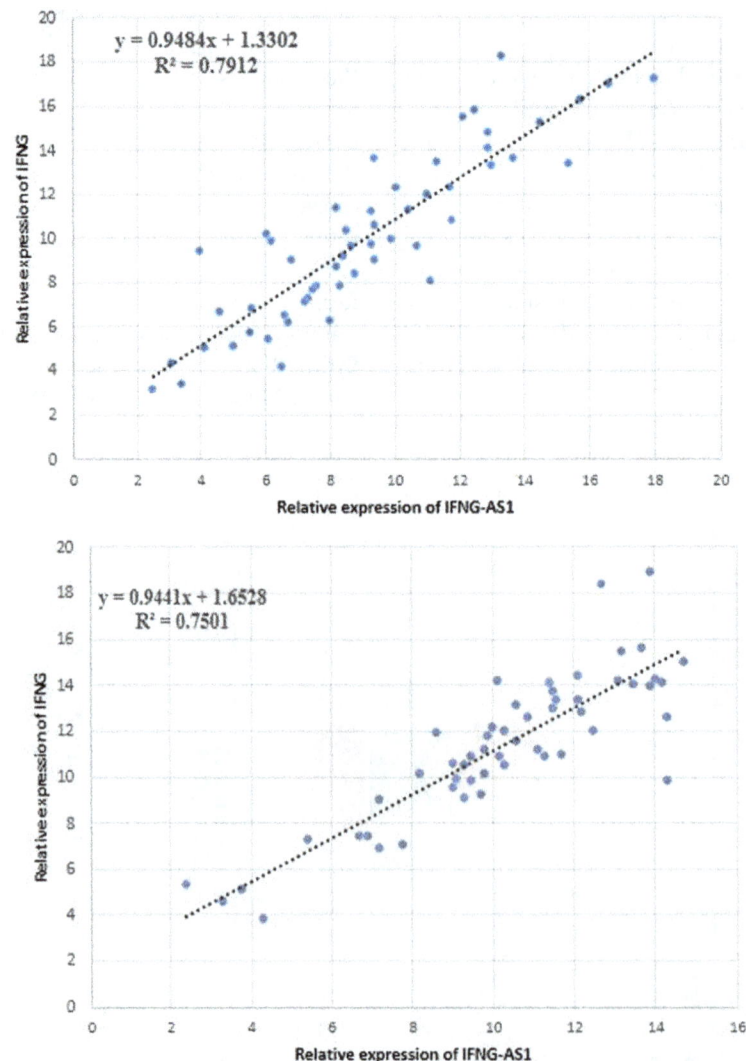

Fig. 2 Correlation between relative expressions of *IFNG* and *IFNG-AS1* in tumoral (**a**) and ANCTs (**b**)

tumoral tissues compared with ANCTs (relative expression = 1.89), it did not reach the level of significance (*P* = 0.07).

Figure 1 shows the –delta CT values (CT housekeeping - CT target gene) in tumoral tissues and ANCTs.

Assessment of correlation between expressions of *IFNG* and *IFNG-AS1* genes revealed strong correlations between their expressions in both tumoral tissues and ANCTs (Fig. 2a, b).

IFNG expression status is associated with clinical features of breast cancer

Table 2 shows the summary of demographic and clinicopathological data of study participants which have been gathered from questionnaires and patients' medical records.

We compared expression level of *IFNG* and *IFNG-AS1* in each tumoral tissue vs. its paired ANCT and classified patients based on these values to upregulation and downregulation groups. *INFG* and *IFNG-AS1* were upregulated in tumoral tissues obtained from 35/54 (64%) and 37/54 (68%) of patients, respectively. Subsequently, we evaluated associations between clinicopathological data and relative expressions of *IFNG* and *IFNG-AS1* genes. No significant associations were found between patients' clinicopathological data and fold changes of expression of these genes in tumoral tissues compared with ANCTs. Table 3 shows the results of association analysis between relative expressions of genes in tumoral tissues compared with ANCTs and patients' clinicopathological data.

Next, we compared relative expression of each gene in tumoral samples between clinicopathological-based groups (Table 4). *IFNG* expression was significantly higher in HER2-negative tumoral tissues compared with HER2-positive ones (*P* = 0.01) and in grade 1 samples compared with grade 2 ones (*P* = 0.03). No other significant difference was found in expressions of genes between other groups.

Assessment of the diagnostic value of *IFNG* and *IFNG-AS1* in breast cancer

Based on the results of ROC curve analysis *IFNG* and *IFNG-AS1* expressions had 83.3% specificity and 85.2% sensitivity for identification of disease status, respectively. The results of ROC curve analysis are shown in Fig. 3 and Table 5.

Discussion

In the present study, we evaluated transcript levels of *IFNG* and *IFNG-AS1* in breast cancer tissues and their paired ANCTs and found significant upregulation of *IFNG-AS1* in tumoral tissues. *IFNG-AS1* has been previously shown to regulate the expression of *IFNG* at both transcriptional and translational level in human CD4+ T cells [5]. Besides, strong positive correlations have

Table 2 General demographic data of study participants

Variables	Values
Age (years) (mean ± SD)	51.79 ± 13.54 (29–81)
Menarche age (years) (mean ± SD)	13 ± 1.65 (10–18)
Menopause age (years) (mean ± SD)	44.91 ± 14.91 (38–60)
First pregnancy age (years) (mean ± SD)	18.04 ± 8.36 (14–32)
Breast feeding duration (months) (mean ± SD)	41.62 ± 34.1 (3–120)
Positive family history for cancer (%)	17%
Cancer stage (%)	
I	30.8
II	28.8
III	30.8
IV	9.6
Overall grade (%)	
I	17
II	49
III	34
Mitotic rate (%)	
I	45.2
II	42.9
III	11.9
Tumor size (%)	
< 2 cm	32
≥ 2 cm, < 5 cm	66
≥ 5 cm	2
Estrogen receptor (%)	
Positive	87.8
Negative	12.2
Progesterone receptor (%)	
Positive	77.1
Negative	22.9
Her2/neu expression (%)	
Positive	25
Negative	75
Ki67 expression (%)	
Positive	100
Negative	0

been detected between the transcript levels of these two genes in thyroid tissues from HT patients [5]. Our data revealed the similar pattern of correlation between transcript levels of these genes in both tumoral tissues and ANCTs.

We could not find significant difference in expression of *IFNG* between tumoral tissues and ANCTs. García-Tuñón et al. have previously evaluated expression of

Table 3 The results of association analysis between relative expressions of genes in tumoral tissues compared with ANCTs and patients' clinicopathological data (up/downregulation of genes was defined based on relative expression of each gene in tumoral tissue compared with the paired ANCT)

	IFNG upregulation	IFNG downregulation	P value	IFNG-AS1 upregulation	IFNG-AS1 downregulation	P value
Age			0.63			0.5
< 40	8 (67.6%)	3 (27.3%)		9 (81.8%)	2 (18.2%)	
40–50	10 (58.2%)	7 (41.2%)		11 (64.7%)	6 (35.3%)	
51–60	10 (76.9%)	3 (23.1%)		10 (76.9%)	3 (23.1%)	
61–70	5 (62.5%)	3 (37.5%)		5 (62.5%)	3 (37.5%)	
> 71	2 (40%)	3 (60%)		2 (40%)	3 (60%)	
Stage			0.95			0.25
1	9 (56.3%)	7 (43.7%)		10 (62.5%)	6 (37.5%)	
2	10 (66.7%)	5 (33.3%)		9 (60%)	6 (40%)	
3	11 (68.8%)	5 (31.2%)		14 (87.5%)	2 (12.5%)	
4	4 (80%)	1 (20%)		3 (20%)	2 (80%)	
Histological grade			0.87			0.91
1	5 (62.5%)	3 (37.5%)		6 (75%)	2 (25%)	
2	16 (69.6%)	7 (30.4%)		15 (62.5%)	8 (34.8%)	
3	10 (62.5%)	6 (37.5%)		12 (75%)	4 (25%)	
Mitotic rate			0.9			0.64
1	13 (68.4%)	6 (31.6%)		14 (73.7%)	5 (26.3%)	
2	11 (61.1%)	7 (38.9%)		11 (61.1%)	7 (38.9%)	
3	3 (60%)	2 (40%)		4 (80%)	1 (20%)	
Tumor size			0.7			0.67
< 2	9 (56.3%)	7 (43.7%)		12 (75%)	4 (25%)	
2–5	22 (66.7%)	11 (33.3%)		21 (63.6%)	12 (36.4%)	
> 5	1 (100%)	0 (0%)		1 (100%)	0 (0%)	
ER status			0.08			0.65
Positive	26 (60.5%)	17 (39.5%)		29 (67.4%)	14 (32.6%)	
Negative	6 (100%)	0 (0%)		5 (16.7%)	1 (83.3%)	
PR status			0.07			0.46
Positive	22 (59.5%)	15 (40.5%)		25 (67.6%)	12 (32.4%)	
Negative	10 (90.9%)	1 (9.1%)		9 (81.8%)	2 (18.2%)	
HER2 status			0.48			0.27
Positive	7 (58.3%)	5 (41.7%)		7 (58.3%)	5 (41.7%)	
Negative	25 (69.4%)	11 (30.6%)		27 (75%)	9 (25%)	

IFNG in fibrocystic lesions, in situ tumors, and infiltrating tumors of breast and found higher expression of IFNG in in situ carcinoma than in benign and infiltrating tumors. They proposed IFNG as a prospective therapeutic modality in breast cancer [9]. In line with their observation, we found higher levels of *IFNG* in grade 1 samples compared with grade 2 ones. It is possible that tumor cells downregulate expression of *IFNG* as a mechanism for escaping from immune surveillance. We also detected higher *IFNG* expression in HER2-negative tumoral tissues compared with HER2-positive ones. IFN-γ has been previously shown to downregulate expression of HER2 in prostate cancer cells [10]. The existence of similar mechanism in breast cancer cells needs to be assessed. However, the direct effect of IFN-γ on HER2-positive breast cancer cells as reported by Nagai et al. [11] supports a similar function in the context of breast cancer.

Consistent with García-Tuñón et al. [9], we did not find any association between *IFNG* expression and ER/ PR status. Mostafa et al. have shown an ERα inhibitory

Table 4 Comparison of expression levels of *IFNG* and *IFNG-AS1* genes in tumoral tissue of breast cancer patients between clinicopathological-based categories (mean and SD values of ($E\hat{}CT_{B2M}/E\hat{}CT_{target\ gene}$) are presented)

	IFNG	P value	IFNG-AS1	P value
Age				
Pre-menopause vs. post-menopause	0.02 (0.04) vs. 0.03 (0.04)	0.59	0.01 (0.01) vs. 0.01 (0.02)	0.78
ER status				
ER(+) vs. ER(−)	0.03 (0.05) vs. 0.02 (0.01)	0.66	0.01 (0.02) vs. 0.01 (0.01)	0.97
PR status				
PR(+) vs. PR(−)	0.03 (0.05) vs. 0.02 (0.02)	0.74	0.01 (0.02) vs. 0.01 (0.01)	0.92
HER2 status				
HER2(+) vs. HER2(−)	0.009 (0.01) vs. 0.03 (0.05)	0.01	0.01 (0.01) vs. 0.01 (0.02)	0.57
Tumor grade				
Grade 1 vs. 2	0.06 (0.08) vs. 0.01 (0.03)	0.03	0.02 (0.02) vs. 0.01 (0.02)	0.73
Grade 1 vs. 3	0.06 (0.08) vs. 0.02 (0.02)	0.1	0.02 (0.02) vs. 0.01 (0.01)	0.69
Grade 2 vs. 3	0.01 (0.03) vs. 0.02 (0.02)	0.89	0.01 (0.02) vs. 0.01 (0.01)	0.99

effect on IFN-γ signaling which results in immune escape in ERα-positive breast cancer cells [12]. However, such inhibitory effects are not necessarily exerted on expression of *IFNG* itself. Future studies are needed to assess the effect of estradiol or its receptor on *IFNG* expression.

We observed higher levels of *IFNG-AS1* in breast cancer tissues compared with ANCTs. This finding might be either the cause or the consequence of the tumorigenesis process. Future functional studies are needed to elaborate the consequence of its overexpression in breast tissues. As previous studies have

linked its overexpression with autoimmune conditions, it is possible that such overexpression is a compensatory mechanism to conquer immune evasion in tumor microenvironment. Critchley-Thorne et al. have evaluated the effectiveness of IFNG in peripheral blood lymphocytes from breast cancer patients and detected diminished IFN-γ-induced signaling in B cells of these patients in spite of normal signaling in T cells or natural killer cells [13]. Noticeably, no difference has been found within stages II, III, and IV breast cancer patients in this regard [13] which is in accordance with our finding regarding similar expression of the *IFNG* gene

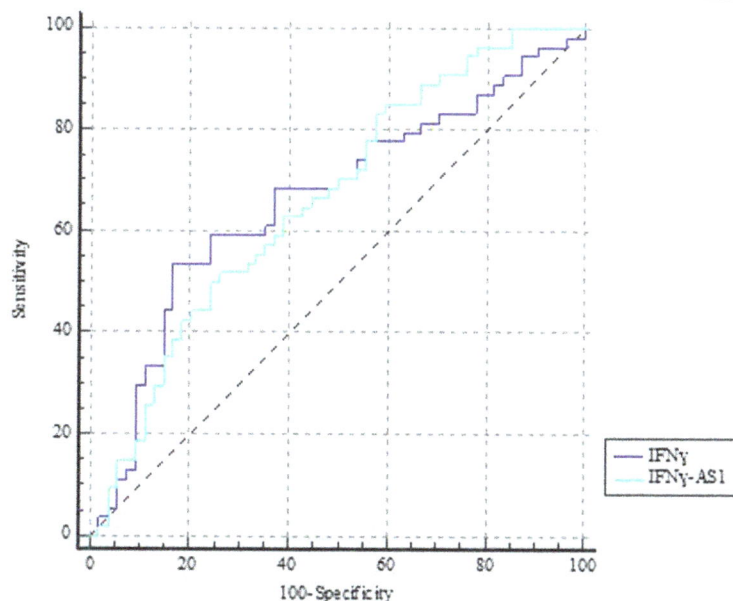

Fig. 3 ROC curve for prediction of disease status based on the expression levels of *IFNG* and *IFNG-AS1*

Table 5 The results of ROC curve analysis

	Estimate criterion	AUC	J^a	Sensitivity	Specificity	P value[b]
IFNG	> 0.007	0.664	0.37	53.7	83.3	0.002
IFNG-AS1	> 0.0001	0.665	0.25	85.2	40.7	0.001
Combination of both genes	> 0.47	0.665	0.33	61.1	72.2	0.001

Estimate criterion: optimal cutoff point for gene expression
[a]Youden index
[b]Significance level P (area = 0.5)

in histopathological-based groups. Consequently, there is a cell type-dependent regulatory mechanism for IFN function. So, future studies are needed to elaborate such mechanism in the epithelial tissues obtained from breast tumors to find whether these functional responses are impaired in the cancer tissue. Moreover, the significance of local expression of *IFNG* and *IFN-G-AS1* in response to systemic IFN-γ therapy of breast cancer patients must be investigated in imminent researches.

Conclusion

Apart from functional consequences of dysregulation of *IFNG-AS1* in breast tumor tissues, transcript levels of this gene might be used for diagnosis purposes in the panels of putative biomarkers comprising both coding and non-coding genes. However, based on the results of ROC curve analysis, none of the assessed genes in the present study fulfill the requirements as an individual biomarker as the AUC values of both genes and their combinations were between 0.6 and 0.7 which means the poor accuracy of a diagnostic test.

Acknowledgements
The current study was supported by a grant from Shahrekord University of Medical Sciences.

Funding
Not applicable

Authors' contributions
MT and SG-F supervised the study. HY and HA did the laboratory assessment. VKO analyzed the data. All authors read and approved the final manuscript.

Competing interests
The authors declare that they have no competing interests.

Author details
[1]Cellular and Molecular Research Center, Basic Health Sciences Institute, Shahrekord University of Medical Sciences, Shahrekord, Iran. [2]Department of Medical Biotechnology, School of Advanced Technologies, Shahrekord University of Medical Sciences, Shahrekord, Iran. [3]Department of Medical Parasitology, School of Medicine, Zabol University of Medical Sciences, Zabol, Iran. [4]Department of Medical Genetics, Shahid Beheshti University of Medical Sciences, Tehran, Iran. [5]Student Research Committee, Shahid Beheshti University of Medical Sciences, Tehran, Iran. [6]Urogenital Stem Cell Research Center, Shahid Beheshti University of Medical Sciences, Tehran, Iran.

References
1. Nikpayam E, Tasharrofi B, Sarrafzadeh S, Ghafouri-Fard S. The role of long non-coding RNAs in ovarian cancer. Iran Biomed J. 2017;21(1):3–15.
2. Eftekharian MM, Ghafouri-Fard S, Soudyab M, et al. Expression analysis of long non-coding RNAs in the blood of multiple sclerosis patients. J Mol Neurosci. 2017;63(3–4):333–41.
3. Collier SP, Collins PL, Williams CL, Boothby MR, Aune TM. Cutting edge: influence of Tmevpg1, a long intergenic noncoding RNA, on the expression of Ifng by Th1 cells. J Immunol. 2012;189(5):2084–8.
4. Smolle MA, Calin HN, Pichler M, Calin GA. Noncoding RNAs and immune checkpoints-clinical implications as cancer therapeutics. FEBS J. 2017;284(13): 1952–66.
5. Peng HY, Liu YZ, Tian J, et al. The long noncoding RNA IFNG-AS1 promotes T helper type 1 cells response in patients with Hashimoto's thyroiditis. Sci Rep. 2015;5:17702.
6. Mandai M, Hamanishi J, Abiko K, Matsumura N, Baba T, Konishi I. Dual faces of IFNgamma in cancer progression: a role of PD-L1 induction in the determination of pro- and antitumor immunity. Clin Cancer Res. 2016; 22(10):2329–34.
7. Legrier ME, Bieche I, Gaston J, et al. Activation of IFN/STAT1 signalling predicts response to chemotherapy in oestrogen receptor-negative breast cancer. Br J Cancer. 2016;114(2):177–87.
8. Nagai Y, Tsuchiya H, Ji MQ, Zhang H, Greene MI. Synergistic effect of IFN-γ on breast cancer targeted therapy. (2017).
9. García-Tuñón I, Ricote M, Ruiz A, Fraile B, Paniagua R, Royuela M. Influence of IFN-gamma and its receptors in human breast cancer. BMC Cancer. 2007; 7(1):158.
10. Kominsky SL, Hobeika AC, Lake FA, Torres BA, Johnson HM. Down-regulation of neu/HER-2 by interferon-gamma in prostate cancer cells. Cancer Res. 2000;60(14):3904–8.
11. Nagai Y, Tsuchiya H, Runkle EA, et al. Disabling of the erbB pathway followed by IFN-γ modifies phenotype and enhances genotoxic eradication of breast tumors. Cell Rep. 2015;12(12):2049–59.
12. Mostafa AA, Codner D, Hirasawa K, et al. Activation of ERα signaling differentially modulates IFN-γ induced HLA-class II expression in breast cancer cells. PLoS One. 2014;9(1):e87377.
13. Critchley-Thorne RJ, Simons DL, Yan N, et al. Impaired interferon signaling is a common immune defect in human cancer. Proc Natl Acad Sci. 2009; 106(22):9010–5.

Permissions

The contributors of this book come from diverse backgrounds, making this book a truly international effort. This book will bring forth new frontiers with its revolutionizing research information and detailed analysis of the nascent developments around the world.

We would like to thank all the contributing authors for lending their expertise to make the book truly unique. They have played a crucial role in the development of this book. Without their invaluable contributions this book wouldn't have been possible. They have made vital efforts to compile up to date information on the varied aspects of this subject to make this book a valuable addition to the collection of many professionals and students.

This book was conceptualized with the vision of imparting up-to-date information and advanced data in this field. To ensure the same, a matchless editorial board was set up. Every individual on the board went through rigorous rounds of assessment to prove their worth. After which they invested a large part of their time researching and compiling the most relevant data for our readers.

The editorial board has been involved in producing this book since its inception. They have spent rigorous hours researching and exploring the diverse topics which have resulted in the successful publishing of this book. They have passed on their knowledge of decades through this book. To expedite this challenging task, the publisher supported the team at every step. A small team of assistant editors was also appointed to further simplify the editing procedure and attain best results for the readers.

Apart from the editorial board, the designing team has also invested a significant amount of their time in understanding the subject and creating the most relevant covers. They scrutinized every image to scout for the most suitable representation of the subject and create an appropriate cover for the book.

The publishing team has been an ardent support to the editorial, designing and production team. Their endless efforts to recruit the best for this project, has resulted in the accomplishment of this book. They are a veteran in the field of academics and their pool of knowledge is as vast as their experience in printing. Their expertise and guidance has proved useful at every step. Their uncompromising quality standards have made this book an exceptional effort. Their encouragement from time to time has been an inspiration for everyone.

The publisher and the editorial board hope that this book will prove to be a valuable piece of knowledge for researchers, students, practitioners and scholars across the globe.

List of Contributors

Hsiang-Ying Lee, Hsin-Chih Yeh, Wen-Jeng Wu and Ching-Chia Li
Department of Urology, Kaohsiung Municipal Ta-Tung Hospital, Kaohsiung, Taiwan

Hsiang-Ying Lee
Graduate Institute of Clinical Medicine, College of Medicine, Kaohsiung Medical University, Kaohsiung, Taiwan

Hsiang-Ying Lee, Hsin-Chih Yeh, Wen-Jeng Wu, Chun-Nung Huang, Hung-Lung Ke, Wei-Ming Li and Ching-Chia Li
Department of Urology, Kaohsiung Medical University Hospital, Kaohsiung, Taiwan

Hsin-Chih Yeh, Wen-Jeng Wu, Chun-Nung Huang, Hung-Lung Ke, Wei-Ming Li and Ching-Chia Li
Department of Urology, School of Medicine, College of Medicine, Kaohsiung Medical University, Kaohsiung, Taiwan.
Graduate Institute of Medicine, College of Medicine, Kaohsiung Medical University, No.100, Tzyou 1st Road, Kaohsiung 807, Taiwan

Jiun-Shiuan He
Department of Public Health, Kaohsiung Medical University, Kaohsiung, Taiwan

Wei-Ming Li
Department of Urology, Ministry of Health and Welfare Pingtung Hospital, Pingtung, Taiwan.

Chien-Feng Li
Department of Pathology, Chi-Mei Medical Center, Tainan, Taiwan
Department of Biotechnology, Southern Taiwan University of Science and Technology, Tainan, Taiwan
National Cancer Research Institute, National Health Research Institutes, Tainan, Taiwan
Institute of Clinical Medicine, Kaohsiung Medical University, Kaohsiung, Taiwan
Department of Internal Medicine and Cancer Center, Kaohsiung Medical University Hospital, Kaohsiung Medical University, Kaohsiung, Taiwan

Junhai Pan, Xiaolong Ge, Wei Zhou, Xin Zhong, Lihu Gu, Hepan Zhu, Xinlong Li, Weilin Qi and Xianfa Wang
Department of General Surgery, School of Medicine, Sir Run Run Shaw Hospital, Zhejiang University, 3 East Qingchun Road, Hangzhou 310016, Zhejiang, China

Heqing Zhang, Li Qiu and Yulan Peng
Department of Ultrasound, West China Hospital, Sichuan University, Chengdu, China

Ryutaro Mori, Manabu Futamura, Kasumi Morimitsu, Yoshimi Asano, Yoshihisa Tokumaru, Mai Kitazawa and Kazuhiro Yoshida
Department of Surgical Oncology, Gifu University Graduate School of Medicine, 1-1 Yanagido, Gifu 501-1194, Japan

Lihong Cao
Department of Ear-nose-throat, Tianjin Medical University General Hospital, No. 154, Anshan Road, Heping District, Tianjin 300052, China

Zheng Liu, Ming Yang, Zhi-xun Zhao, Xu Guan, Zheng Jiang, Hai-peng Chen, Song Wang, Ji-chuan Quan, Run-kun Yang and Xi-shan Wang
Department of Colorectal Surgery, National Cancer Center/National Clinical Research Center for Cancer/Cancer Hospital, Chinese Academy of Medical Sciences and Peking Union Medical College, Beijing, China

Li-Jun Wang, Xiao-Luan Yan and Bao-Cai Xing
Key laboratory of Carcinogenesis and Translational Research (Ministry of Education/Beijing), Department of Hepatopancreatobiliary Surgery Unit I, Peking University Cancer Hospital and Institute, 52 Fucheng Road, Haidian District, Beijing 100142, China

Wang, Zhong-Yi Zhang, Wei Yang and Kun Yan
Key laboratory of Carcinogenesis and Translational Research (Ministry of Education/Beijing), Department of Ultrasound, Peking University Cancer Hospital and Institute, 52 Fucheng Road, Haidian District, Beijing 100142, China

Pauline Duconseil, Ugo Marchese and Jacques Ewald
Department of Surgery, Institut Paoli-Calmettes, Marseille, France

Marc Giovannini
Department of Endoscopy, Institut Paoli-Calmettes, Marseille, France

Djamel Mokart
Department of Intensive Care, Institut Paoli-Calmettes, Marseille, France

Olivier Turrini
Department of Surgery, Aix-Marseille University, Institut Paoli-Calmettes, CNRS, Inserm, CRCM, Marseille, France

Young Jae Ryu, Jin Seong Cho, Jung Han Yoon and Min Ho Park
Department of Surgery, Chonnam National University Medical School, 322 Seoyang-ro Hwasun-eup, Hwasun-gun Jeonnam, Gwangju 58128, South Korea

Hiroshi Urakawa and Yoshihiro Nishida
Department of Orthopaedic Surgery, Nagoya University, 65 Tsurumai, Showa-ku, Nagoya, Aichi 466-8550, Japan

Tsukasa Yonemoto
Division of Orthopaedic Surgery, Chiba Cancer Center, Chiba, Japan.

Seiichi Matsumoto
Department of Orthopaedic Surgery, Cancer Institute Hospital, Japanese Foundation for Cancer Research, Tokyo, Japan

Tatsuya Takagi
Department of Orthopaedic Surgery, Juntendo University, Tokyo, Japan

Kunihiro Asanuma
Department of Orthopaedic Surgery, Graduate School of Medicine, Mie University, Tsu, Japan

Munenori Watanuki
Department of Orthopaedic Surgery, Tohoku University Hospital, Sendai, Japan

Akira Takemoto
Department of Orthopaedic Surgery, School of Medicine, Yokohama City University, Yokohama, Japan

Norifumi Naka
Musculoskeletal Oncology Service, Osaka International Cancer Institute, Osaka, Japan

Yoshihiro Matsumoto
Department of Orthopaedic Surgery, Kyushu University, Fukuoka, Japan

Akira Kawai
Department of Orthopaedic Surgery, National Cancer Center, Tokyo, Japan

Toshiyuki Kunisada
Department of Medical Materials for Musculoskeletal Reconstruction, Graduate School of Medicine, Dentistry, and Pharmaceutical Sciences, Okayama University, Okayama, Japan

Tadahiko Kubo
Department of Orthopaedic Surgery, Hiroshima University, Hiroshima, Japan

Makoto Emori
Department of Orthopaedic Surgery, Sapporo Medical University, Sapporo, Japan

Hiroaki Hiraga
Department of Orthopaedic Surgery, Hokkaido Cancer Center, Sapporo, Japan

Hiroshi Hatano
Department of Orthopaedic Surgery, Niigata Cancer Center Hospital, Niigata, Japan

Satoshi Tsukushi
Department of Orthopaedic Surgery, Aichi Cancer Center, Nagoya, Japan

Toshihiro Akisue
Department of Orthopaedic Surgery, Kobe University, Kobe, Japan

Takeshi Morii
Department of Orthopaedic Surgery, Kyorin University, Mitaka, Japan

Mitsuru Takahashi
Department of Orthopaedic Surgery, Shizuoka Cancer Center, Shizuoka, Japan

Akihito Nagano
Department of Orthopaedic Surgery, Gifu University, Gifu, Japan

Hideki Yoshikawa
Department of Orthopaedic Surgery, Osaka University, Osaka, Japan.

Kenji Sato
Department of Orthopaedic Surgery, Teikyo University, Tokyo, Japan

Masanori Kawano
Department of Orthopaedic Surgery, Oita University, Oita, Japan

Koji Hiraoka
Department of Orthopaedic Surgery, Kurume University, Kurume, Japan

Kazuhiro Tanaka
Department of Endoprosthetic Surgery, Oita University, Oita, Japan

Yukihide Iwamoto
Kyushu Rosai Hospital, Kitakyushu, Japan

Toshifumi Ozaki
Department of Orthopaedic Surgery, Graduate School of Medicine, Dentistry, and Pharmaceutical Sciences, Okayama University, Okayama, Japan

Liangbo Dong, Jun Lu, Bangbo Zhao, Weibin Wang and Yupei Zhao
Department of General Surgery, Peking Union Medical College Hospital, Chinese Academy of Medical Science and Peking Union Medical College, Beijing 100730, People's Republic of China

Zhou Yang, Guo Chunhua, Yuan Huayan, Yang Jianguo and Cheng Yong
Department of Gastrointestinal Surgery, First Affiliated Hospital of Chongqing
Medical University, Chongqing 400010, China

Minglei Yang, Nanzhe Zhong, Chenglong Zhao, Wei Xu, Shaohui He, Jian Zhao, Xinghai Yang and Jianru Xiao
Department of Orthopedic Oncology, Changzheng Hospital, Second Military Medical University, 415 Fengyang Road, Shanghai 200003, China

Chih-Yi Chen
Division of Thoracic Surgery, Department of Surgery, Chung Shan Medical
University, Chung Shan Medical University Hospital, Taichung, Taiwan

Chia-Chin Li and Chun-Ru Chien
Department of Radiation Oncology, China Medical University Hospital, Taichung, Taiwan

Chun-Ru Chien
Department of Radiation Oncology, China Medical University Hsinchu Hospital, Hsinchu, Taiwan
School of Medicine, College of Medicine, China Medical University, No.91 Hsueh-Shih Road, North District, Taichung 40402, Taiwan

Minxun Lu, Jie Wang, Fan Tang, Li Min, Yong Zhou, Wenli Zhang and Chongqi Tu
Department of Orthopedics, West China Hospital, Sichuan University, No. 37 Guoxue Street, Chengdu 610041, People's Republic of China

Cong Xiao
Department of Orthopedics, The Third Hospital of Mianyang, No. 190 The East Jiannan Road, Mianyang 621000, Sichuan, People's Republic of China

Giuseppe Nigri, Livia Maria Mangogna, Anna Crovetto, Giovanni Moschetta, Raffaello Persechino, Paolo Aurello and Giovanni Ramacciato
Department of Medical and Surgical Science and Translational Medicine, St. Andrea Hospital Rome, Sapienza University of Rome, Via di Grottarossa 1035, 00189 Rome, Italy

Niccolò Petrucciani
Digestive Surgery, Hepatobiliopancreatic Surgery and Liver Transplantation, UPEC University, Henri Mondor Hospital, Creteil, France

Tarek Debs
Department of Digestive Surgery and Liver Transplantation, Nice University Hospital, Nice, France
Krzysztof Kaliszewski, Paweł Kiełb, Jerzy Maksymowicz, Aleksander Krawczyk and Otto Krawiec
First Department and Clinic of General, Gastroenterological, and Endocrine Surgery, Wroclaw Medical University, 66 Maria Skłodowska-Curie Street, 50-369 Wrocaw, Poland

Agnieszka Zubkiewicz-Kucharska
Department of Endocrinology and Diabetology for Children and Adolescents, Wroclaw Medical University, Wroclaw, Poland

Chunyang Li, Xiaoxi Zeng, Haopeng Yu, Yonghong Gu and Wei Zhang
West China Biomedical Big Data Center, West China Hospital, Sichuan University, Chengdu, China
Medical Big Data Center, Sichuan University, Chengdu, China

Li Zhu, Huaidong Tu and Yanmei Liang
Department of Gynecologic Oncology, The People's Hospital of Taojiang County, Taojiang, China

Dihong Tang
Department of Gynecologic Oncology, Hunan Cancer Hospital, No.283 Tongzipo Road, Yuelu District, Changsha 410006, Hunan Province, China

Liang Tang, Peng Zhao and Dalu Kong
Department of Colorectal Cancer, Tianjin Medical University Cancer Institute and Hospital, Key Laboratory of Cancer Prevention and Therapy, National Clinical Research Center of Cancer, Huanhuxi Road, Hexi District, Tianjin, People's Republic of China

Shuzhen Wei, Xiaoli Zhu and Shuhua Han
Department of Respiratory, Zhongda Hospital, Southeast University, Nanjing, China

Yang Chen, Xiyong Wang, Xiaoli Zhu and Shuhua Han
Medical School of Southeast University, Nanjing, China

Yi Hou, Xudong Wang and Jing Chen
Department of Gastrointestinal Surgery, The Fourth Affiliated Hospital of China Medical University, Chongshan road 4th, Huanggu district, Shenyang 110032, Liaoning, China

Xudong Zhang, Hongfei Li, Qian Li, Ying Li, Chao Li, Minmin Zhu and Bing Zhao and Guowen Li
Radiotherapy inpatient Ward II, The First Affiliated Hospital of Zhengzhou University, No.1 Eastern Jianshe Road, Zhengzhou 450000, Henan, China

Gian Andrea Prevost, Manfred Odermatt, Markus Furrer and Peter Villiger
Department of Surgery, Kantonsspital Graubünden, Loëstrasse 170, CH-7000 Chur, Switzerland

Gian Andrea Prevost and Markus Furrer
Private University of the Principality of Liechtenstein, Triesen, Principality of Liechtenstein

Daiki Ikarashi, Yoichiro Kato, Mitsugu Kanehira, Ryo Takata, Akito Ito, Mitsutaka Onoda, Renpei Kato, Tomohiko Matsuura, Kazuhiro Iwasaki and Wataru Obara
Department of Urology, Iwate Medical University School of Medicine, 19-1, Uchimaru, Morioka-shi, Iwate 020-8505, Japan

Hajar Yaghoobi
Cellular and Molecular Research Center, Basic Health Sciences Institute, Shahrekord University of Medical Sciences, Shahrekord, Iran
Department of Medical Biotechnology, School of Advanced Technologies, Shahrekord
University of Medical Sciences, Shahrekord, Iran

Hakim Azizi
Department of Medical Parasitology, School of Medicine, Zabol University of Medical Sciences, Zabol, Iran

Vahid Kholghi Oskooei and Soudeh Ghafouri-Fard
Department of Medical Genetics, Shahid Beheshti University of Medical Sciences, Tehran, Iran.

Mohammad Taheri
Student Research Committee, Shahid Beheshti University of Medical Sciences, Tehran, Iran Urogenital Stem Cell Research Center, Shahid Beheshti University of Medical Sciences, Tehran, Iran

Index

www.ingramcontent.com/pod-product-compliance
Lightning Source LLC
Chambersburg PA
CBHW080625200326

41458CB00013B/4514